Advances and Technical Standards in Neurosurgery

Volume 40

Editor-in-Chief

Johannes Schramm

Volume Editors

Concezio Di Rocco
Nejat Akalan

For further volumes
http://www.springer.com/series/578

Sponsored by the
European Association of Neurosurgical Societies

Concezio Di Rocco • Nejat Akalan
Editors

Pediatric Craniovertebral Junction Diseases

Surgical Management of Craniovertebral Junction Diseases in Children

Springer

Editors
Concezio Di Rocco
INI-International Neuroscience Institute
Hannover
Germany

Nejat Akalan
Department of Neurosurgery
Hacettepe University
Sihhiye, Ankara
Turkey

ISBN 978-3-319-34655-7 ISBN 978-3-319-01065-6 (eBook)
DOI 10.1007/978-3-319-01065-6
Springer Cham Heidelberg New York Dordrecht London

Printed on acid-free paper

Springer is part of Springer Science+Business Media (www.springer.com)

Preface

The management of the congenital and acquired diseases of the craniovertebral junction (CVJ), that is, the occipital bone which surrounds the foramen magnum, the atlas, and the axis vertebrae, constitutes one of the more complex chapters of neurosurgery. This is particularly true in the pediatric population in which the neurosurgeon is faced with a large variety of congenital developmental anomalies and acquired diseases; the treatment of which is weighted by further problems possibly related to the necessity of not interfering with still-growing structures significantly.

The CVJ is essentially a bone enclosure which encompasses the medulla oblongata, the cervicomedullary junction, and the upper cervical spinal cord. Its anomalies may result in compression of the underlying neuronal structures along the entire circumference, in vascular compromise requiring surgical or medical therapy, and in abnormalities of the cerebrospinal fluid dynamics.

The basis for understanding surgical and medical problems generated by the diseases of this bone complex relies on a perfect knowledge of its embryology and the clear understanding of its functional anatomy and biomechanics. Pediatric neurosurgeons are called to face this stimulating region; the diseases of which may be nowadays managed with rewarding results even in the first years of age due to the progress of neurosciences, availability of advanced neuroimaging diagnostic tools, as well as improved surgical and anesthesiological techniques.

This dedicated volume of the series *Advances and Technical Standards in Neurosurgery* provides a comprehensive approach to the CJV diseases and their management based on the multidisciplinary cooperation of neurosurgeons, anatomists, neuroradiologists, and neuroanesthesiologists. The contributing authors represent the European and also the world's most renowned clinical and surgical experts.

According to the traditional architecture of *Advance and Technical Standards in Neurosurgery*, the 12 chapters of the volume are organized in two parts of 7 (Advanced) and 5 (Standard) chapters, respectively.

The main topics highlighted concern the embryology, the normal and abnormal development of the CVJ, including the related vessels, the modern radiological contributions to the diagnosis, the genetic and metabolic factors which may impact on the surgical strategies, the opportunities offered by the traditional operative techniques, and the recently introduced minimal and endoscopic surgical modalities. A special emphasis is also placed on to the evolution of the principles of surgical treatment as matured by the last-decade experiences in a still-open field of pediatric neurosurgery.

Bonn, Germany J. Schramm
Rome, Italy C. Di Rocco
Ankara, Turkey N. Akalan

Contents

Technical Standards

Nosographic Identification and Management of Pediatric Craniovertebral Junction Anomalies: Evolution of Concepts and Modalities of Treatment

Arnold H. Menezes

Contents

Abstract The clinical significance of abnormalities of the craniocervical junction has gained tremendous momentum with the increasing interest in the area as a result of better neurodiagnostic imaging. Abnormalities of the bone, soft tissue, and neural structures are easily recognized and there is a better understanding of the biomechanics of this complex region as well as the embryology. A database of symptomatic patients, children, and adults with neurological symptoms and signs secondary to abnormalities at the craniocervical junction have been evaluated by the author at the University of Iowa Hospitals and Clinics. This large database comprises 6,000 patients and provides a better awareness of the natural history of abnormalities as well as diseases affecting this area.

A surgical physiological approach to pathology at this region was proposed in 1977 and still holds true. However, with the advent of better imaging as well as surgical approaches and instrumentation, treatment of problems in this region can be divided into the clinical syndromes, surgical approaches, and techniques of stabilization. A brief outline of the evolving nature of this is provided in this manuscript.

Keywords Craniovertebral junction • Chiari malformation • Occipitoatlantoaxial stabilization • Brain stem compression • Atlantoaxial arthrodesis

A.H. Menezes, MD, FACS, FAAP, FAANS
Department of Neurosurgery, University of Iowa Hospitals and Clinics,
Iowa City, IA 52242, USA
e-mail: arnold-menezes@uiowa.edu

C. Di Rocco, N. Akalan (eds.), *Pediatric Craniovertebral Junction Diseases*,
Advances and Technical Standards in Neurosurgery 40,
DOI 10.1007/978-3-319-01065-6_1, © Springer International Publishing Switzerland 2014

Introduction

Toward the latter part of the nineteenth century, the clinical significance of abnormalities of the craniocervical junction was brought to light with autopsy reports describing the anatomical and embryological abnormalities [14]. This gained clinical importance with the advent of radiographic imaging. Chamberlain, in 1939, presented his treatise on basilar invagination and platybasia. In 1941 Carl List described the neurological syndromes accompanying the developmental anomalies of the occipital bone, the atlas, and the axis vertebrae. He also recognized that cervical traction could result in restoration of anatomical alignment and also relieve compression on the neural structures. The initial treatment of bony lesions at the craniocervical junction consisted of posterior decompression of the foramen magnum and removal of the posterior arch of the atlas and axis vertebra, whether or not there was compression from a dorsal or ventral aspect. Occasionally, a fusion procedure accompanied this. There were unfortunate results when an irreducible ventral lesion at the craniocervical junction caused cervicomedullary compression.

Neurodiagnostic imaging at the craniocervical border has undergone very significant changes in the last three decades [14]. Abnormalities of the bone, soft tissue, and neural structures are easily recognized, and in combination with advances in microsurgical instrumentation, treatment of abnormalities at the craniocervical junction has undergone a great change. There is an increased understanding of the biomechanics of this complex region as well as the embryology. Refinements in computerized technology have better defined, with three-dimensional reconstructions, the normal and abnormal anatomy as well as the visualization of the vascular structures (Fig. 1). Magnetic resonance imaging (MRI) provides information of all the structures and also is capable of being incorporated with dynamic studies to study the motion and vasculature around the craniocervical border (Fig. 2).

A surgical physiological approach to abnormalities at the CVJ in children was proposed in 1977, based on an understanding of the dynamics, the stability, the site of encroachment, and associated neural abnormalities at the craniocervical junction [12, 14]. Since then, more than 6,000 patients, children, and adults with neurological symptoms and signs secondary to abnormalities at the craniocervical junction have been evaluated by the author at the University of Iowa Hospitals and Clinics. This large database has led to a better awareness of the natural history of bony abnormalities as well as diseases affecting this region.

Epidemiology and Classification

A myriad of pathological diagnoses affect the craniocervical junction (Table 1). This has been classified and the reader is referred to other previous publications [12, 14]. A wide variety of congenital, hereditary, developmental, and acquired anomalies exists both individually and in combination.

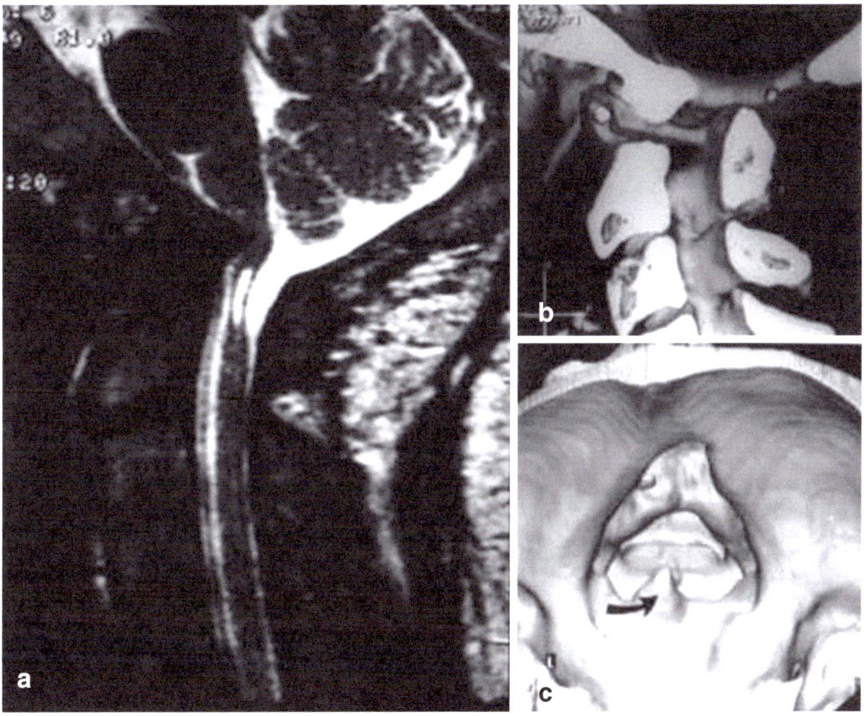

Fig. 1 Composite of (**a**) midsagittal T2-W MRI of CVJ, (**b**) midsagittal 3D CT reconstruction of CVJ, and (**c**) 3D CT of CVJ viewed from within foramen magnum. There is a third occipital condyle "pro-atlas" (*arrow*) remnant that caused the quadriparesis and cervicomedullary atrophy and changes in (**a**)

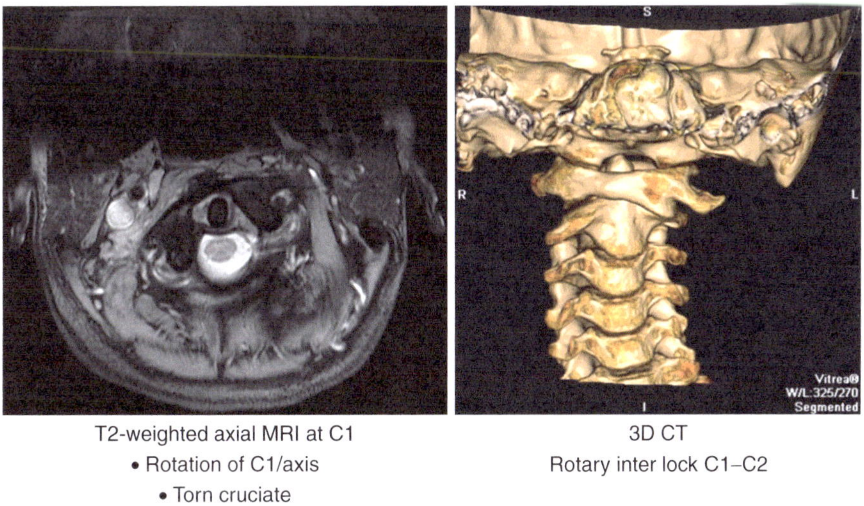

Fig. 2 C1–C2 rotary dislocation in a 9-year-old gymnast

Table 1 Pathology encountered at foramen magnum and upper cervical spinal canal requiring surgical treatment

Location	Congenital	Acquired	Primary neoplastic	Secondary neoplastic	Intra/extradural	Neural tumors
Clivus and foramen magnum	1. Occipital sclerotome segmentation failures 2. Neurenteric cysts	Basilar invagination Basilar impression (Padgets, Rickets, Osteogenesis imperfecta, Acro-osteolysis, Rheumatoid arthritis) Paramesial invagination as in achondroplasia	Eosinophilic granuloma Fibrous dysplasia Chordoma Chondroma Chondrosarcoma Plasmacytoma	Metastasis Nasopharyngeal malignancy Ectopic pituitary	Neurofibroma Meningioma Chordoma Glomus tumor Rhabdomyosarcoma	Brain stem and cerebellar tumors Aneurysms Arachnoid and ependymal cysts Chiari malformation
Atlas vertebra	Assimilation with segmentation failures	Stenosis as in achondroplasia; secondary to chronic dislocations in Morquio syndrome, Down's syndrome, rheumatoid arthritis and arthropathies, etc.	Chordoma Chondroma Giant cell tumor Osteoid osteoma Osteoblastoma	Metastasis Plasmacytoma Local malignancy extensions	Neurofibroma Meningioma Chordoma	Glioma of spinal cord Syringohydromyelia Chiari malformation
Axis vertebra	Segmentation failure, Os odontoi-deum Neurenteric cysts	1. Basilar invagination 2. Basilar impression e.g. osteogenesis imperfecta, Padgets, skeletal dysplasias, rheumatoid arthritis, hyperparathyroidism arthropathies 3. Chronic dislocation 4. Osteomyelitis	Aneurysmal bone cyst Plasmacytoma Chordoma Giant cell tumor Osteoblastoma Chondroma	Metastasis, Local tumor extension	Meningioma Neurofibroma	Glioma of spinal cord Syringohydromyelia

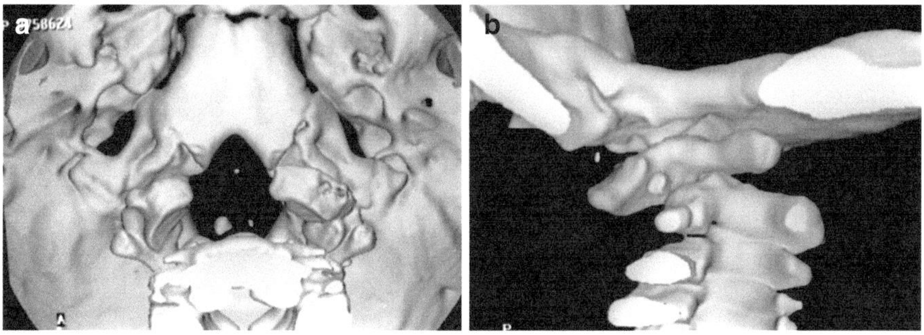

Fig. 3 Composite of 3D CT viewed from skull base (**a**) and in lateral projection (**b**). Note the grossly abnormal anatomy and dislocation

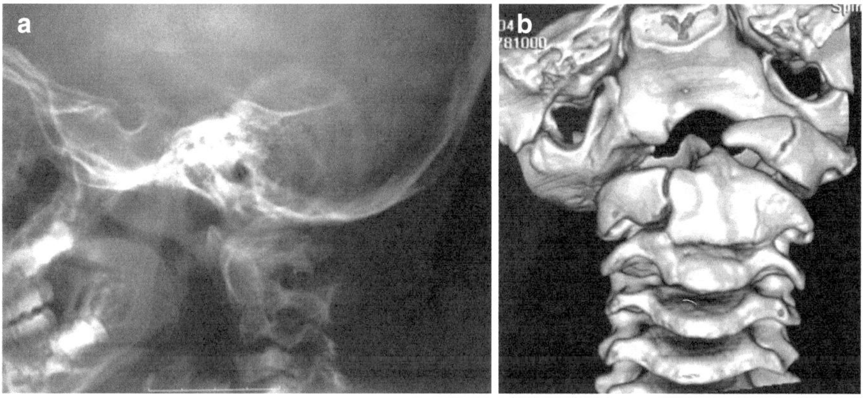

Fig. 4 Lateral cervical radiographs (**a**) and frontal view 3D CT of CVJ in a 4 year old with torticollis (**b**). The right lateral C1 mass is absent

One has to suspect abnormalities of the CVJ in syndromes such as skeletal dysplasias and Goldenhar's syndrome. These can be recognized from the time of birth and the infant's neck supported with custom-built cervical collars (Figs. 3 and 4). Diseases such as Down syndrome, glycogen-storage diseases, and atlas assimilation have a high incidence of craniocervical junction abnormalities [15, 18]. The symptomatic abnormalities in this region present with a constellation of symptoms and signs that reflect dysfunction of the brain stem, cerebellum, cervical spinal cord, cranial nerves, and the cervical roots as well as compression or compromise of the neural structures and their vascular supply. The clinical presentation may be gradual and insidious or rapid in onset.

Imaging of the craniocervical junction starts with magnetic resonance imaging and CT (Figs. 5a–d and 6). The factors taken into consideration for treatment of

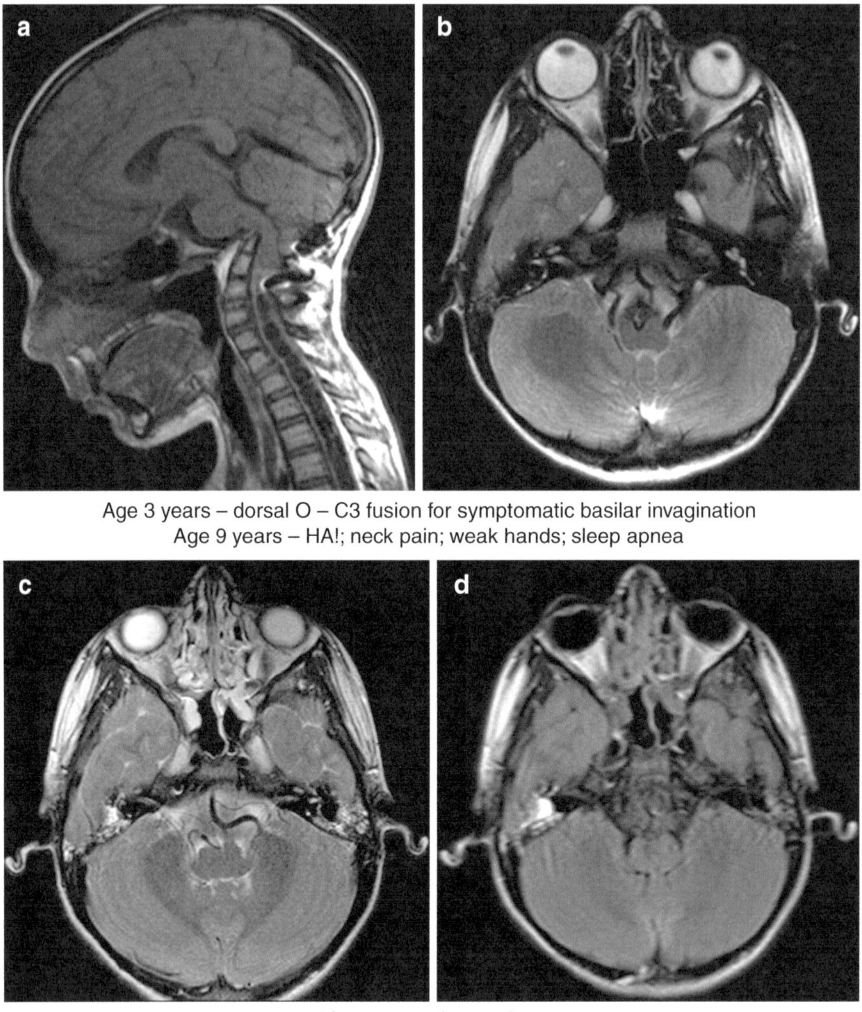

Fig. 5 Composite of midsagittal T1-W MRI of CVJ (**a**) and axial view just above foramen magnum (**b**). The odontoid has invaginated into the medulla (**b**). T2-W MRI (**c**) and T1-W MRI in (**d**) axial views after odontoid resection

bony abnormalities of the craniocervical junction in children consist of the following: [14] (1) reducibility, (2) mechanism of encroachment, (3) the underlying embryological abnormality, and (4) the relationship to the vascular and CSF spaces. A reducible lesion is one where there is restoration of anatomical alignment thereby relieving compression of the neural structures. This could be by head and neck positioning, cervical traction, or intraoperative reduction.

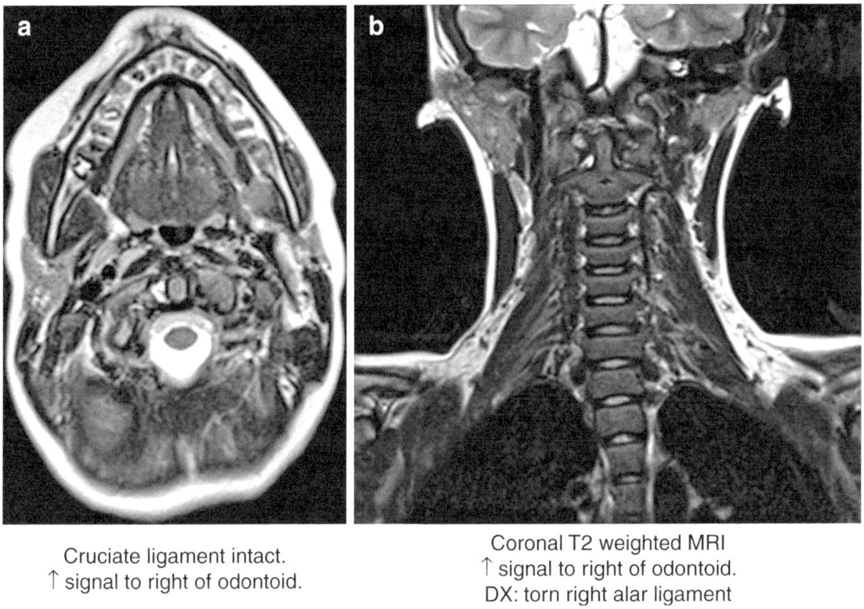

Fig. 6 Composite of axial T2-W MRI at C1 (**a**) and coronal image through plane of odontoid (**b**). Note the torn alar ligament as a hyperintense signal lateral to the odontoid process

In a reducible lesion, stabilization is paramount [15]. In irreducible states, decompression is first accomplished followed by attention to the stability. Thus the surgical treatment could be divided into approaches for decompression and those that are used for fusion at the craniocervical border. This implies correction of occipitoatlantoaxial instability or separate components within.

Reducibility

It is evident when one can restore craniocervical alignment with head and neck position or with traction. A recent development has been intraoperative traction facilitated by pharmacological muscle relaxation under general anesthesia and positioning with documentation using intraoperative CT [6]. This has proven useful in 60 % of children with what was felt to be "irreducible" lesions. One has to differentiate between reducibility and distraction. Meer "pulling down" of the spine from the cranium does not correspond to a reducible lesion unless there is restoration of alignment and relief of compression on the neural structures. One also has to keep in mind the stretch on vascular structures. This is done under halo cervical traction accompanied with somatosensory evoked potentials (SSEP) and motor evoked potentials (MEP) (reference). Once the abnormality is felt to be reducible in the supine position, the procedure is carried out again in the prone position which would be the position for posterior decompression and fusion (Fig. 7a–c). Intraoperative reduction with distraction is also possible as illustrated (Fig. 8a, b).

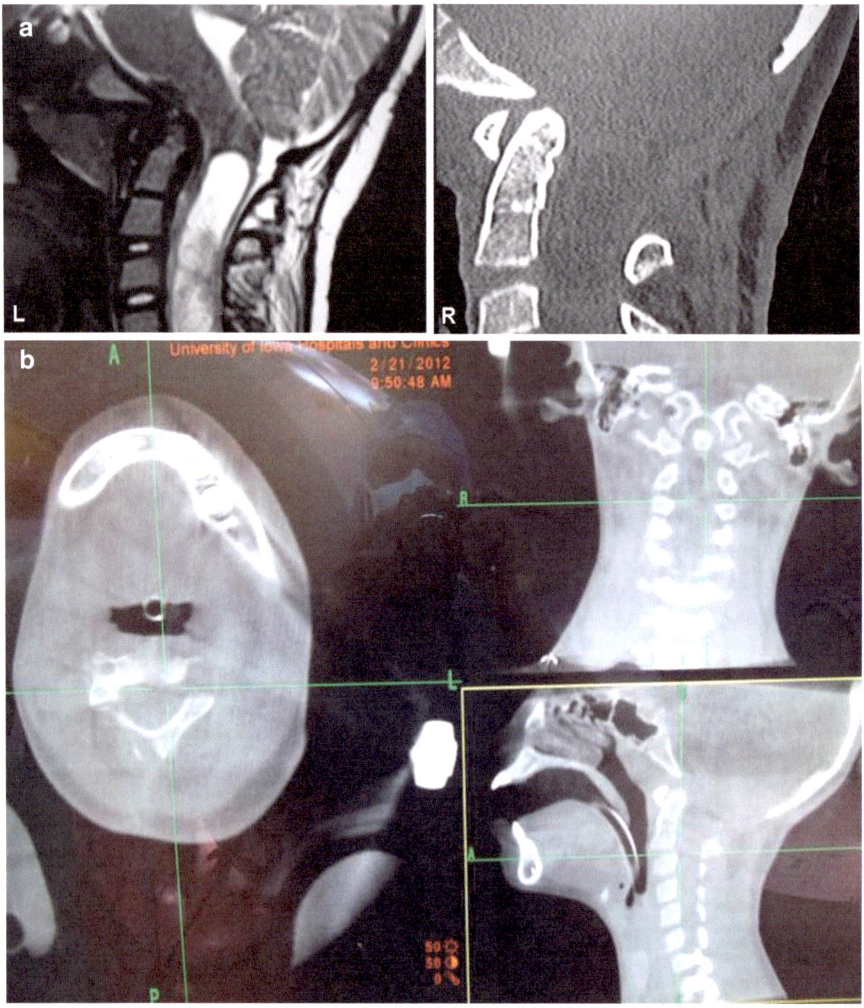

Fig. 7 (**a**) Composite of T2-W MRI of CVJ (*L*) and midsagittal 2D CT at CJV (*R*). This child underwent dorsal decompression for Chiari I 16 months prior. Note the new syringohydromyelia and 95° clivus-canal angle indenting into the medulla. (**b**) CT scans obtained in halo traction with muscle paralysis under anesthesia with intraoperative CT. This documents realignment of the clivus-canal angle to 140°. (**c**) Operative view of occipitocervical fusion (O–C2–C3) with screw/plate and rods and into grafts

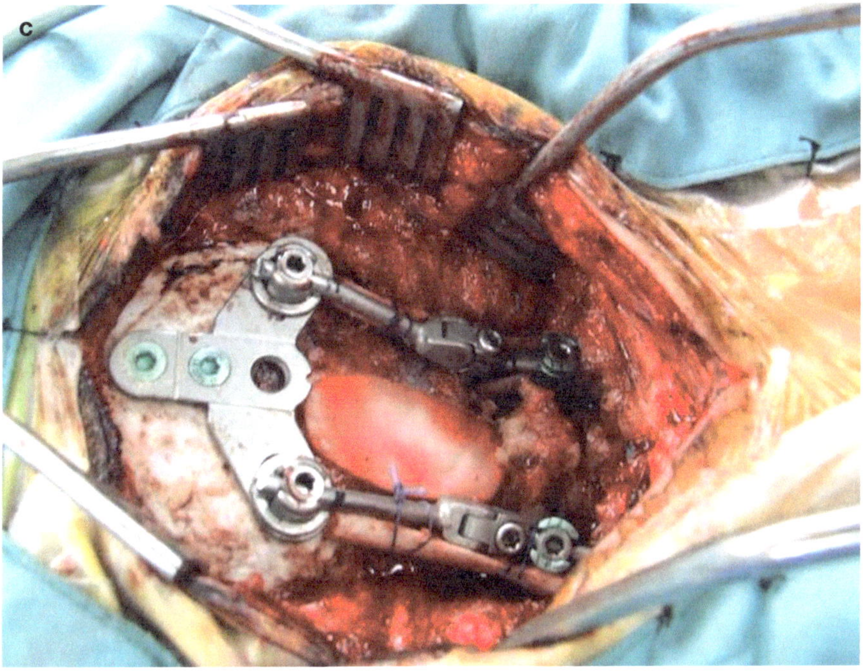

Fig. 7 (continued)

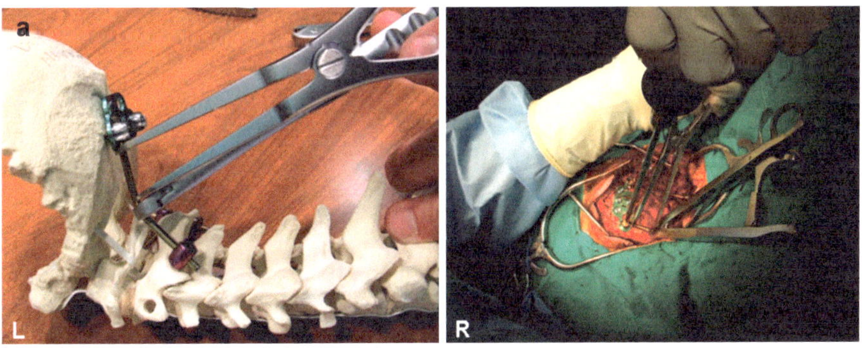

Fig. 8 (**a**) Demonstration of reduction/distraction of O-C2 fusion construct in a "sawbone" model (*L*) and at surgery (*R*). (**b**) O–C1–C2 instability viewed through lateral fluoroscope in a patient with atlas assimilation who had undergone a posterior foramen magnum decompression (*L*); and after reduction and fusion (*R*)

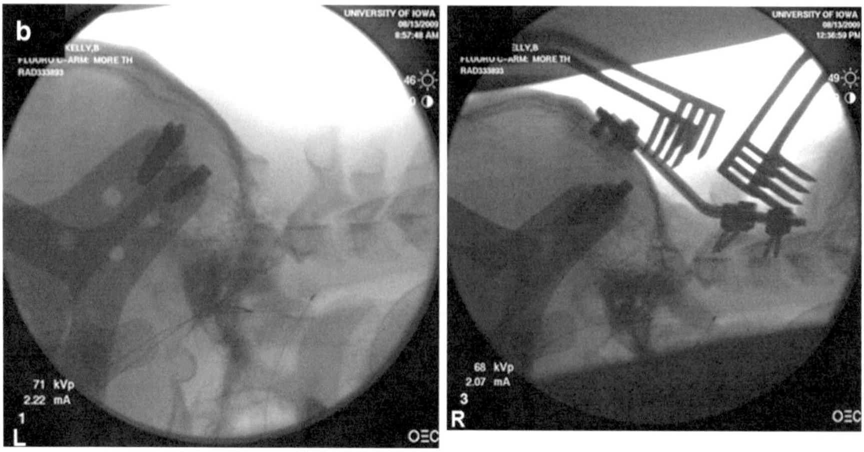

Fig. 8 (continued)

Surgical Approaches (Table 2) [14]

1. Ventral – this comprises of the transoral-transpalatine approach, the mandibular split, and the lateral extrapharyngeal approach. All these have separate indications.
2. Endoscopic transnasal and lateral extrapharyngeal approach
3. Lateral transcondylar posterolateral approach to craniocervical border
4. Posterolateral partial transcondylar approach
5. Dorsal approach

Fusions at the Craniocervical Junction

In the very young, below the age of 5–6 years, a bony fusion between the dorsal atlas and the axis has been the mainstay with this author [1, 5, 13]. A similar extension to the occiput has been described. The author has used rib grafts for this. Having said this, the youngest child for craniocervical instrumentation has been 6 years of age. This is dependent on the size and thickness of the occiput, its midline keel, the width of the lateral atlantal masses, the thickness of the pars, and the lamina at C2.

Instrumentation for craniocervical fusions has made a radical change due to the design and concepts as well as information of the biomechanics and long-term effects [1, 2, 4, 9, 11].

In the author's experience, the transarticular C2–C1 fixation has been useful (Fig. 9a, b) but is now circumvented by the lateral atlantal mass screw with a pars

Table 2 Surgical approaches to the craniocervical cervical junction

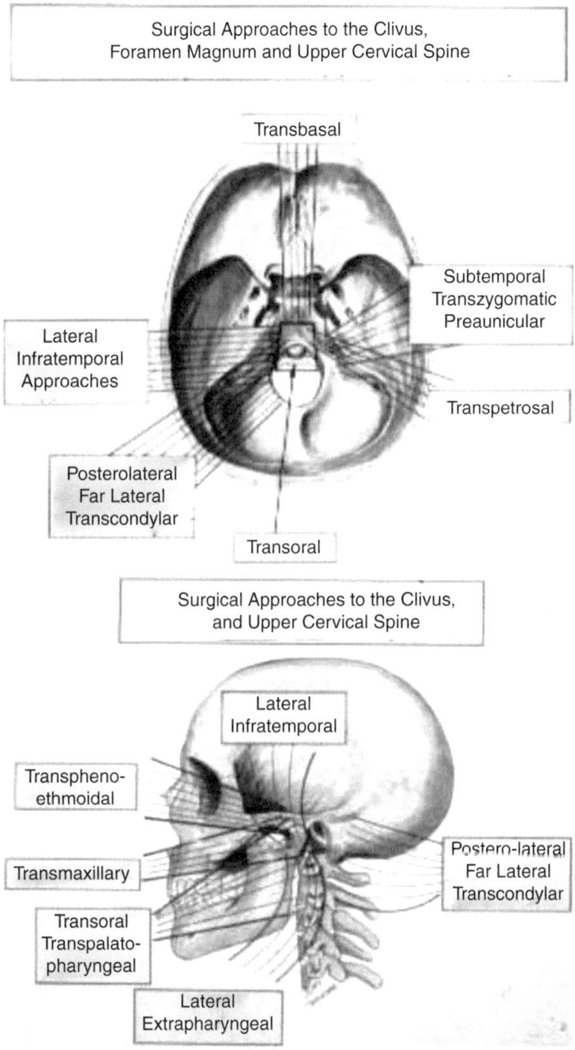

screw at C2 and an inter-rod fixation for atlantoaxial instrumented arthrodesis. In the face of narrow pars at C2, a translaminar screw is possible [1, 11]. The occipital keel provides a very satisfactory fixation of occipital screws and plates to be incorporated with craniocervical fixation. It is now evident that occiput-C2 fusion does not actually require a screw at C1 lateral mass with both class III and class II evidence [4, 9].

The natural history of diseases and abnormalities affecting the craniocervical region in the pediatric population is extremely important to predict the long-term outlook and to take steps to avoid unfortunate results. An example of this is posterior fossa decompression for hindbrain herniation (Chiari I) in the face of atlas assimilation and segmentation failure of C2–C3. These patients require a dorsal occipitocervical fixation simultaneous with the decompression. A similar situation arises with the collagen diseases such as Ehlers-Danlos disease which may be associated with a symptomatic Chiari I abnormality. "Irreducible" craniocervical junction abnormalities with pediatric basilar invagination may be treated with only a dorsal procedure if intraoperative reduction is possible and documented. Decompression procedures available from the ventral approach have been a gold standard with the open approaches (Fig. 10a, b). The endoscopic procedures have certain indications and limitations. Pharyngeal closure via a strictly endoscopic procedure is not possible [8]. We have used this in a limited manner for bony abnormalities but have relied on it for petroclival midline tumors with good results (Fig. 11a, b). Interest at the craniocervical border has brought about a greater understanding of the anatomy as well as its identification on neurodiagnostic imaging [3, 7, 10, 16, 17]. The ligamentous abnormalities, disruptions of the cruciate, the alar

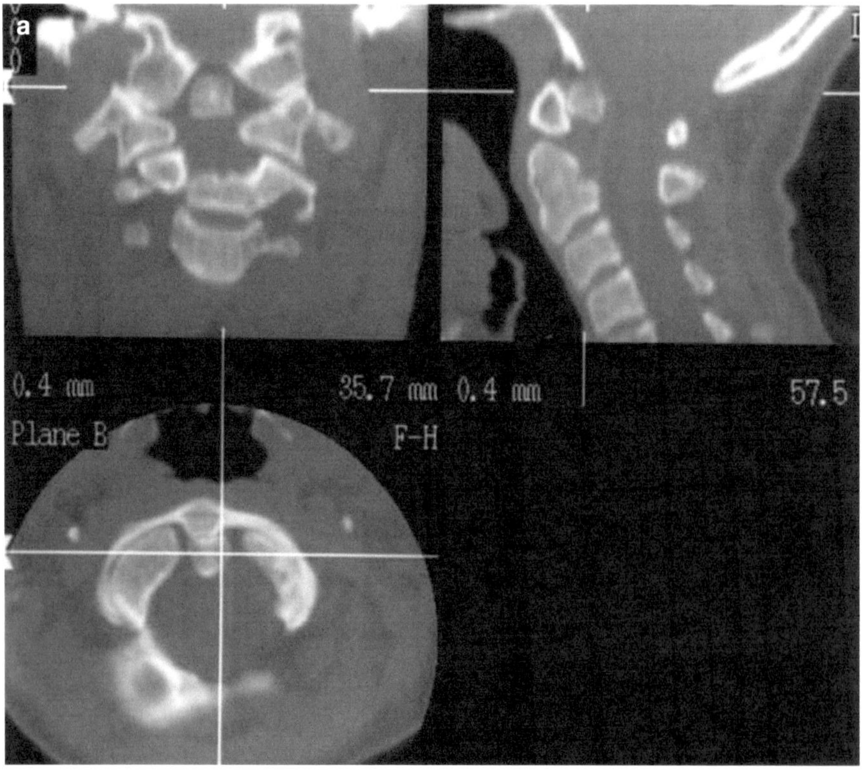

Fig. 9 (**a**) Composite of coronal, sagittal, and axial 2D CT at CVJ in a 12-year-old male with unstable CVJ secondary to dystopic os odontoideum. (**b**) Lateral cervical radiograph after transarticular C2–C1 screw fixation and interlaminar fusion

Fig. 9 (continued)

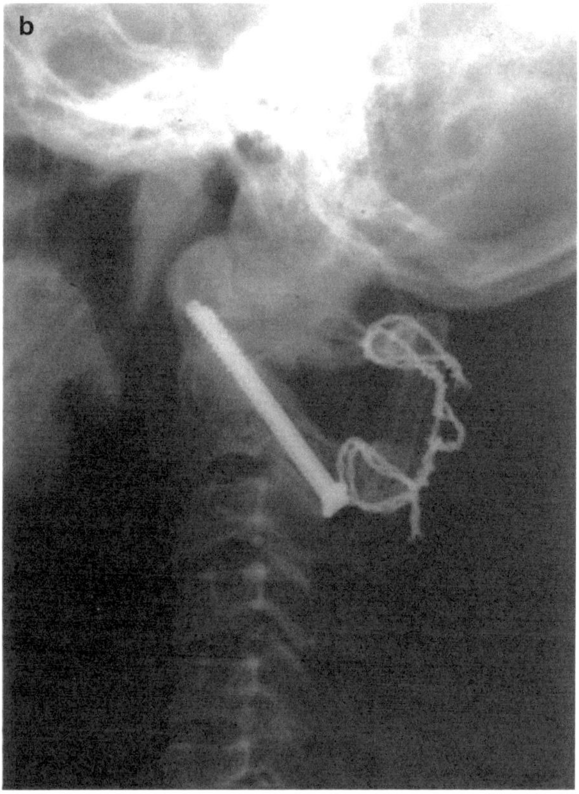

ligaments, and the tectorial membrane are easily recognized on specific image modalities with magnetic resonance imaging. Once cruciate ligament rupture has been recognized, this automatically calls for stabilization. The craniocervical region can no longer be called as "no man's land" as significant strides are being made in management of disorders in this location.

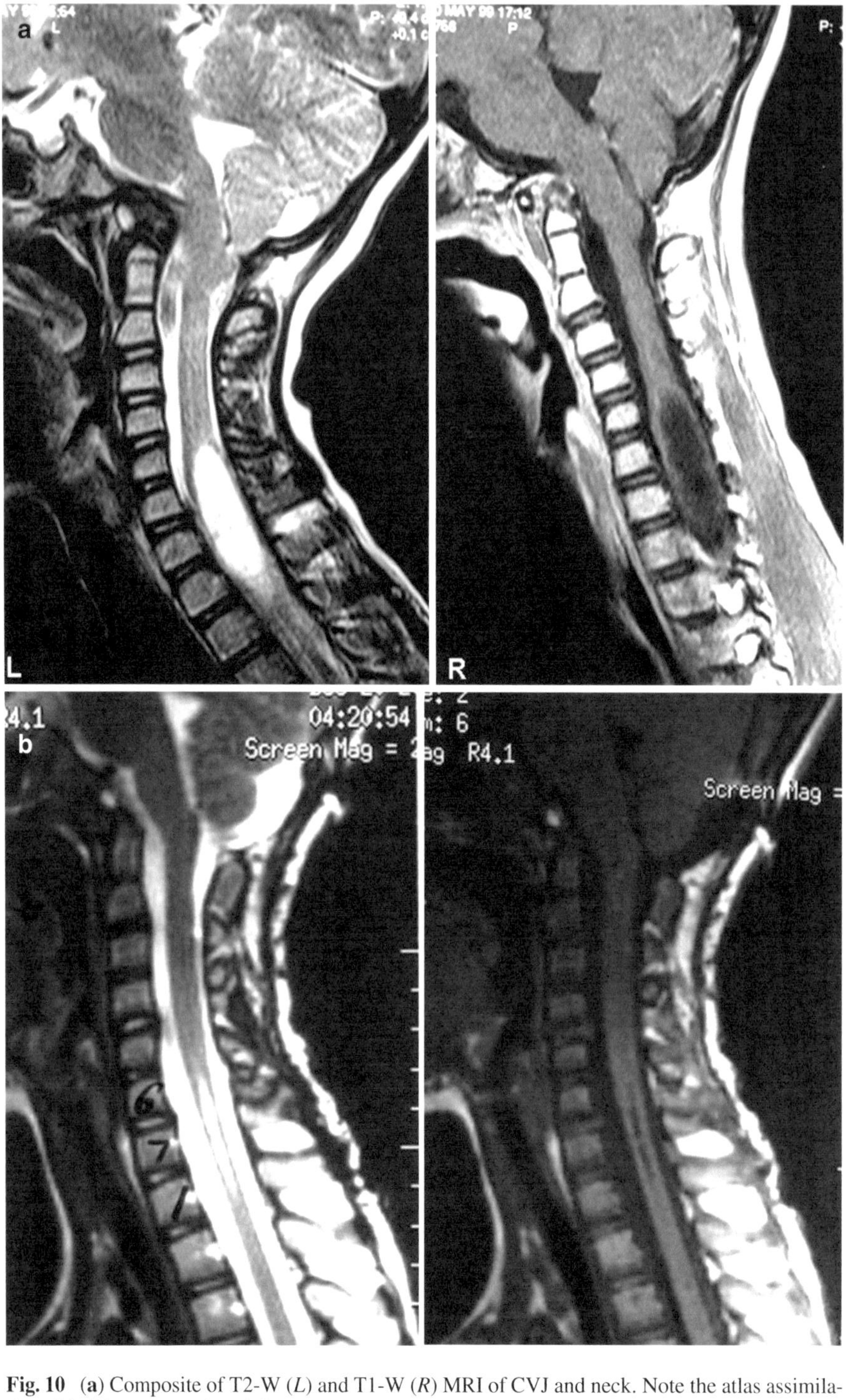

Fig. 10 (**a**) Composite of T2-W (*L*) and T1-W (*R*) MRI of CVJ and neck. Note the atlas assimilation, C2–C3 segmentation failure, ventral medulla compression, tonsillar ectopia, and cervical syringomyelia. (**b**) Composite as in Fig. 10a; after ventral CVJ decompression. Note the syrinx deflation and tonsillar ascent

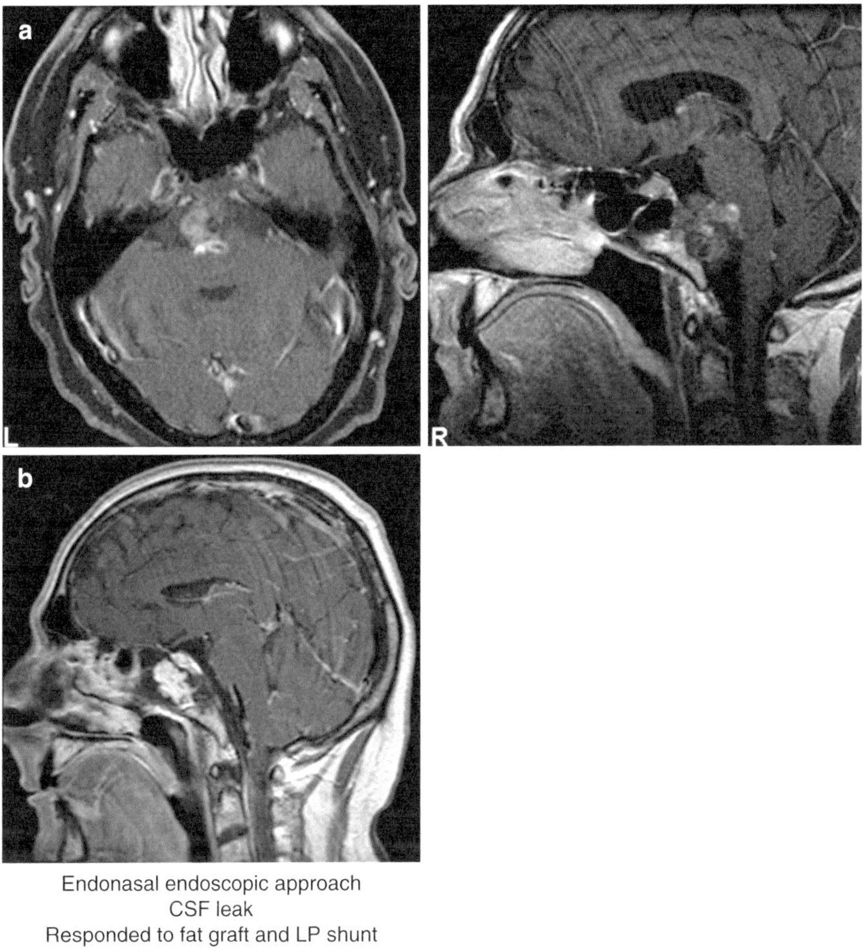

Fig. 11 (**a**) Axial (*L*) and midsagittal MRI with gadolinium reveals retroclival chordoma. (**b**) Midsagittal T1-W MRI with contrast; made after endonasal endoscopic resection of the retroclival chordoma

References

1. Ahmed R, Traynelis VC, Menezes AH (2008) Fusions at the craniovertebral junction. Childs Nerv Syst 24:1209–1224
2. Anderson RCE, Ragel BT, Mocco J, Bohman LE, Brockmeyer DL (2007) Selection of a rigid interval fixation construct for stabilization at the craniovertebral junction in pediatric patients. J Neurosurg Pediatr 107:36–42
3. Arvin B, Fournier-Gosselin MP, Fehlings MG (2010) Os odontoideum: etiology and surgical management. Neurosurgery 66:22–31
4. Brockmeyer DL (2007) Editorial: lateral mass screw fixation of C1. J Neurosurg Pediatr 107:173–177
5. Cohen MW, Drummond DS, Flynn JM, Pill SG, Dormans JP (2001) A technique of occipitocervical arthrodesis in children using autologous rib grafts. Spine 26(7): 825–829

6. Dahdaleh NS, Dlouhy BJ, Menezes AH (2012) Application of neuromuscular blockade and intraoperative 3D imaging in the reduction of basilar invagination. J Neurosurg Pediatr 92:119–124
7. Deichmueller CM, Welkoborsky HJ (2010) Grisel's syndrome – a rare complication following "small" operations and infections in the ENT region. Eur Arch Otorhinolaryngol 267(9):1467–1473
8. Frempong-Boadu AK, Faunce WA, Fessler RG (2002) Endoscopically assisted transoral-transpharyngeal approach to the craniovertebral junction. Neurosurgery 51:S60–S66
9. Hankinson TC, Avellino AM, Harter D et al (2010) Equivalence of fusion rates after rigid internal fixation of the occiput to C2 with or without C1 instrumentation. J Neurosurg Pediatr 5(4):380–384
10. Kotil K, Kalayci M (2005) Ventral cervicomedullary junction compression secondary to condylus occipitalis (median occipital condyle): a rare entity. J Spinal Disord Tech 18:382–384
11. Leonard JR, Wright NM (2006) Pediatric atlantoaxial fixation with bilateral crossing C2 translaminar screws. Technical note. J Neurosurg Pediatr 104:59–63
12. Menezes AH (2008) Craniocervical developmental anatomy and its implications. Childs Nerv Syst 24:1109–1122
13. Menezes AH (2012) Craniocervical fusions in children. J Neurosurg Pediatr 9(6):573–585
14. Menezes AH, Albert GW (2011) Acquired abnormalities of the craniocervical junction. In: Winn R (ed) Youmans neurological surgery. Saunders, Philadelphia, pp 2961–2972
15. Menezes AH, Fenoy KA (2009) Remnants of occipital vertebrae: proatlas segmentation abnormalities. Neurosurgery 64:945–953
16. Nader-Sepahi A, Casey ATH, Hayward R, Crockard HA, Thompson D (2005) Symptomatic atlantoaxial instability in Down syndrome. J Neurosurg Pediatr 103:231–237
17. Pang D, Thompson DP (2011) Embryology and bony malformations of the craniovertebral junction. Childs Nerv Syst 27:523–564
18. Taggard DA, Menezes AH, Ryken TC (2000) Treatment of Down syndrome – associated craniovertebral junction abnormalities. J Neurosurg Spine 93:205–213

Embryology, Classification, and Surgical Management of Bony Malformations of the Craniovertebral Junction

Dachling Pang and Dominic N.P. Thompson

Contents

D. Pang, MD, FRCS(C), FRCS(Eng), FACS (✉)
Department of Paediatric Neurosurgery, University of California, Davis, CA, USA

Department of Paediatric Neurosurgery, Regional Centre of Pediatric Neurosurgery, Kaiser Foundation Hospitals of Northern California, Oakland, CA, USA

Department of Paediatric Neurosurgery, Kaiser Permanente Medical Center, 280 W. MacArthur Blvd., Oakland, CA 94611, USA
e-mail: pangtv@aol.com

D.N.P. Thompson, MBBS, BSc, FRCS(SN)
Department of Paediatric Neurosurgery, Great Ormond Street Hospital for Children NHS Trust, Great Ormond Street, London, UK

C. Di Rocco, N. Akalan (eds.), *Pediatric Craniovertebral Junction Diseases*, Advances and Technical Standards in Neurosurgery 40,
DOI 10.1007/978-3-319-01065-6_2,

Abstract The embryology of the bony craniovertebral junction (CVJ) is reviewed with the purpose of explaining the genesis and unusual configurations of the numerous congenital malformations in this region. Functionally, the bony CVJ can be divided into a central pillar consisting of the basiocciput and dental pivot; and a two-tiered ring revolving round the central pivot, comprising the foramen magnum rim and occipital condyles above, and the atlantal ring below. Embryologically, the central pillar and the surrounding rings descend from different primordia, and accordingly, developmental anomalies at the CVJ can also be segregated into those affecting the central pillar and the surrounding rings, respectively. A logical classification of this seemingly unwieldy group of malformations is thus possible based on their ontogenetic lineage, morbid anatomy, and clinical relevance. Representative examples of the main constituents of this classification scheme are given, and their surgical treatments are selectively discussed.

Keywords Congenital malformation • Craniovertebral junction • Genetic control • Hox genes • Instability • Neural compression • Occipital-cervical fusion • Primary somitogenesis • Sclerotomal resegmentation

The bony craniovertebral junction (CVJ) can be conceptually divided into two components with respect to the governance of intersegmental movements and functional space for the nervous system. The first component consists mainly of a central pivot made up of the dens and the C_2 vertebral body, but the basiocciput, though anatomically part of the foramen magnum, is embryologically and functionally in vertical linearity with the dens and is thus part of the central pillar. The second component consists of two ringed structures surrounding the central pivot, albeit eccentrically. They are the foramen magnum ring, comprising the lateral portion of the basiocciput (clivus), the exocciput including the occipital condyles, and the opisthion; and the atlantal ring, with its anterior and posterior arches and lateral masses. These two superimposing rings transmit the lower brainstem and upper cervical spinal cord, while permitting limited rotatory and flexion-extension motions upon each other and round the dental pivot. Straddling these two rings and anchoring upon them are the stabilising ligaments between the pivot and the rings: the alar and apical dental ligaments at the upside of the pivot, the transverse atlantal ligament (TAL) across the main dental shaft, and the arching mantle of the tectorial membrane and cruciate ligament, strapping the clivus to the whole of the dens-axis assembly.

Not surprisingly, the anatomical division of the CVJ into axial and flanking components has close analogy in the embryology of this region. The constituents of the central pillar are all derived from the axial portion of the occipital and upper two cervical sclerotomes, whereas the ring structures all come from the lateral portion of these same sclerotomes as well as from a small sclerotomal offshoot ventral to the notochord called the hypochordal bow (see below). Accordingly, disturbance in the axial sclerotomes produces anomalies of the dens-pivot and the basiocciput; the former comprise the various forms of odontoid dysgenesis, and the latter, the less familiar types of clival abnormalities. A testament to the proximate origins of the dental and clival primordia is readily proclaimed by the large archive of associative syndromes of platybasia, brachybasia, basilar kyphosis, basilar impression, retroflexed dens, and cerebellar ectopia. In contrast, disturbance in the lateral portion of the occipital and upper cervical sclerotomes and hypochordal bow results in anomalies of the "rings", including dysplasia of the lateral clival rim, occipital condyles, the anterior and posterior atlantal arches, and the lateral masses of C_1 and C_2. Table 1 segregates these anomalies by ontogenetic lineages and shows that this seemingly confusing and unwieldy group of malformations are in fact steep in embryological logic.

This chapter deals first with the normal development and genetic control of the bony CVJ, followed by descriptions of congenital malformations of this region with emphasis on their embryogenesis and clinical relevance. Special considerations of the techniques and pitfalls of fusion and decompression of the occiput-C_1–C_2 complex in young children are provided when applicable.

Embryology of the Craniovertebral Junction

The Pre-somitic Stage

At gastrulation, epiblastic cells from the embryonic plate caudal to the head process invaginate through the primitive streak to form mesoderm on each side of the neural plate, while cells from both sides of the dorsal lip of Hensen's node migrate through the primitive pit to integrate into the midline notochord. The embryonic plate thus elongates by new additions to its rear (caudal) aspect [24].

The anterior-posterior (rostrocaudal) polarity of the embryo is determined very early during gastrulation. The prechordal mesoderm rostral to the otic vesicle (and notochord) forms most of the bones and muscles of the head and face without ever developing somites. Caudal to this tissue is the somitic region which extends along the body axis down to the tip of the tail (Fig. 1). The anterior somitic region from the otic vesicle to the blastopore (future anus) corresponds to the future body axis from the occiput to the anus. Here, the epiblastic cells condense to form the parachordal mesoderm on each side of the notochord following systematic ingression movements through the primitive streak. This initially homogenous column of cells, also called pre-somitic mesoderm (PSM) or segmental plate, subsequently segregates into segmental clusters called somites, which will eventually give rise to the smooth muscle of the dermis, the axial musculature, the vertebral column, and support structures of the peripheral nervous system. After blastopore closure and complete regression of the primitive streak, the gastrulating region for the tail is restricted to a

Table 1 Classification of bony malformations of the CVJ according to embryogenesis

Malformations of central pillar		Malformations of surrounding rings	
Disturbance of axial component of occipital sclerotome, proatlas and C_1 resegmented sclerotome		Disturbance of lateral component and hypochordal bows of proatlas and C_1 resegmented sclerotome	
Odontoid dysgeneses	Basioccipital dysgeneses	Proatlas anomalies	C_1 sclerotome anomalies
Aplasia/hypoplasia of odontoid components	Failed midline integration of basioccipital primordium	Hyperplasia of hypochordal bow of proatlas	Aplasia of hypochordal bow of C_1
Disturbance of odontoid synchondroses (IBZ)	Bifid clivus	Third occipital condyle	Aplasia and hypoplasia of anterior C_1 arch
Os odontoideum	Basioccipital dysplasia	Pre-basioccipital arch	Aplasia/hypoplasia of lateral sclerotome of C_1
Ossiculum terminale	Basilar impression	Hyperplasia of lateral (exoccipital) sclerotome of proatlas	Aplasia and hypoplasia of posterior C_1 arch
Abnormal resegmentation of proatlas centrum	Platybasia	Hypertrophic occipital condyle	Aplasia of lateral mass of C_1
Os avis	Retroflexed dens	Non-resegmentation of proatlas (anterior homeotic transformation)	Combined C_1 hypochordal bow and lateral sclerotome dysplasia
Failed midline integration of basal dental segment	Basilar invagination	Atlas assimilation	Aplasia of lateral mass and anterior C_1 arch
Bifid dens	Basilar kyphosis	Posterior homeotic transformation	Combined anterior and posterior C_1 arch defects
	Short clivus		Bifid anterior and posterior C_1 arch

small region called the tail bud, located at the caudal tip of the primitive streak. The tail bud functions as a blastema of undifferentiated cells [20, 21]. The pre-somitic mesoderm and later somites of the caudal and tail regions are therefore not formed by epiblastic ingression but by progenitor condensation in situ.

Primary Segmentation: Somitogenesis

Prior to the appearance of somites, the PSM remains a loose mesenchyme without specific cellular polarity or stratification pattern alongside the lengthening notochord and neural plate [75]. During somitogenesis, the loose mesenchymal cells of

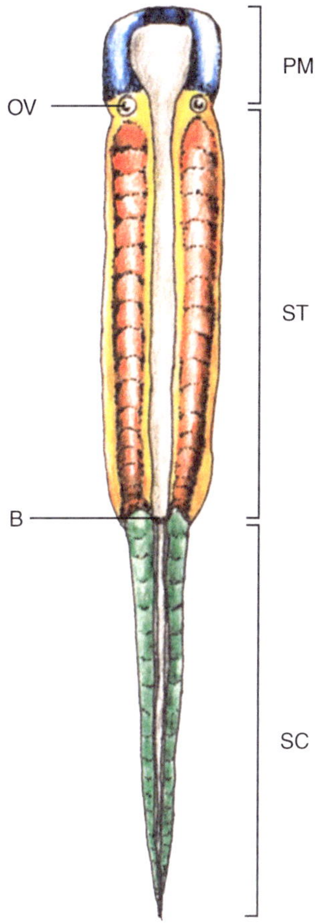

Fig. 1 Vertebrate embryonic plate around gastrulation showing the three main regions of the body plan: The prechordal mesoderm (*PM*) is anterior to the otic vesicle (*OV*). Posterior to the OV to the blastopore (*B*) is the somitic region of the trunk (*ST*), caudal to which is the caudal (tail) somitic region (*SC*)

the PSM undergo transformation into tightly-apposed epithelial cells with definite polarity and orientation. A newly formed somite is a compact epithelial sphere ("somitomere") composed of a single layer of radially arranged cells with apices pointing towards a central lumen (somitocoele), which contains a few mesenchymal cells [45] (Fig. 2). The epithelial cells have polarised Golgi zones, basally aligned nuclei, and actin molecules near the luminal border, the entire sphere being enveloped by a collagen-containing basal lamina [4]. This epithelial conversion of the PSM is aided by an increase in cell-cell adhesion mediated by a sharp but transient rise in the levels of the calcium-dependent adhesion molecule N-cadherin, of fibronectin and possibly cytotactin [88].

Somitogenesis begins soon after internalisation of the prochordal (head) mesoderm and continues through subsequent production of the body axis. The first somite forms immediately caudal to the otic vesicle [38], followed by sequential transformation such that a new pair of somites is regularly added in a rostrocaudal direction until a fixed species-specific number of somites is reached (Fig. 3). Thus, depending on the stage of gastrulation, the growing column of body mesoderm

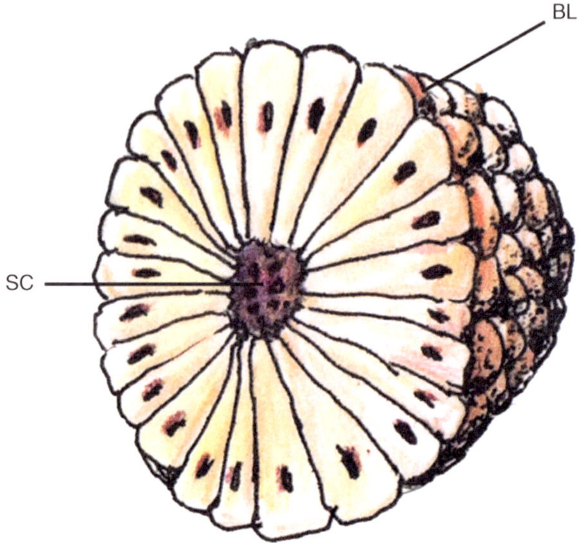

Fig. 2 Somite with radially arranged and polarised epithelial cells surrounding a central cavity, the somitocoele (*SC*) and enveloped by a basal lamina (*BL*)

consists of a rostral section of mature somites already undergoing differentiation into sclerotomes and dermomyotomes, a middle section of new pre-differentiated epithelial somites, and a caudal section of pre-somitic mesoderm just rostral to the remaining primitive streak, the whole enterprise necessarily evolving in parallel with the neurulating neural plates (Fig. 4).

Current thinking regarding the mechanism of metameric transformation of the PSM follows what is called the "Clock and Wavefront" model, first proposed by Cooke and Zeeman in 1976. In this model, PSM cells oscillate between a permissive and a nonpermissive state for somite formation. These oscillations are phase-linked and controlled cell-autonomously by a "Segmentation Clock". Somitic formation is triggered when cells of the rostral PSM, while in the permissive phase of the Clock, are hit by a wavefront of maturation (or determination) that slowly moves caudally along the embryonic axis (Fig. 5). At this exact site, a transverse column of "boundary cells" forms across the width of the PSM, such that at the next periodic activation of the "Segmentation Clock", a consecutive column of boundary cells, together with the previous boundary, now segregates out a segment of PSM that will ultimately evolve into a somite. Thus, the Clock generates a temporal periodicity that is translated spatially into the periodic boundaries of the somites [75] (Fig. 6).

At the molecular level, the phasic oscillation of the Segmentation Clock is reflected by rhythmic expressions of a class of genes called cycling genes [74]. These genes include the *c-hairy1* family in fish, chick, frog, and mouse, which encode transcription factors such as the split (HES) family and the glycosyltransferase Lunatic Fringe [28, 56], all tightly involved in the Notch signalling pathway and its ligands, suggesting that periodic Notch activation plays a critical role in the oscillator (Fig. 7). Also, these genes oscillate largely in synchrony in the PSM, suggesting they are downstream of a common cycling activator.

In chick and mouse embryos, the maturation or determination wave is generated by the expression of genes which include the fibroblast growth factor gene

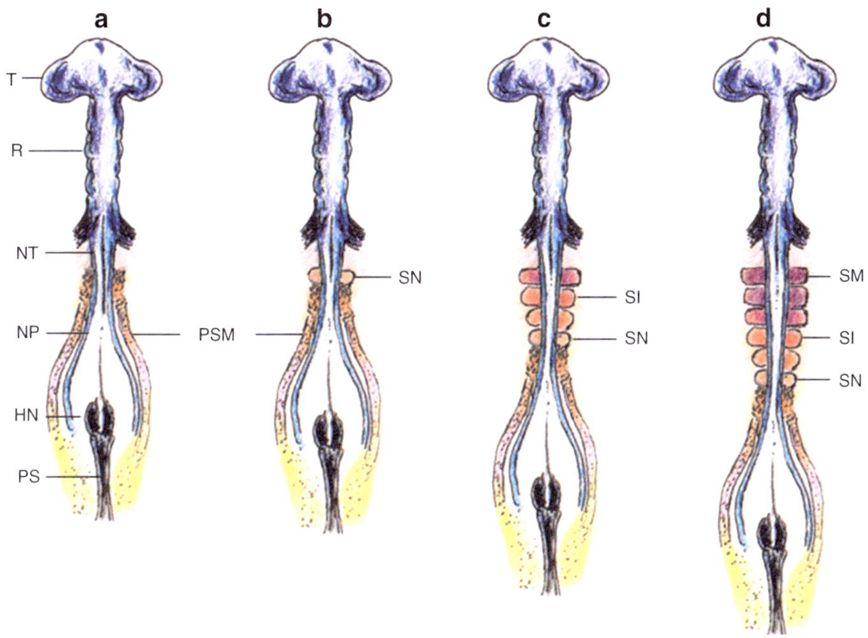

Fig. 3 Primary somitogenesis in a chick embryo. (**a**) At very early gastrulation, the mostly unneurulated neural plate caudal to the prochordal plate (head process) is flanked on each side by the pre-somitic (pre-segmented) mesoderm or PSM. (**b**) The first pair of somites is formed just caudal to the otic vesicles. The PSM column elongates from addition of new cells from the caudal embryonic pole rostral to Hensen's node. (**c**) The new somites (*SN*) are formed in a rostrocaudal direction so that the older more matured somites (*SM*) are rostral, i.e., closer to the cephalic end of the embryo. (**d**) The older matured somites (*SM*) have undergone dorsoventral differentiation (*purple colour*) into sclerotome and dermomyotome. The intermediate-aged somites (*SI*) (*orange colour*) are pre-differentiated units without dorsoventral specification. The PSM is always at the most caudal end closest to Hensen's node. Rostrocaudal sequential somitogenesis parallels progression of primary neurulation. *HN* Hensen's node, *PS* primitive streak, *T* telencephalon, *R* rhombencephalon, *NT* neural tube, *NP* neural plate

fgf8 [82]. It is known that the caudal domain of the PSM is very high in the factor FGF8, which seems to actively maintain the mesenchymal identity of caudal PSM cells. The FGF8 gradient decreases towards the rostral axis, so that at the rostral domain of the PSM where somitogenesis is taking place, FGF8 level is very low. Also, overexpression of *fgf8* in this region results in inhibition of somitogenesis. Thus, the activation of epithelisation of PSM cells is *negatively* regulated by FGF8, whose absence allows the PSM cells to become competent to respond to the clock signal and initiate somitic boundary formation [26]. The limit between the two domains of high (in the caudal PSM) and low (in the rostral PSM) *fgf8* expression therefore marks the determination wavefront of somitogenesis [75] (Fig. 8).

Due to the constant caudal elongation of the body axis during gastrulation and the addition of new PSM cells with strong *fgf8* expression to the rear, the FGF8 gradient is continuously displaced caudally. Accordingly, the determination wavefront also

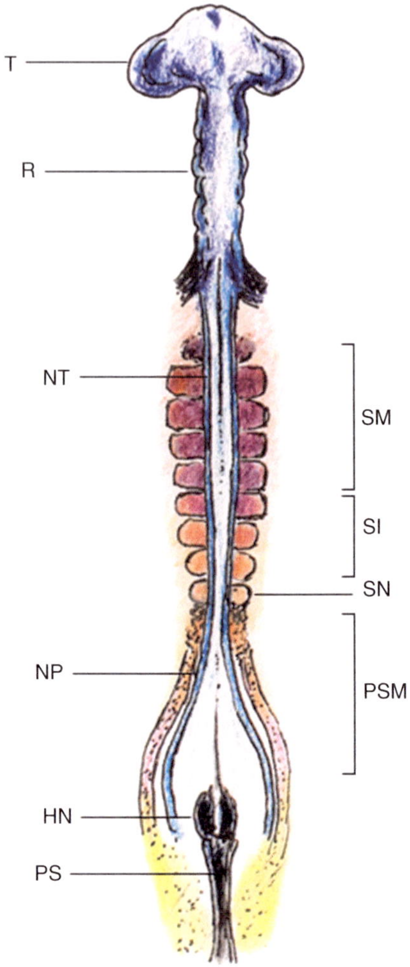

Fig. 4 Chick embryo during sequential somite formation close to the end of gastrulation. The rostral-most mesoderm consists of matured somites (*SM*) already having undergone dorsoventral differentiation into dermomyotome and sclerotome, flanking the formed neural tubes (*NT*); followed by the newer intermediate-aged pre-differentiated epithelial somites (*SI*), the new somites (*SN*), and the pre-somitic mesoderm (*PSM*) on each side of the unneurulated neural plate (*NP*). *HN* Hensen's node, *PS* primitive streak, *T* telencephalon, *R* rhombencephalon

moves slowly in a caudal direction along the body axis. This ensures that the old and new metameric boundaries, at both ends of a new somite, are separated by a distance corresponding to the caudal displacement of the determination wavefront during one period of oscillation of the Segmentation Clock [74] (Fig. 8). The speed of new somite production is thus linked to the Clock period, which is species specific: 30 min for zebra fish, 90 min for chick, and 120 min for mouse [70].

Differentiation of the Somitic Mesenchyme

Within hours after its formation, each somite starts differentiating along its dorsoventral axis. Cells from its ventromedial part lose their epithelial arrangement and migrate towards the notochord to form, with the luminal cells, the mesenchymal

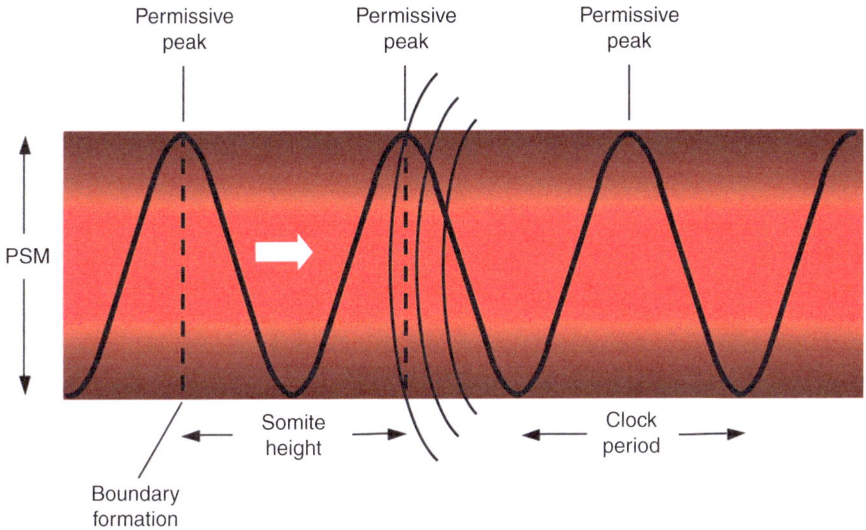

Fig. 5 The clock and wavefront theory of primary somitogenesis. The Segmentation Clock is a pattern of cell-autonomous, phase-linked oscillations of certain "cycling" gene expression within the PSM cells, producing a sinusoidal wave of peaks and troughs of gene products which render the cell either "permissive" or "nonpermissive" to changes when "hit" by a moving wavefront. *Block arrow* shows direction of wavefront. When the wavefront (*curved lines*) hits the "permissive" peak of the gene cycle, the cells at that region of the PSM undergo changes which demarcate them from the surrounding uncommitted mesenchyme, causing formation of a boundary zone (*dotted vertical lines*) cutting across the whole width of the PSM column because the clock periods (time lapses between wave peaks) in the PSM are in synchrony. The distance between two boundary lines thus represents the height of a somite, which, in turn, depends on the clock period and, to a certain extent, the velocity of the moving wavefront. Thus, in the clock and wavefront model of primary somitogenesis, time, in terms of the clock period, is transformed into space, in terms of the somite size. The Clock periodicity is species specific

sclerotomes [12, 45]. Together with the notochord, the sclerotomes provide exclusive material for the vertebral column. Cells from the dorsolateral part of the somite retain their epithelial arrangement to produce the dermomyotomes (Fig. 9a, b). The dermomyotomes later subdivides into the dorsal dermatome immediately beneath the ectoderm to give rise to the dermis and its smooth muscles, while the disaggregated cells between the dermatome and the sclerotomes remain closely packed as the myotome, forming ultimately the axial skeletal muscles [10, 12, 24] (Fig. 9c, d).

While specification of the anterior-posterior pattern of the somite appears to be determined very early [1, 39, 46], the dorsoventral values are not intrinsic to the somites. Thus, if the somite were to be surgically rotated dorsoventrally by 180°, sclerotomes still develop in the ventromedial position while the dermomyotomes remain dorsolateral. Moreover, a dorsally implanted notochord represses dermatomal differentiation but encourages sclerotomal formation dorsally, while notochord ablation completely prevents sclerotomal appearance [24] (Fig. 10). These findings suggest that the dorsoventral differentiations of the somite depend on appositional instructions from the notochord, very possibly through sonic hedgehog (*Shh*) expression [48] (Fig. 11).

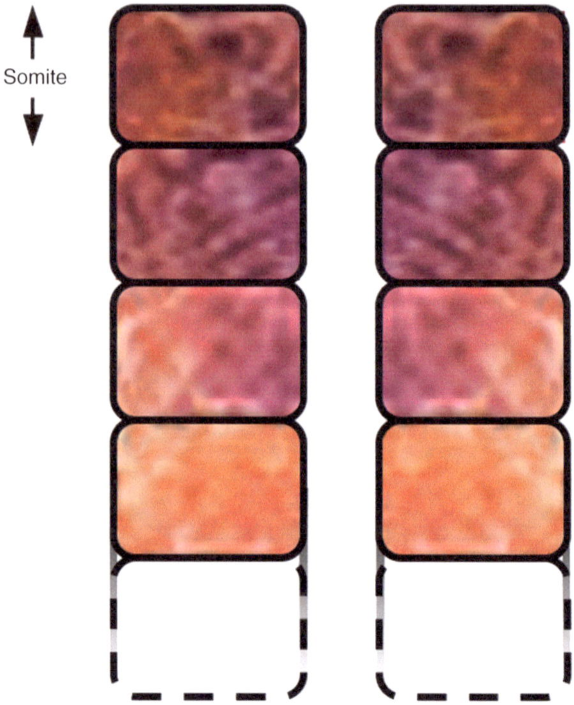

Fig. 6 Periodic boundary formation across the width of the PSM column along its rostrocaudal axis causes segregated somites to form sequentially. The distance between two adjacent boundaries represents the longitudinal dimension of a somite

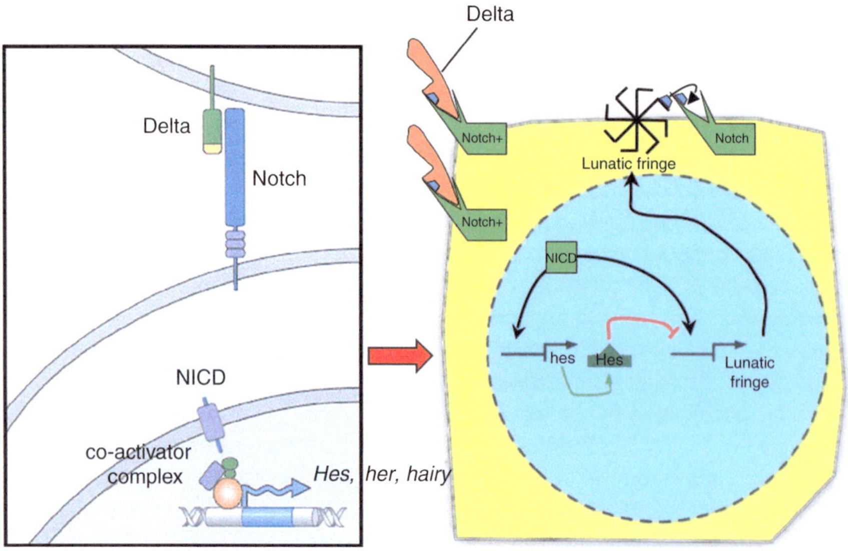

Fig. 7 The molecular basis of the Segmentation Clock. A ligand (e.g., Delta) is bound to the surface Notch signalling receptor, whose intracellular domain (*NICD*) then detaches from the cell membrane and enters the nucleus, where it coactivates cycling genes of the *C-hairy 1* family, encoding transcription factors such as HES, HER, HAIRY, and Lunatic Fringe. In chick, Lunatic Fringe is known to recycle back to the cell surface, where it "enables" the surface Notch signalling receptor to accept another ligand. The repetitive working of this simplified cycling gene model is the underlying mechanism of the oscillating Segmentation Clock

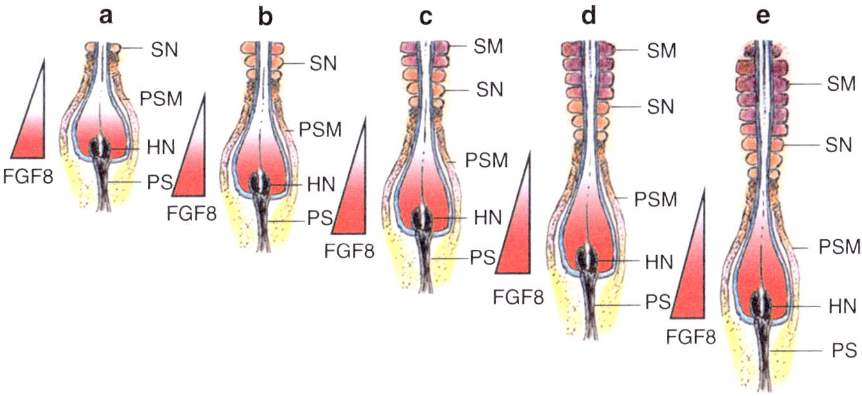

Fig. 8 The molecular basis of the somitogenesis wavefront. Boundary formation at the PSM is linked to expressions of fibroblast growth factor genes, especially *fgf8*. High concentrations of FGF8 maintains PSM cells in a primitive mesenchymal state, but a low concentration of FGF8 permits PSM cells to form boundary during the Segmentation Clock peak. Thus, the epithelial transformation (into somites) of PSM cells is negatively regulated by *fgf8*. High concentration of FGF8 is expressed by newly formed PSM cells at Hensen's node, and low concentration is expressed in "older" PSM cells near the somitogenesis front. Thus, the limit between the high- and low-*fgf8* domains near the site of active somitogenesis represents the somitogenesis wavefront (Represented by the apex of the FGF8 *triangle*). Figure **a–e** represent progressive stages of somite formation, elongation of the embryo, and caudal movement of the FGF8 wavefront. Because new PSM cells are continually being formed near Hensen nodes and the PSM column constantly elongates and gets ever "older" near the last formed somite, the wavefront also moves caudally. High concentration of FGF8 is indicated by deep red colour and low concentration by pale grey to white. The moving FGF8 gradient is also displayed by the coloured triangle. *HN* Hensen's node, *PS* primitive streak, *PSM* pre-somitic mesoderm, *SN* new somite, *SM* mature somite. Significance of somite colours as in Fig. 3

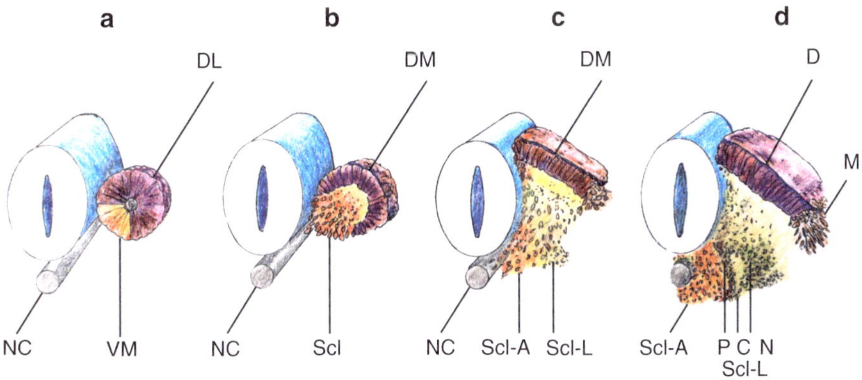

Fig. 9 Dorsoventral differentiation of somite. (**a**) Epithelial somite shows ventromedial cells (*VM*) destined to form the sclerotome. (**b**) Ventromedial sclerotome cells (*Scl*) de-epithelise from the somite and migrate towards the ventral notochord (*NC*). (**c**) Sclerotomal cells further subdivide into an axial cluster (*Scl-A*) surrounding the notochord and lateral paired clusters (*Scl-L*) flanking the perichordal axial sclerotome. Dorsolateral somite retains its epithelial pattern to become the dermomyotome (*DM*). (**d**) The lateral sclerotome (Scl-L) forms a triangle next to the axial sclerotome. The three sides of the triangle become anlagen for the pedicle (*P*), neural arch (*N*), and the costal process (*C*), respectively. The dermomyotome also subdivides into the dermatome (*D*) and the lateral migrating myotome (*M*)

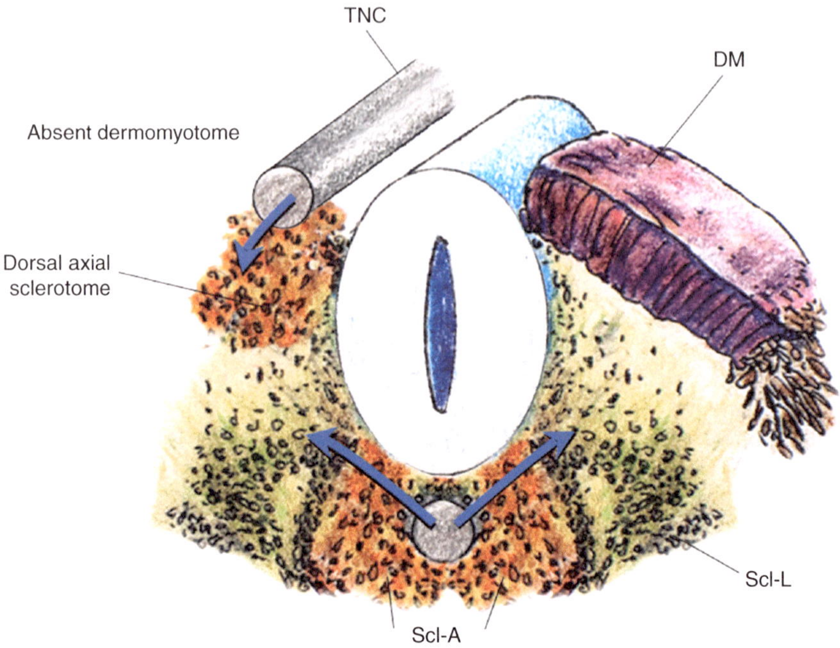

Fig. 10 A transplanted notochord (*TNC*) to the dorsal aspect of the somite induces sclerotomal differentiation dorsally and represses dermomyotomal formation on the side of the transplant, indicating inducers from the notochord direct dorsoventral specification of the somite. *DM* dermomyotome, *Scl-A* axial sclerotome, *Scl-L* lateral sclerotome

Fig. 11 Expressions of sonic hedgehog gene (*shh*) (*blue arrows*) from the notochord and floor plate of the neural tube signal sclerotomal differentiation and ventral migration from the somite. Bone morphogenetic protein (*BMP*) (*yellow arrow*) expressed by the roof plate and Wnt signalling (*green arrow*) from the ectoderm (*grey mantle*) induce dermomyotome differentiation. Other lateralising signals (*red arrow*) further encourage myotomal cell development

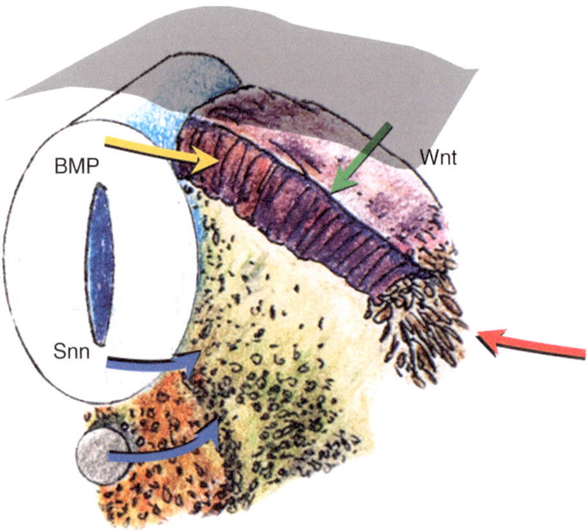

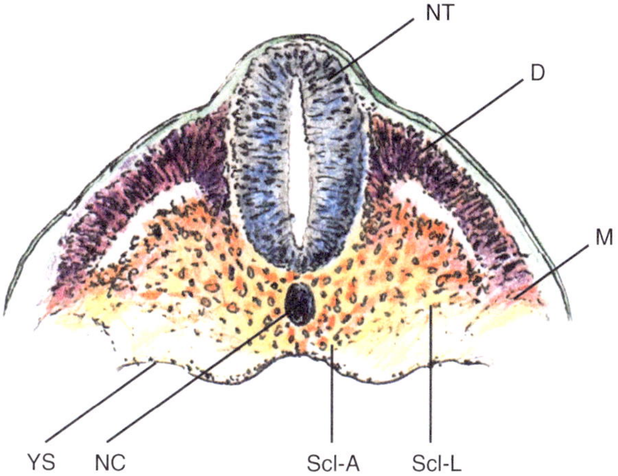

Fig. 12 Coronal section of chick embryo after dorsoventral differentiation of somites, showing axial or perichordal sclerotome (*Scl-A*) surrounding the notochord (*NC*) and lateral sclerotome (*Scl-L*) on both sides of the neural tube (*NT*). *D* dermatome, *M* myotome, *YS* yolk sac membrane

"Resegmentation" of the Sclerotome

The term "resegmentation" was originated by Remak in 1855 ("Neugliederung") [81] and remains still a subject of controversies [16, 24]. It refers to the fact that the early metameric boundaries between the somites are once again changed and "reshuffled" during the development of the sclerotome, so that the later boundaries between the vertebral bodies do not match up with the original intersomitic clefts [12].

During somitic differentiation, the ventromedial cells destined to become sclerotome subdivide into paired lateral clusters flanking the ventral aspects of the neural tube, and an unpaired median (axial) cluster surrounding the midline notochord (Fig. 12). The formation of the vertebral column takes place first in the lateral sclerotome, where a conspicuous subdivision into a densely packed caudal half and a more loosely cellular cranial half soon appear, separated by a fissure (of von Ebner [27]). The loose cranial half attracts, promotes, and supports the growth and expansion of peripheral nervous tissue from the neural tube and neural crests, but itself never chondrifies into vertebral parts (Fig. 13, middle). In contrast, the caudal densely-packed mesenchyme of the lateral scleroderm soon takes on a triangular shape. The side of the triangle facing the axial perichordal sclerotome, which will become the future vertebral body, gives rise to the pedicle. The side facing dorsolaterally away from the axial sclerotome forms rudiments of the neural arch, and the side of the triangle facing ventrolaterally becomes the costal process (Fig. 9d).

Shortly after the specifications of the lateral sclerotome into its arcual, costal, and pedicular components, the initially loosely-meshed mesenchyme within the perichordal axial sclerotome also begins to show compartmentalisation. A cell-dense zone develops at the same level as the dense caudal half of each lateral sclerotome, partly due to medial expansion of the lateral band of condensed tissues from the lateral sclerotome. The axial sclerotome in between these median dense zones remains loosely cellular. Later, the cranial-most layer of the axial dense zone, in line with von Ebner's fissure in the lateral sclerotome, becomes even more tightly packed

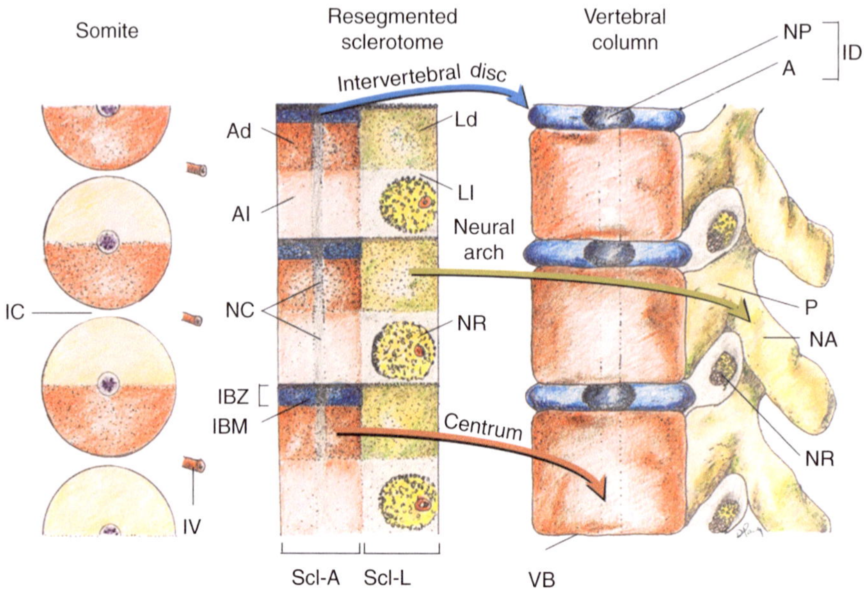

Fig. 13 Resegmentation of somites to form sclerotomes and changes of sclerotomal primordia to mature vertebral parts. The somitic and primordial origins of vertebral parts and phenotypic parts are colour-matched, and the locations of the somites, resegmented sclerotomes, and vertebrae along the embryonic axis are approximately counter-registered. During resegmentation, the sclerotome is formed from the caudal and rostral halves of two adjacent somites, such that the middle of the resegmented sclerotome lines up with the intersomitic cleft (*IC*). Both the axial sclerotome (*Scl-A*) and lateral sclerotome (*Scl-L*) develop dense and loose zones. The dense zone of the lateral sclerotome (*Ld*) becomes the neural arch (*NA*) and pedicle (*P*), which is attached to the rostral part of the vertebral body (*VB*) formed from chondrification of the loose (*Al*) and part of the dense zones (*Ad*) of the axial sclerotome. The rostral layer of the dense zone of the axial sclerotome soon forms the intervertebral boundary zone (*IBZ*) containing intervertebral boundary mesenchyme (*IBM*), which ultimately forms the annulus (*A*) and, together with notochord remnants (*NC*), the nucleus pulposus (*NP*) of the intervertebral disc (*ID*). The loose zone of the lateral sclerotome (*Ll*) does not form bone but promotes emergence of the nerve roots (*NR*). Thus, the neural arch is derived from a single somite, but the vertebral body receives contributions from two adjacent somites. *IV* intersomitic vessel. *Arrows* indicate developmental fates of the sclerotomes

and forms the intervertebral boundary zone (IBZ) (Fig. 13, middle). This intervertebral boundary mesenchyme (IBM) ultimately forms the ringlike annulus fibrosus of the intervertebral disc, permanently enclosing a looser central core of nucleus pulposus made partly of notochordal remnants. The vertebral body itself is mainly made from chondrogenesis in the loose-cell zone of the perichordal sclerotome, now called the prevertebra [11, 12, 24, 67], although contributions from the condensed tissue adjacent to the IBZ have been observed [16, 23]. As a final step, the pedicular anlagen from the lateral sclerotomes fuse with the chondrifying prevertebra of the axial sclerotome, while the neural arches surround the neural tube to complete the vertebral ring (Fig. 13, right). The costal component becomes the future transverse process but only in the thoracic region is it predestined to form ribs.

Thus, the neural arch of the vertebra is derived from the caudal-lateral part of a single somite [16]. However, labelling and transplantation experiments of half-somites have repeatedly demonstrated that each vertebral body is made up of cells from the axial zones of two adjacent somites [2, 3]. Although the exact boundary of individual somite participation is not known [12], the juxtapositioning of axial and lateral sclerotomal components suggests that each vertebra probably comes from the caudal half of one somite and the rostral half of the somite below [67]. This will explain the slightly off-step registration between the levels of the somite and the resegmented sclerotome [12, 17, 67] on the embryonic axis such that the middle of the resegmented sclerotome lines up with the original intersomitic cleft (Fig. 13, left and middle). Also, since the dense portion of the lateral sclerotome is in line with the dense zone of the axial sclerotome adjacent to the IBZ, it makes perfect sense that the mature pedicle is joined to the cranial and not the caudal half of the vertebral body [12]. It also follows that the spinal nerve, ganglion, and blood vessel from the corresponding somitic segment, being associated with the loose cranial half of the lateral sclerotome, must cross above its own neural arch and that the corresponding segment of the spinal cord is always slightly more rostral to its companion vertebral body (Fig. 13, right). Given there are eight cervical somites but only seven resegmented axial sclerotomes and consequently seven cervical vertebrae, the C_1 nerve root emerges above the C_1 neural arch, and the C_8 nerve root comes through below the C_7 neural arch and above the T_1 neural arch, which in fact is derived from the C_8 somite. Finally, resegmentation of the sclerotome explains why the original "pre-resegmented" intersomitic vessel ultimately enters the midpoint of the vertebral body as the segmental nutrient artery.

Special Developmental Features of the CVJ

The CVJ is the product of the occipital somites and the first three cervical somites. There is controversy regarding the proper number of occipital somites in vertebrates. Wilting et al. and others [14, 80, 99] thought there were five occipital somites in the chick and mouse but conceded that the first somite either disappeared early or was an insignificant clan of cells that lacked sclerotomal lineage. Müller and O'Rahilly [67] studied staged human embryos and concluded that, in humans, there are only four occipital somites that participate in formation of the skull base. The transitional zone between the skull and the cervical spine is thus taken to be between the 4th and 5th somites. During the fourth week of gestation, there are consequently 4 occipital, 8 cervical, 12 thoracic, 5 lumbar, 5 sacral, and 8–10 coccygeal somites, 42 pairs all told.

Occipital Somites (Somites 1–4) and the Proatlas

Following the general scheme, the first three occipital somites give rise to an axial perichordal sclerotome and a lateral sclerotome, but no resegmentation takes place here. The axial sclerotomes never subdivide into dense and loose zones and

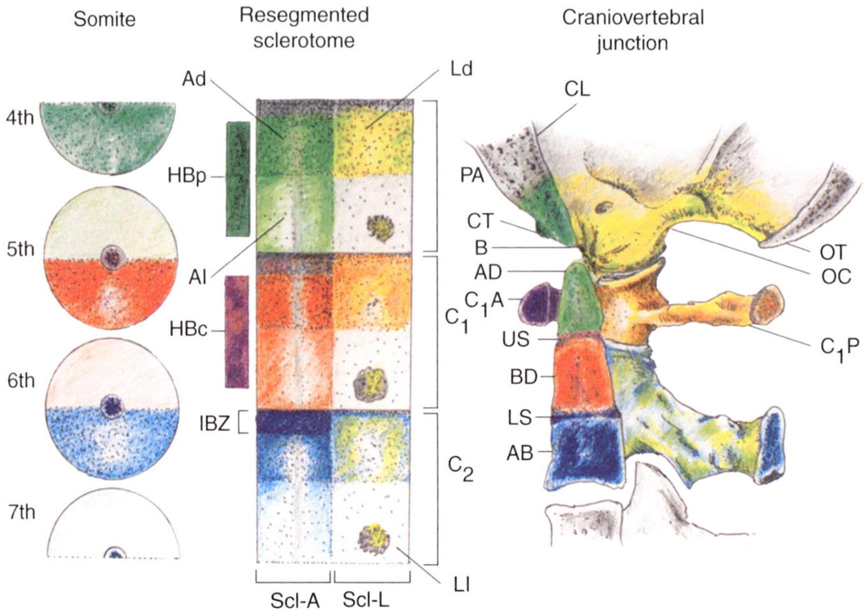

Fig. 14 Formation of the human craniovertebral junction. Sclerotomal primordia and their vertebral phenotypes are colour-matched. During resegmentation, the caudal half of the 4th somite (4th occipital somite) and rostral half of the 5th somite combine to form the proatlas sclerotome (*PA*). Derived from the proatlas are the axial zones (*Ad* and *Al*) which become the basion (*B*) of the basioccipital or clivus (*CL*) and the apical segment of the dens (*AD*), the lateral dense zone (*Ld*) becomes the exoccipital comprising the occipital condyle (*OC*), and lateral rim and opisthion (*OT*) of the foramen magnum; the proatlas' hypochordal bow (HB_p) forms the ventral clival tubercle (*CT*). The C_1 resegmented sclerotome (C_1) comes from adjacent halves of the 5th and 6th somites. Derived from the C_1 sclerotome are: the axial zones form the basal segment of the dens (*BD*); the lateral zone forms the posterior atlantal arch (C_1P); and the hypochordal bow (HB_c) forms the anterior atlantal arch (C_1A). The C_2 resegmented sclerotome (C_2) comes from the 6th and 7th somites. From the C_2 sclerotome: the axial zone forms the C_2 vertebral body (*AB*); the lateral zone forms the neural arch of C_2 vertebra. The intervertebral boundary zone (*IBZ*) between the proatlas and C_1 sclerotome forms the upper dental synchondrosis (*US*), and the IBZ between the C_1 and C_2 sclerotomes forms the lower dental synchondrosis (*LS*)

therefore no intervertebral boundary mesenchyme exists. They all eventually fuse into a unit which later chondrifies to become the rostral basioccipital [67]. The first three lateral occipital sclerotomes, like the vertebral sclerotomes, form dense and loose zones, and the loose zones of the second and third lateral occipital sclerotomes foster expansion of the upper and lower hypoglossal nerve roots and artery, while the corresponding dense zones form the bony hypoglossal canal.

Unlike the first three occipital somites, the fourth occipital (O_4) somite does show resegmentation. Its caudal dense zone combines with the cranial loose half of the first cervical somite to produce the transitional sclerotome called the proatlas [17, 53, 61, 62, 66, 67] (Fig. 14, left and middle). The cranial region of the axial sclerotome of the proatlas soon fuses with the other three axial occipital sclerotomes to become the basion of the basioccipital [66], but its most caudal portion, probably derived from the 1st cervical

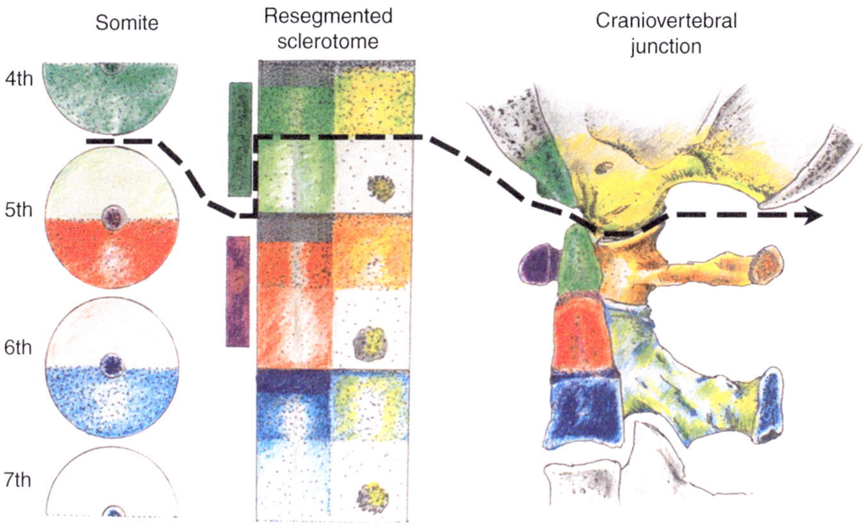

Fig. 15 The severance line, which results in final cellular separation of the skull from the cervical spine, runs through the original resegmentation fronts of the adjacent somites 4 and 5, corresponding to the junction between the basion and apical segment of the dens, and between the exoccipital, or future occipital condyle, and the lateral mass of C_1, which is derived from the lateral portion of the C_1 resegmented sclerotome

somite (somite 5), forms the anlage for the apical segment of the dens. Late in resegmentation, a boundary zone appears between this apical dental centrum and the loosely cellular prevertebra of the basioccipital, and the former soon detaches from the basioccipital and eventually becomes joined to the basal segment of the dens to complete the dental pivot (see below) [67, 99] (Fig. 14). Herein lies the most unique feature of the transitional zone of the CVJ between somites 4 and 5: unlike other IBZs that form intervertebral discs, downstream activity of the proatlas' IBZ includes a physical severance of cells from the immediately adjacent loose perichordal zone of the basioccipital. The severance line appears to go through the original resegmentation fronts of the adjacent somites 4 and 5, so that the final cellular separation occurs right through the junction between the basion and the apical segment of the dens, both derived from the axial portion of the proatlas, which in turn comes from a combination of the caudal half of somite 4 and the rostral half of somite 5 (Fig. 15). This action, no doubt mediated by special cleavage genes (see below), not only allows the skull to become independent from the vertebral column, but also the separation and descent of the primordium for the apical dens from the basiocciput, to complete the final installation of the dens-axis assembly.

The lateral dense region of the proatlas becomes the two exoccipitals, which later form the two occipital condyles and the remainder of the anterolateral rim of the foramen magnum (Fig. 14). The lateral loose region promotes emergence of the C_1 nerve root. In humans, an additional arcuate cluster of dense proatlas cells ventral to the notochord, likely an offshoot of the axial sclerotome and aptly called the hypochordal bow, gives rise to the bony anterior clival tubercle on the ventral surface of the basioccipital [66, 67] (Fig. 14).

First Three Cervical Somites (Somites 5–7)

Axial Sclerotomes

During resegmentation, the caudal half of somite 5 and the cranial half of somite 6 combine to produce the first cervical sclerotome; likewise, the second cervical sclerotome is made up of corresponding parts of somites 6 and 7. In the axial region of these sclerotomes destined to form vertebral centra, dense and loose zones appear in regular succession as in the lower cervical sclerotomes. The loose prevertebral zone of the first cervical sclerotome gives rise to the basal segment of the dens, and that of the second cervical sclerotome becomes the body of the axis (Fig. 14). Unlike in the more caudal sclerotomes, however, where the dense IBZ ultimately becomes the annulus and nucleus pulposus of an intervertebral disc, the dense zones in the first two cervical sclerotomes do not form true intervertebral discs and soon disappear [67]. Their intervertebral boundary mesenchyme gradually turns into the upper and lower dental synchondroses that ultimately cement the apical to the basal dens and the basal dens to the body of C_2, respectively (Fig. 14).

Thus, after resegmentation, the human membranous axis consists of three median constituents that have been designated the apical dental segment from the caudal proatlas, the basal dental segment from the first cervical sclerotome, and the body of the axis from the second cervical sclerotome [6, 7, 37, 80, 84]. These three constituents chondrify simultaneously round 6 weeks gestation but remain segregated by the more cellular upper and lower dental synchondroses. Ossification of the cartilaginous axis occurs in three chronological waves (Fig. 16). The first wave appears as a single ossification centre within the axial body round 4 months gestation. The second wave begins at 6 months gestation as two separate ossification centres on each side of the basal dental segment [71, 76, 90, 100]. At birth, these two centres integrate and fuse, and the main component of the dens should at least have begun to show bony fusion with the axis body, even though a clear rarification may still be discernible at the lower synchondrosis till the 5th or 6th postnatal year (Figs. 16 and 17). Occasionally, the basal dens remains bifid (dens bicornis) when the third wave of ossification arrives within the apical dens round 3–5 years of age [6, 55, 76] (Figs. 16, 17, and 18). Ossification of the dental tip and bony fusion of the upper synchondrosis are not completed until adolescence [57, 58, 91, 96].

Lastly, the apical ligament is almost certainly derived from the axial proatlas, and the alar and transverse atlantal ligaments are from the axial component of the first cervical sclerotome in association with the basal dental segments [67].

Lateral Sclerotomes

The lateral dense zone of the first cervical sclerotome develops into the posterior arch of the atlas, while the lateral dense zone of the second cervical sclerotome forms the arch of the axis. Their respective loose zones promote outgrowths of the

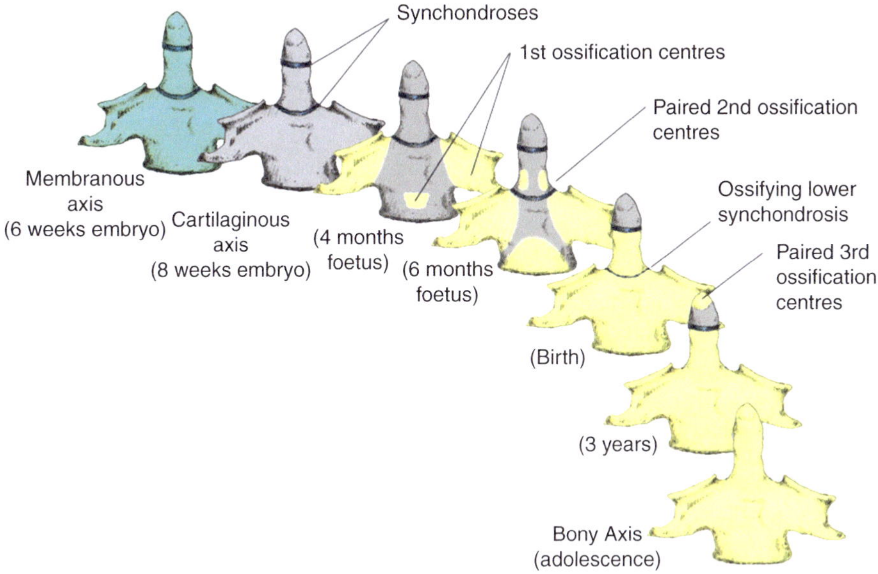

Fig. 16 The three developmental phases of the axis (C_2) and the three waves of ossification. The primordia for the dens components are assembled during the membranous phase. Upper and lower dental synchondroses are shown as dense lines. First wave of ossification at 4th foetal month consists of bilateral centres for the neural arches and a single centre for the centrum. Second wave at 6th foetal month consists of bilateral ossification centres for the basal dental segment. At birth, the basal dental centres should have integrated in the midline and begun to be fused to the centrum. Third wave of C_2 ossification occurs from 3 to 5 years postnatal life at the apical dental segment, which does not become fused to the basal dens till the 6th–9th year and fully formed during adolescence

second and third cervical nerves and segmental arteries. The hypochordal bow of the first cervical sclerotome ventral to the notochord subsequently forms the anterior arch of the atlas (Fig. 14, middle and right) [65–67, 84]. No definite hypochordal bows are seen caudal to this level, and equivalent cells in the lower segments appear to play no role in the formation of the vertebral column.

Genetic Control of CVJ Development

Hox Genes: The Control of Rostrocaudal Specification

Following primary segmentation, the determination of the positional identity of the prevertebral segments along the embryonic axis, which in turn ordains the regional developmental specifications of the vertebral phenotypes, is controlled by Hox genes. The mammalian Hox genes encode transcription factors used in regulating the establishment of the body plan. They contain the phylogenetically highly

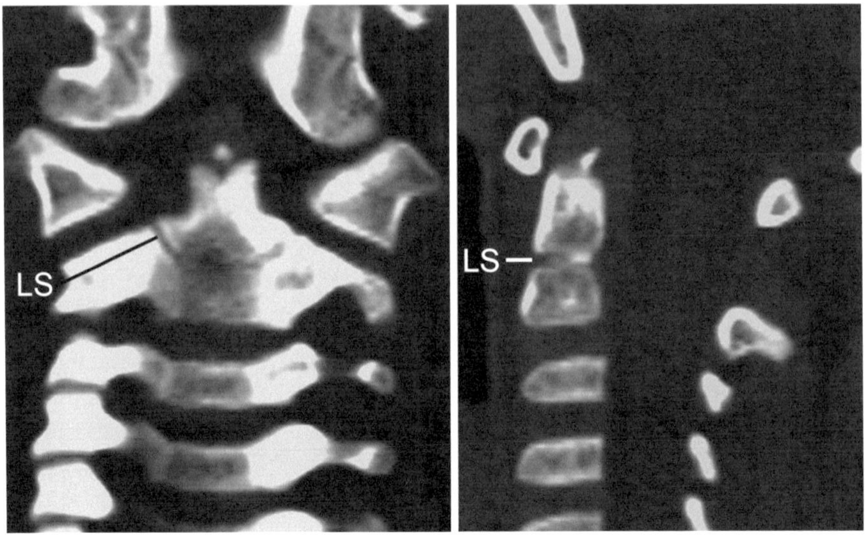

Fig. 17 State of ossification of the dens of a 4-year-old child. The tip of the basal dental segment is bicornuate from bilateral secondary ossification centres. Small density above this represents early third wave of ossification within the apical dental segment. Note lower dental synchondrosis (*LS*) in the coronal and sagittal views

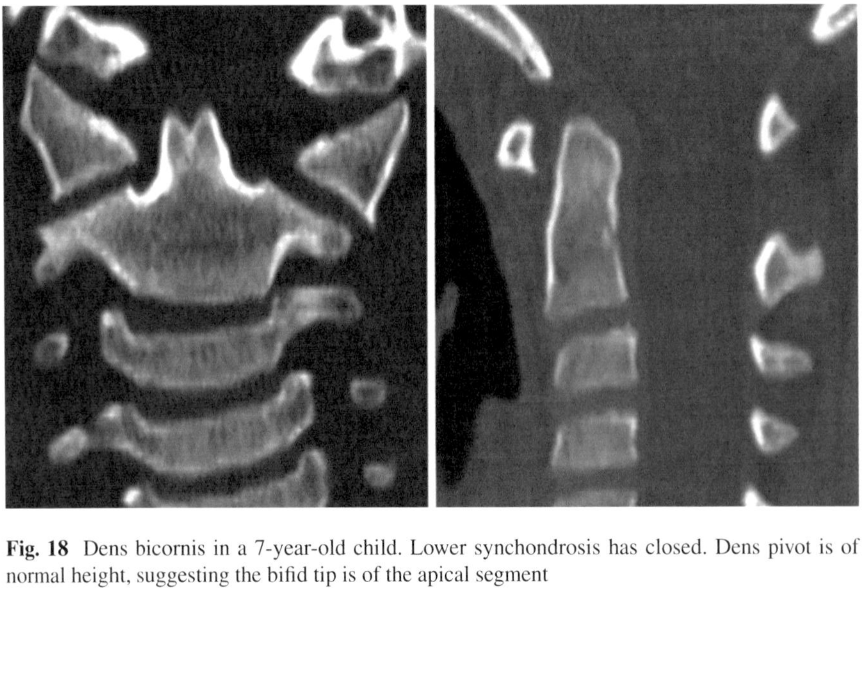

Fig. 18 Dens bicornis in a 7-year-old child. Lower synchondrosis has closed. Dens pivot is of normal height, suggesting the bifid tip is of the apical segment

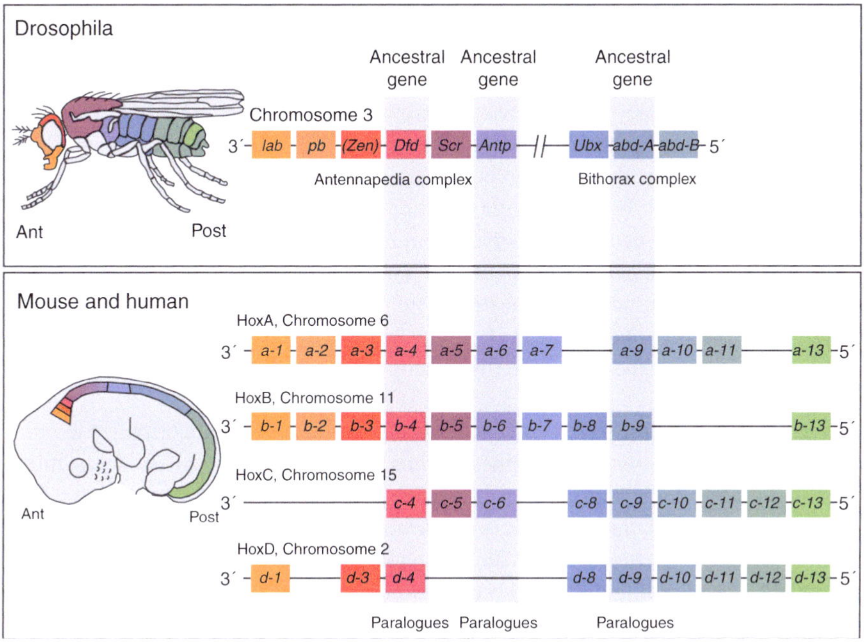

Fig. 19 *Hox* genes in mouse and human with their phylogenetic counterparts in *Drosophila*. Thirty-nine *Hox* genes are involved in the mouse and human vertebral column, found in four clusters of Hox A, B, C, and D on four chromosomes [2, 6, 11, 15], designated by Arabic numbers within each cluster and arranged as paralogues, so that the lower numbered Hox paralogues such as *Hox a-1* and *Hox d-1* are located on the anterior 3′ position of the chromosomes, and the higher numbered paralogues such as *Hox a-13* and *Hox d-13* are on the 5′ posterior position of the chromosomes. There is also temporal and structural colinearity with the embryonic axis so that the lower numbered paralogues are expressed earlier and more anterior on the embryonic axis than the higher numbered paralogues. (See colour match between genes and their expression domains on the embryonic axis.) Three sets of paralogues and their corresponding ancestral genes are designated by the *grey bars*

conserved homeobox domain [24, 43, 44]. In mouse and humans, there are 39 Hox genes distributed in four linkage clusters, Hox A, B, C and D, on four different chromosomes (chromosomes 6, 11, 15 and 2) (Fig. 19). The members of each cluster, designated by Arabic numerals, are also grouped vertically along the clusters because analogous members of each group are linked by common origin from a single ancestral gene. For example, *Hox* a_{-4}, b_{-4}, c_{-4}, and d_{-4} of the mouse, called paralogues, are held kin by all being the phylogenetic descendants of the much older *Dfd* gene of the *Drosophila*, and *a-6*, *b-6*, and *c-6* are similarly related to the *Antp* gene of the *Drosophila*'s antennapedia complex (Fig. 19). Topographically, the lower numbered paralogues are located on the anterior 3′ axis of the chromosome, and the higher numbered ones are on its posterior 5′ locations (Fig. 19).

Hox genes are expressed in mesodermal and ectodermal cells along the body axis. Each gene has a characteristic and distinct anterior boundary of expression. A temporal and structural colinearity exists between the position of a gene in a cluster and its expression pattern. Thus, genes from the more anterior 3′ locations in the Hox clusters are expressed earlier and always occupy more anterior (cranial) expression domains than genes closer to the posterior 5′ location in the clusters (Fig. 19). For example, Hox *a-3* has a more anterior expression domain than *Hox a-9* and similarly between *Hox d-4* and *Hox d-10*.

Functionally, only the anterior boundary of the Hox expression is important. Since multiple genes have the same anterior expression boundary along the pre-vertebral axis, each metameric segment can be identified by its own characteristic combination of Hox gene expression domains, i.e., its own Hox code (Fig. 20). A specific Hox code acts as a master switch in determining the exact positional identity of a mesodermal segment along the body axis, and via regional idiosyncrasies in development, the Hox code thus becomes translated into a specific vertebral anatomy [24, 34, 44].

The importance of the Hox code is illustrated by the severe abnormality in numbers and structures of vertebral segments when the code is altered by Hox gene mutations and teratogenic disturbance of Hox gene expressions. One example at the CVJ is the inactivation in mice of *Hox d-3*, an important component of the Hox code for the first cervical prevertebra. This results in a more caudal anterior boundary of *Hox d-3* expression, shifting the transitional sclerotomal properties from C_1 to C_2 prevertebra and transforming the C_1 prevertebra to a more anterior (i.e., occipital) identity, producing mutant mice with atlas assimilation to the basioccipital [13]. This is called anterior homeotic transformation (Fig. 21). Conversely, extension of an expression domain rostrally can transform prevertebral segments into a more caudal (posterior) identity, a phenomenon known as posterior homeotic transformation. This is exemplified in "gain-of-function" transgenic mutation of the murine *Hox d-4* gene, also a component of the Hox code for the C_1 prevertebra, such that its expression domain is forced to extend towards the occipital somites. The exoccipital region of the transgenic mutant shows no occipital condyles but instead ectopic neural arches resembling cervical neural arches, and the basioccipital is fused to the apical dens, "imitating" the behaviour of the atlas centrum [53]. In the human analogue of posterior homeotic transformation, the basion, from the O_4 somite, "imitates" the C_1 prevertebra by being detached from the upper clivus, and the anterior C_1 arch, from the hypochordal bow of the C_1 sclerotome, is fused to the apical dens as if C_1 is trying to become C_2 by acquiring a "true centrum" (Fig. 22). Thus, an altered interpretation of axial position cues in the developing occipital somites leads to an imposition of cervical-vertebral phenotype upon the occipital bones. These various observations suggest that Hox gene abnormality may underlie many malformations in the CVJ [17].

Pax 1: The Resegmentation Gene

The Pax family of regulatory genes is implicated in sclerotomal resegmentation. *Pax* genes in vertebrates all contain the highly conserved DNA sequence called "paired-box", in essence a paired domain with a partial or complete homeodomain.

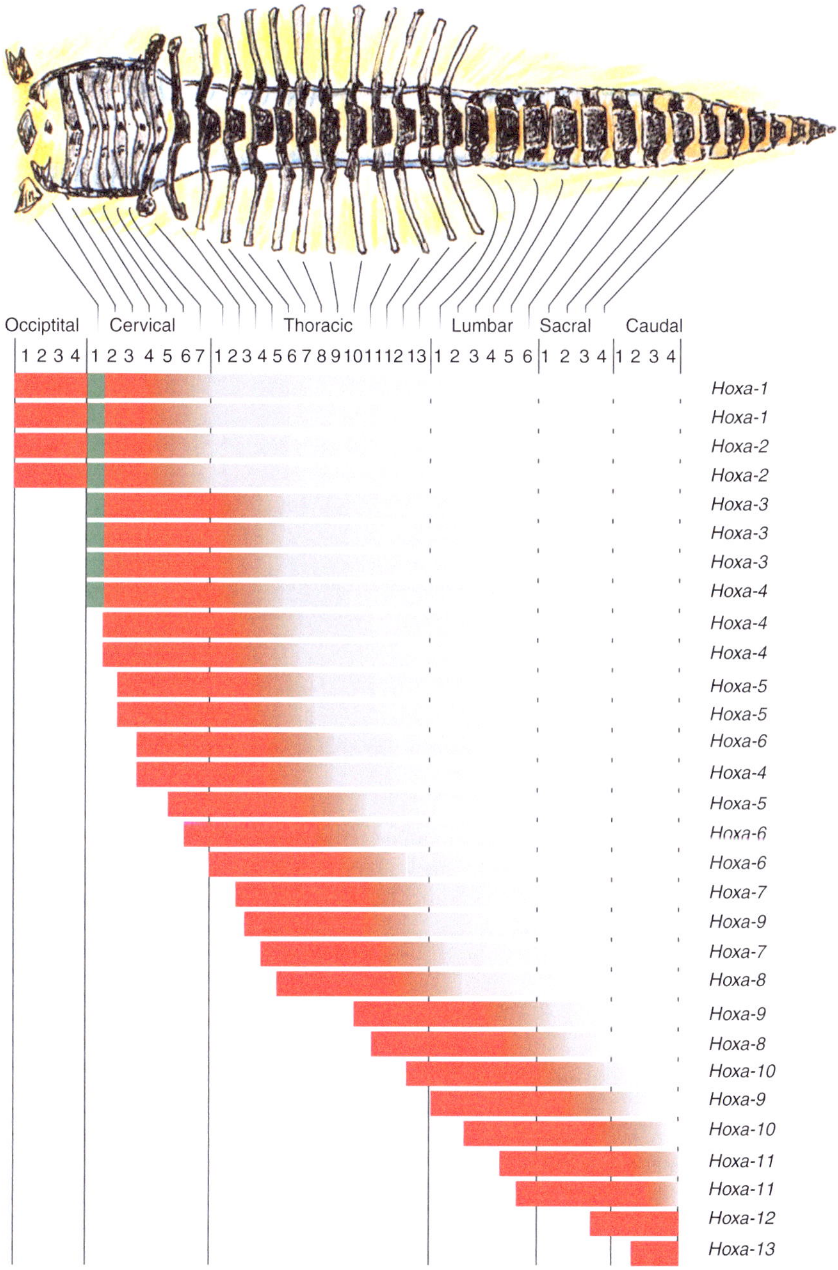

Fig. 20 Expression domains of *Hox* genes lined up with the mouse embryonic vertebral column. Only the anterior expression boundary (in *red*) is important, and since multiple genes have the same anterior expression boundary along the prevertebral axis, each prevertebral segment has its own combination of *Hox* gene expression domains (Hox code). For example, the Hox code for C_1 is Hox *a-1*, *b-1*, *a-2*, *b-2*, *a-3*, *b-3*, *d-3*, and *d-4* (designated by the *vertical green bar*)

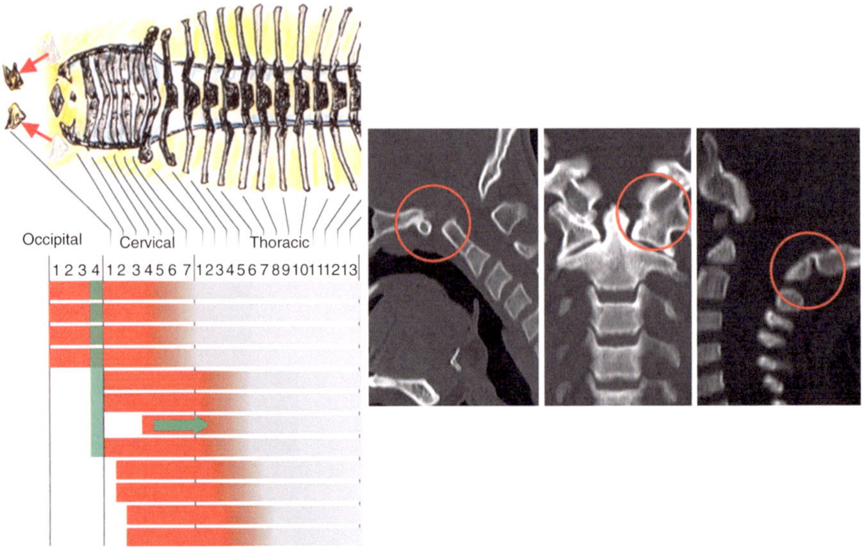

Fig. 21 Anterior homeotic transformation. Mutation of the Hox *d-3* gene in the mouse causes a caudal recession of its anterior expression domain (*green arrow*), allowing the Hox code of the C_1 segment (*green bar*) to resemble that of an occipital somite (Note *green bar* representing C_1 Hox code has moved up to occipital sclerotome position). This renders the C_1 sclerotome to "behave" like an occipital segment (symbolised in the figure by rostral movements of the C_1 sclerotomes to a cranial position; see *red arrows*) and the anterior and posterior arches of C_1 become fused to the basioccipital and exoccipital. *Inset* shows the human version of anterior homeotic transformation with assimilation of C_1 to the occiput

There are nine *Pax* genes in the mammalian family; all except *Pax-1* and *Pax-9* are involved in development of the central neuraxis. These two exceptions, especially *Pax-1* (*PAX-1* in the human homologue) [85, 97], control boundary formation between tissues by keeping two cell populations separate, presumably because the transcription factor encoded by *Pax-1* differentially regulates cell surface molecules expressed by these two cell populations, thereby divergently influences their respective fates. This scenario of cellular partitioning is a necessary condition for resegmentation, and *Pax-1* action at the future IBZ thus helps to demarcate the site and extent of sclerotomal segregation. The downstream target gene for *Pax-1* is unknown but may involve cell adhesion molecules such as NCAM or cytotactin or molecules that promote cell-cell communication such as connexins [41, 42, 68, 85].

Pax-1 expression is detected very early in the pre-differentiated somites before their dorsoventral specification. Signals from the notochord and ventral floor plate of the neural tube, mediated by the SHH protein, induce the somite to divide into dermomyotome and the ventromedial sclerotome. This coincides with intense expression of *Pax-1* ventrally within the sclerotomal field, suggesting that the earliest role of *Pax-1* is mediating the dorsoventral specification of somites [48, 99].

After somitic differentiation, *Pax-1* expression plays a more clearly segregating role within both the lateral and axial sclerotomes, where its timing and fluctuating

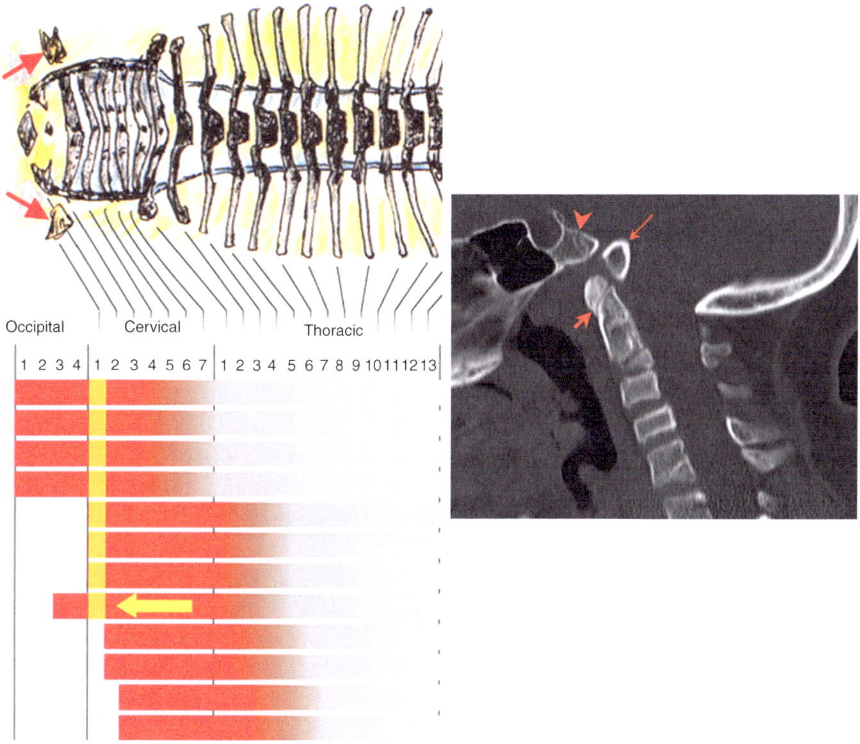

Fig. 22 Posterior homeotic transformation. "Gain-of-function" mutation of the murine Hox *d-4* gene causes its anterior expression domain to extend cranially (*yellow arrow*), allowing the Hox code for the O_4 segment (*yellow bar*) to resemble that of the C_1 and C_2 sclerotomes (*yellow bar* moved to C_1 Hox code position) and render the basiocciput to "imitate" the C_1 segment (symbolised in the figure by caudal movement of the C_1 sclerotomes; see *red arrows* on the drawing). The *inset* shows the human version of posterior homeotic transformation: the basion (*long arrow*) is detached from the upper clivus (*arrow head*), and the C_1 anterior arch (*short arrow*) is fused to the apical dens as if C_1 is trying to become C_2 by acquiring a "true centrum"

levels coincide with crucial events of resegmentation; i.e., the opposite functions of partitioning and aggregation of adjacent sclerotomal clusters are matched to high and low *Pax-1* expression, respectively. For example, during condensation of the axial sclerotome into the loose and dense halves, *Pax-1* expression is weak within the loosely cellular prevertebrae but intense within the dense IBZ [85, 99]. Later, with chondrification of the prevertebra to form the homogeneous vertebral body, *Pax-1* is further actively repressed in this location, but persists in high levels at the IBZ where partition of centra takes place, until formation of the intervertebral disc is well underway [99]. *Pax-1* level is also enhanced during condensation of the lateral sclerotome to form the neural arch [23, 25, 98].

Conversely, normal fusion of certain adjacent sclerotomes takes place only when *Pax-1* expression is turned off. At the CVJ of chick embryos, *Pax-1* repression is timed exactly when the occipital sclerotomes fuse to form the basiocciput. The

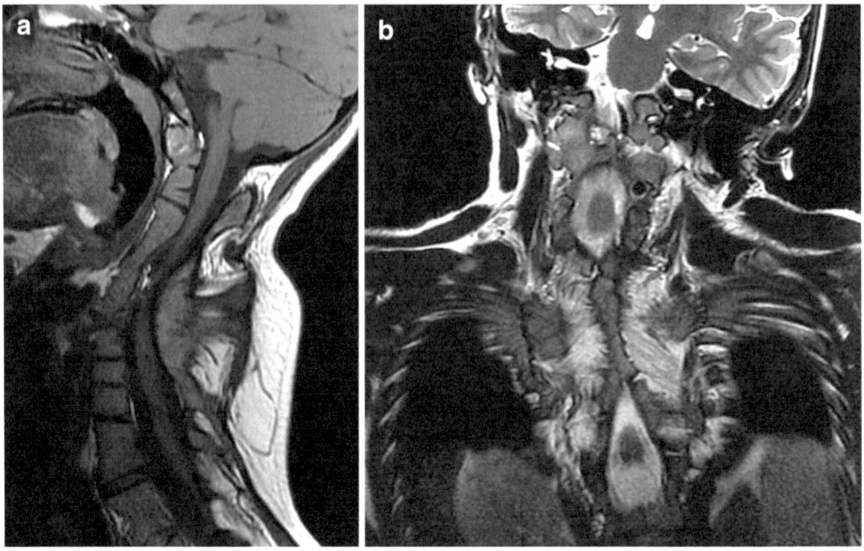

Fig. 23 Fourteen-year-old girl with spondylocostal dysostosis. (**a**) Sagittal MRI shows fusion of the clivus to the entire cervical and upper half of the thoracic spine. C_1 and C_2 are no longer identifiable by any of their unique features but had become part of a homogeneous rigid column. (**b**) Coronal MRI shows bilateral extensive fusion of the ribs, worse on the right thorax where almost all 12 ribs are fused

fusion of the two dens primordia with the axis body also coincides with the down-regulation of the *Pax-1* gene [99]. Ectopic *Pax-1* expression disrupts normal assemblage of the dens-axis and basiocciput, producing mutants with mobile dental fragments and loosely beaded clivus [98]. *Pax-1* is also highly expressed within the transitional zone between the proatlas and the first cervical sclerotome; it may thus also play a role in the separation of the head from the trunk.

Murine *Pax-1* mutants *undulated* show multiple fusion of vertebral bodies and fusion of the dens with the anterior atlantal arch [98]. Extreme cases of complete fusion of the basiocciput-prevertebral column, literally from the clivus to the thoracolumbar spine, have been seen in human spondylocostal dysostosis (Fig. 23). These and the milder form of Klippel-Feil syndrome have been postulated to reflect severe *PAX-1* loss-of-function mutations [85, 86]. It is therefore conceivable that hyper- and hyposegmentation defects in human may be explained by over- and under-expression of *PAX-1* during vertebral development.

Classification of Bony Malformations of the CVJ

The large and seemingly disenfranchised rabble of bony malformations at the CVJ can now be grouped under the orderly logics of embryogenesis (Table 1). The first subdivision is between malformations of the central pillar and those of the surrounding rings, respectively due to a disturbance of the axial and lateral components of the relevant resegmented sclerotomes. Between the two main subclasses of central pillar malformations, the various types of odontoid dysplasias are better known because the odontoid pivot functions as the main axis for almost all motion planes at the CVJ, and its anomalous development severely disrupts the governance of safe motility of the craniocervical hinge. On the other hand, dysgenesis of the basioccipital block profoundly alters both the position and orientation of the odontoid and can lead to no less lethal impingement of the brainstem.

Within the other subclass of malformations of the surrounding rings, the teratogenic insult may be symmetrical or asymmetrical causing bilateral or unilateral dysplasia, involve the hypochordal bow and the lateral sclerotome individually or together, or affect the proatlas and the C_1 resegmented sclerotome individually or simultaneously. Also, because the hypochordal bow may in fact be an early offshoot of the axial sclerotome from the same somite (or half-somite) and share sympathetic developmental fates, dysplasias of the anterior atlantal arch are not infrequently associated with centrum anomalies and together they result in extreme clinical instability.

Our knowledge of the genetic control of the embryology of the region is admittedly limited, but it is assumed that the known "master" transcription genes such as members of the Hox and Pax families each controls a crop of unknown regulator genes, and they, in turn, influence their own arbour of downstream progenitor genes. Mutation in any member gene within this enormous but interlinking tree, particularly higher up in the hierarchy, will likely affect multiple component phenotypes, and the permutations of associated CVJ anomalies may be asymptotic. The catalogue of anomalies in the present classification is therefore expected to expand or amend with future discoveries.

Disturbance of the Axial Component of Occipital Sclerotomes, Proatlas, and C_1 and C_2 Sclerotomes: Anomalies of the Central Pivot

There are two classes of central pivot anomalies: one concerns the dens-axis complex and includes the various forms of odontoid dysgenesis; the other afflicts primarily the basiocciput leading to an abnormal relationship between the odontoid and the skull base, comprising such entities as bifid clivus, platybasia, basilar kyphosis, basilar impression and a retroflexed dens.

Odontoid Dysgeneses

The making of any part of the vertebral column requires the successful completion of three developmental phases: First, the mesodermal primordium has to be properly formed and, in some cases, assembled during the membranous phase; second, the mesodermal primordium undergoes chondrification in the cartilaginous phase; and finally, in the osseous phase, ossification takes place within the cartilaginous mould to complete the end product. In the case of the dens-axis, there is a fourth phase which involves bony fusion of the upper and lower dental synchondroses (Fig. 16).

The various forms of odontoid dysplasia are classifiable according to their probable pathogeneses, which, in turn, are traceable to failure of one or more of the four developmental phases. As with other types of bony malformations of the CVJ, four main developmental errors are encountered in odontoid anomalies:

1. Hyperplasia of primordium
2. Aplasia/hypoplasia of primordium
3. Disturbance of resegmentation
4. Failure of midline integration of primordium

Hyperplasia of odontoid primordium has so far not been recognised.

Aplasia/Hypoplasia of the Axial Sclerotome of Proatlas and First Cervical Sclerotome: Agenesis and Hypogenesis of Odontoid Components

The odontoid process, or dens, develops from the axial sclerotome of the proatlas and first cervical sclerotome. Primordia of the apical and basal dental segments fuse with each other and to the C_2 centrum. Complete agenesis of both dental components is rare and usually occurs in the context of collagenopathy syndromes such as spondyloepiphyseal and spondylometaphyseal dysplasias (Fig. 24). Agenesis or hypogenesis of just the basal segment results in a stumpy dental pivot with a floating apical ossicle (Fig. 25). Both types are associated with instability. Agenesis of the apical segment is the most common variety by comparison. Radiographically the dens is short although there is usually adequate pivot height for the transverse atlantal ligament and there is thus no instability (Fig. 26).

Complete odontoid agenesis in patients with collagenopathy or mucopolysaccharidosis such as Morquio's disease may not always be due to primordial failure since a completed cartilaginous mould of the dens has been seen in situ, where ossification was found to be defective because of the abnormal connective tissue production. Non-syndromic cases of odontoid agenesis, however, are usually due to aplasia or hypoplasia of centrum primordia.

Treatment of symptomatic cases is usually C_1–C_2 fusion.

Disturbance of the Intervertebral Boundary Mesenchyme of Proatlas and First Two Cervical Sclerotomes: Os Odontoideum and Ossiculum Terminale Persistens

Aetiology

Abrogation of the IBZ during early resegmentation such as in the transgenic mutant mice *undulated* (produced by *Pax-1* deletion) causes exuberant fusion between sclerotomal units rather than lack of fusion [85, 99]. Thus when there is non-fusion of discrete individual dental components as in os odontoideum and ossiculum terminale

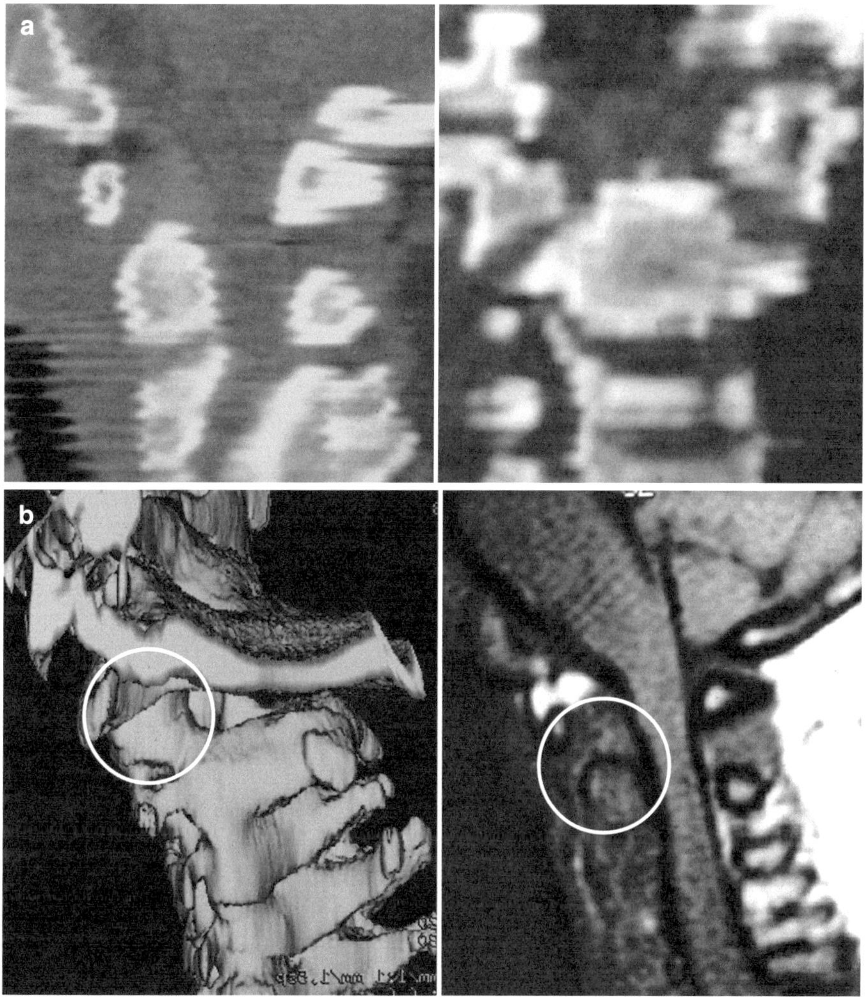

Fig. 24 Complete agenesis of the dens in a 10-year-old child with spondyloepiphyseal dysplasia. (**a**) CT sagittal and coronal views show no dental pivot although the centrum with a flat top does rise up above the 'expected' level of the lower dental synchondrosis. (**b**) 3-D CT reconstruction and MR show the flat top of the centrum and potential for instability

persistens, one may safely assume that the respective IBZ between the proatlas and the first two cervical sclerotomes were initially demarcated, but subsequent development of the upper and lower dental synchondroses was unconsummated.

Os Odontoideum

There are endless debates in the literature about whether os odontoideum is truly a developmental anomaly or an ununited odontoid fracture. Proponents for the traumatic theory argue that the inferior surfaces of most os odontoideum are above the

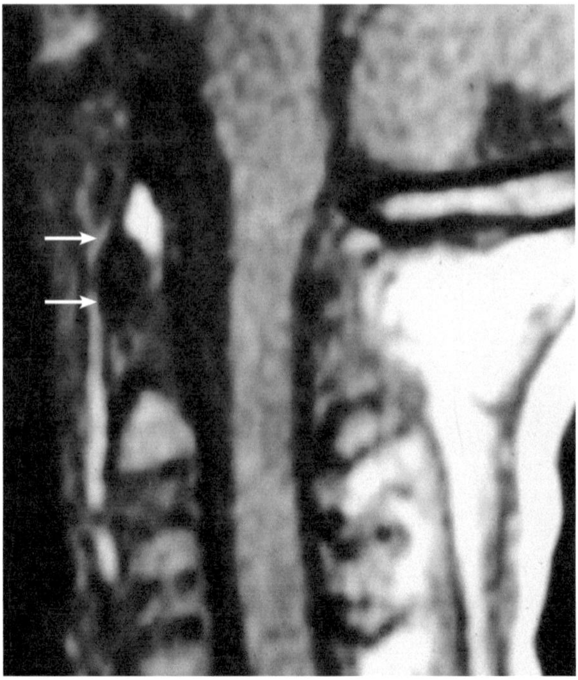

Fig. 25 Agenesis of basal dental segment with a stumpy C_2 centrum and a high-riding "floating" apical ossiculum (between *arrows*)

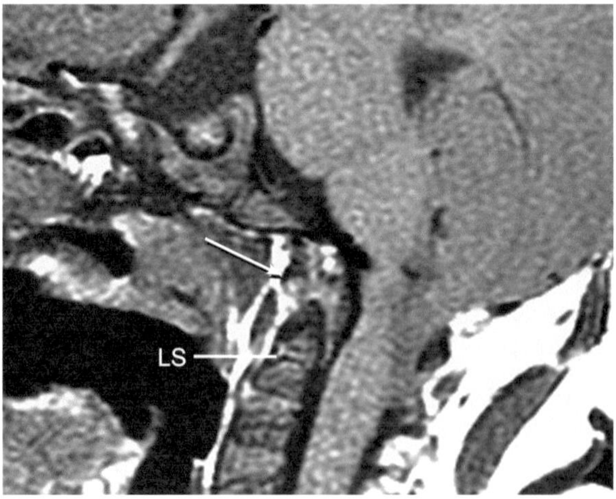

Fig. 26 Agenesis of apical dental segment, with a slightly short dental pivot but a definite basal segment (pointed) and a lower dental synchondrosis (*LS*). *Arrow* points to anterior arch of C_1. Note platybasia and Chiari I malformation

"expected base" of the normal dens, which is supposed to be below the level of the C_2 lateral masses [15, 17, 35–37, 60, 63, 91], and that there is often a "cupola" bulging cranially from the axis stump that represents the bottom half of a fractured dens [91]. In countering, the developmentalists point out that transgenic mutant experiments repeatedly show vertebral primordia that have undergone aberrant development seldom evolve into the orthodox configuration of the normal phenotype, but instead become oddly shaped due to over-, under-, or even erratic growth depending on the activities of local inducers [76, 85, 99]. The often expanded roundness of the os odontoideum with its corrugated horn-like corners (Fig. 27a) can hardly be the expected visage of an unhealed odontoid fracture, with its compromised blood supply. In addition, os odontoideum has been found in identical twins [47] and families [64], as well as amongst children with collagenopathies, and it frequently coexists with other developmental bony anomalies of the skull base, all reinforcing the congenital theory. We believe that what has been called os odontoideum is a heterogeneous designation of both the congenital and post-traumatic varieties, but there may also be cases with mixed aetiologies. For example, the mesenchyme at the IBZ may have failed to chondrify and therefore cannot ultimately undergo ossification and fusion. As the two dental components ossify on opposite sides of the IBZ and lengthen their respective moment arm, the persisting weak mesenchymal tissue of the IBZ eventually succumbs to the stress caused by foetal movements, and the upper part separates as the loose os odontoideum. The evidence for either theory is selectively circumstantial although the clinical implications are the same.

Ossiculum Terminale Persistens

There is little dispute about the developmental origin of ossiculum terminale persistens. The ossiculum represents an unfused and detached apical dental segment, which comes from the proatlas centrum [18, 19, 37, 91] (Fig. 28). The detachment is probably due to upper dental synchondrosis failure although late disturbance of

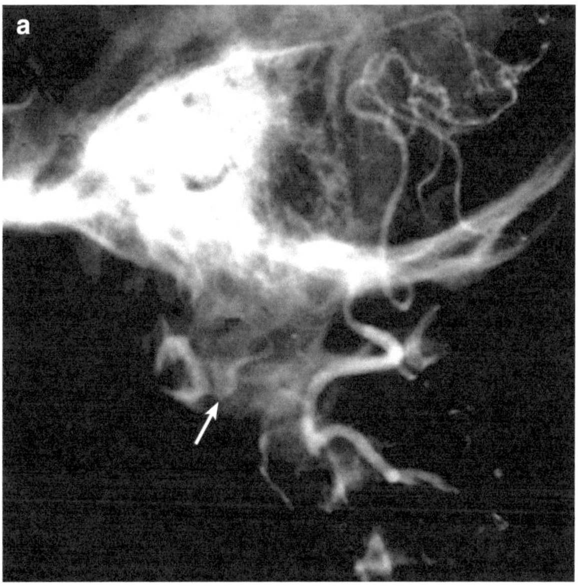

Fig. 27 Os odontoideum in an 8-year-old child presented with multiple cerebellar and thalamic strokes. (**a**) Cerebral angiogram shows os odontoideum with a corrugated horn-like inferior edge (*arrow*) with anterior C_1–C_2 subluxation and stretch injury to the vertebral artery. (**b**) CT scans show multiple small infarcts of left cerebellar hemisphere and thalamus secondary to multiple vertebrobasilar emboli

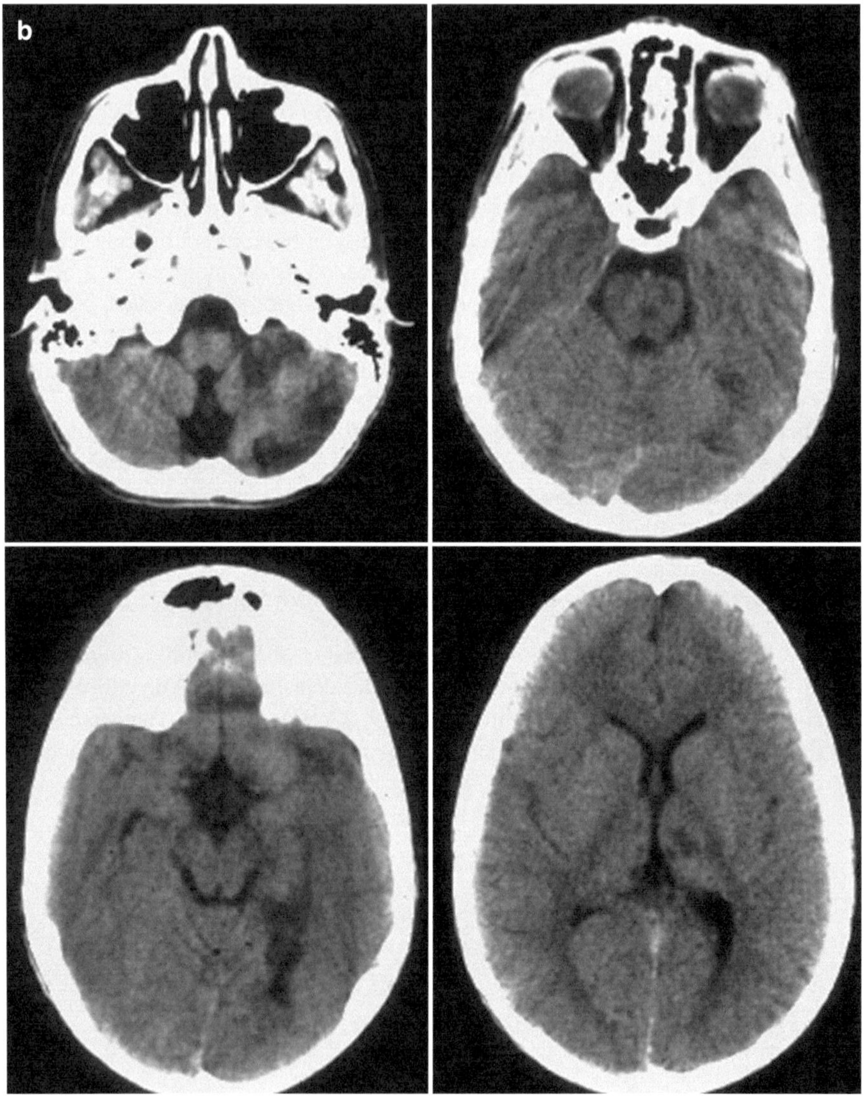

Fig. 27 (continued)

the third wave of odontoid ossification may be responsible. The ossiculum is usually non-syndromic although cases are seen with Morquio's disease.

Clinical Significance

Because the TAL straps round the basal segment of the dens, os odontoideum is at least potentially unstable (Fig. 29). Symptoms vary from persistent neck pain, torticollis, transient quadriparesis, and lower cranial neuropathies, to recurrent brainstem strokes caused by stretching of the vertebral arteries and basilar artery embolism (Fig. 27b).

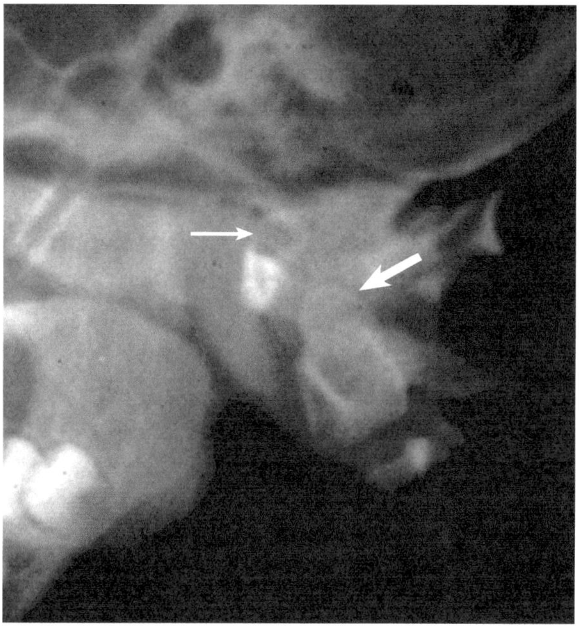

Fig. 28 Ossiculum terminale persistens (*thin arrow*), detached from the slightly shortened dental pivot formed by the basal dental segment (*thick arrow*)

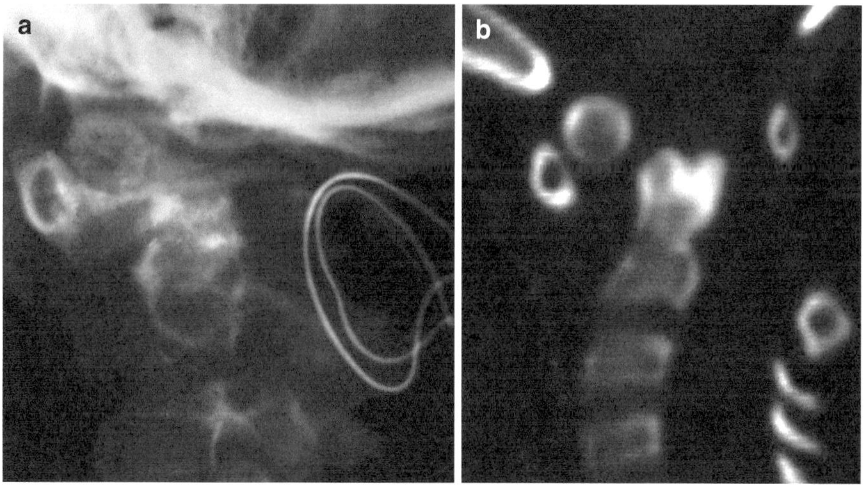

Fig. 29 Unstable os odontoideum with C_1–C_2 subluxation. (**a**) Shows widened ADI (13 mm) and a failed posterior C_1–C_2 fusion. (**b**) Shows another os with tall but jagged remaining dental pivot suggesting a traumatic aetiology

Although most ossiculum terminales are stable anomalies [17, 91] because the TAL's anchorage is not affected, we have encountered cases in which the basal dental segment is hypoplastic and the dental pivot is short, illustrative of associated hypogenesis of both the proatlas and the C_1 centrum sclerotomes. Some of these are conducive to atlantoaxial subluxation and high cord compression (Fig. 30a, b). Posterior

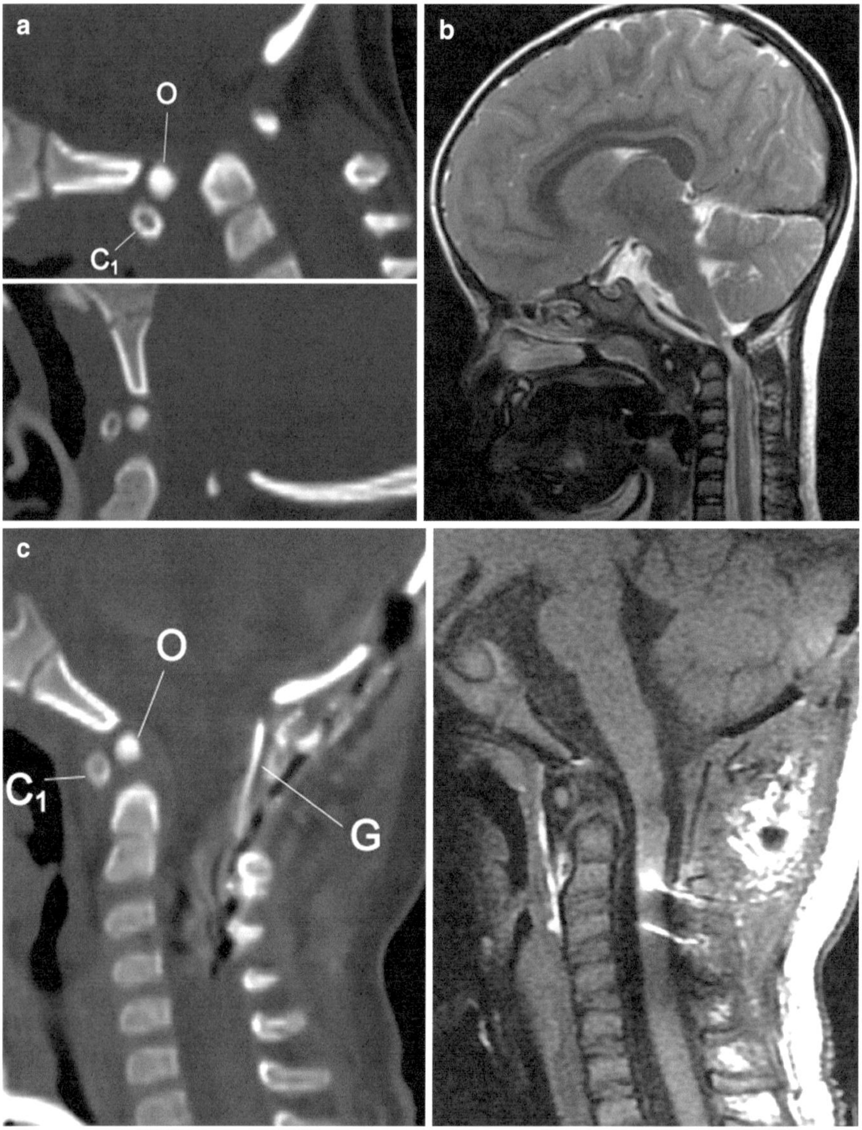

Fig. 30 Unstable ossiculum terminale in a 2-year-old child with intermittent quadriparesis. (**a**) Flexion (*upper*) and extension (*lower*) sagittal-reconstructed CTs showing highly mobile ossiculum (*O*) and C_1 with obvious translational subluxation. (**b**) Sagittal T_2 MRI shows C_1 cord compression and T_2 signal changes in the cord. (**c**) Post-operative sagittal CT (*left*) and MRI (*right*) showing resection of C_1 posterior arch, reduced C_1–C_2 subluxation after bone grafts (*G*) and Inside-Outside Screw-plate occipital-C_2–C_3 fusion. MRI (*right*) shows restored width of the upper cervical canal and relief of cord compression. *O* ossiculum terminale, C_1 anterior arch of C_1

C_1–C_2 fusion is adequate treatment if complete reduction is achievable. If there is persistent anterior dislocation of C_1, its posterior arch may have to be removed for decompression, in which case occipital C_2–C_3 fusion is necessary (Fig. 30c).

Case 1

A 10-year-old girl presented with intermittent quadriparesis and neck pain. Dynamic sagittal CT reconstruction shows an ossiculum terminale with anterior subluxation and only partial reduction on extension and persistent cord compression by the posterior arch of C_1 (Fig. 31a). The nearly spherical ossiculum forms a synovial joint with the posterior aspect of the anterior C_1 arch, and the two structures move together (Fig. 31a). The basal dental segment looks dysplastic but seems to have adequate height, although the TAL evidently interfaces with the loose ossiculum and not with the dental pivot. Sagittal MRI shows an extremely narrow spinal canal at C_1 (Fig. 31b). C_1 laminectomy and instrumentation fusion of occiput to C_2–C_3 was performed. Her occiput had a robust midline keel so that a regular cruciate occipital plate was secured to the skull with three 6 mm screws (Fig. 31c) and then to two upright rods contoured to the region. The rods were affixed by interlocking links to bilateral C_1–C_2 transarticular screws and C_3 lateral mass screws (Fig. 31d).

Abnormal Resegmentation of Proatlas Centrum: Os Avis

In this rare anomaly, the apical dental segment remains attached to the basioccipital and is not fused to the main dental stem. The pivot is thus shortened but firmly fixed to the axis centrum, where a semilucent line representing the lower synchondrosis marks the successful integration of the two lower dens-axis components. This anomaly has been called "dystopic os odontoideum" by von Torklus and Prescher [76, 78, 91] to distinguish it from the "orthotopic os odontoideum" used by these authors to designate the common variety of os odontoideum. Their use of the term os odontoideum differs from ours in that they have included both the unfused basal and apical dental segments.

Embryogenesis

In human malformations, it is not uncommon to find errant ontogeny reverting to a morphology reminiscent of an organ's phylogenetic past. As case in point, a separate bone between the dens and the basioccipital resembling the attached ossiculum in the human anomaly is found in some fish and reptiles and many birds [30, 32, 40, 76, 78, 87, 100], hence, our terminology os avis. In higher vertebrates, this bone, the primordium of the apical dens, normally becomes detached from the basioccipital rim, which shares with it a common origin in the proatlas centrum. Lack of proper resegmentation of the proatlas centrum, in essence

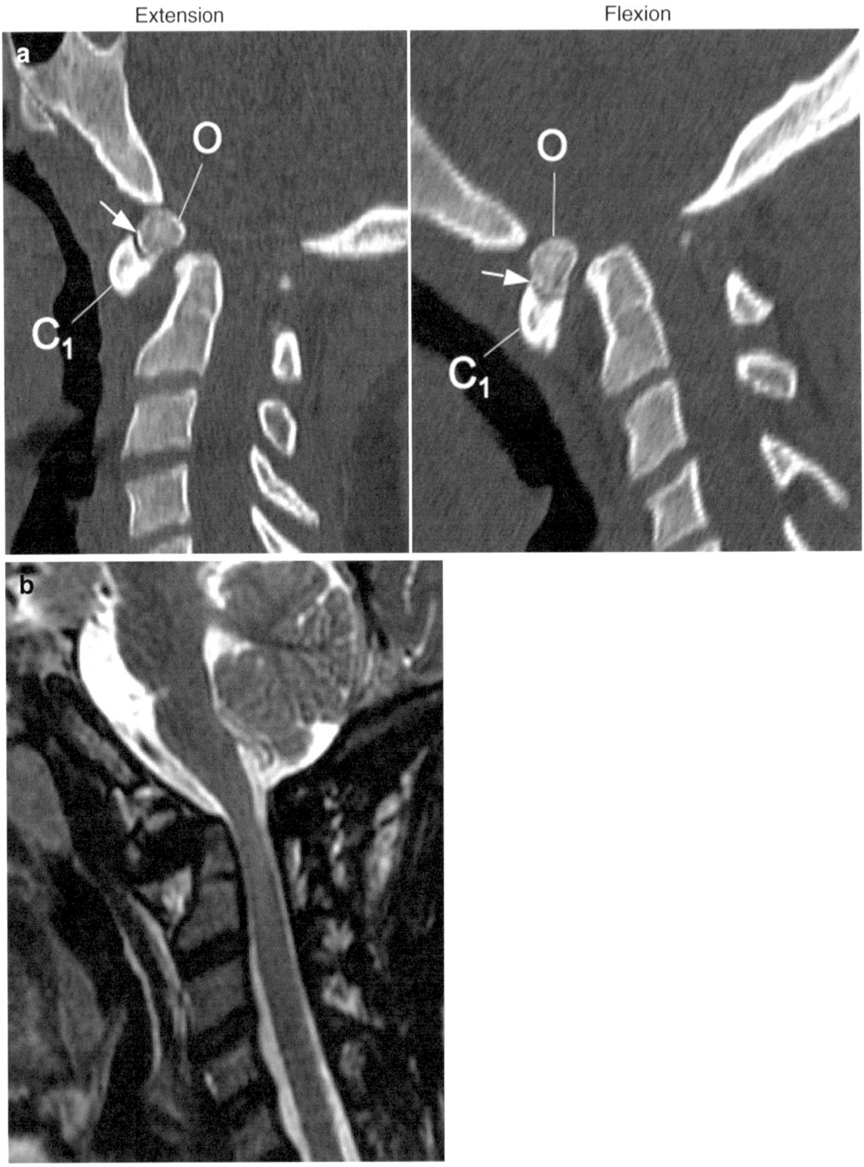

Fig. 31 Case 1: 10-year-old boy with ossiculum terminale. (**a**) Flexion-extension CT shows highly mobile ossiculum and anterior subluxation. The ossiculum terminale (*O*) forms a joint (*arrow*) with the posterior surface of the anterior arch of C_1 (C_1). Both C_1 and ossiculum move together as one unit. (**b**)Sagittal MR in neutral position shows narrowing of upper cervical canal. (**c**)After maximum intraoperative reduction and partial resection of the C_1 posterior arch, the occiput is fused to C_2 and C_3 using a screw-plate and contoured-upright rods. (**d**)Post-operative plain film (*left side*) and CTs (*right side*) show the C_2 transarticular screws to include the lateral mass of C_1, and the C_3 lateral mass screws. Note the three occipital screws through the thick mid-occipital keel for the occipital plate

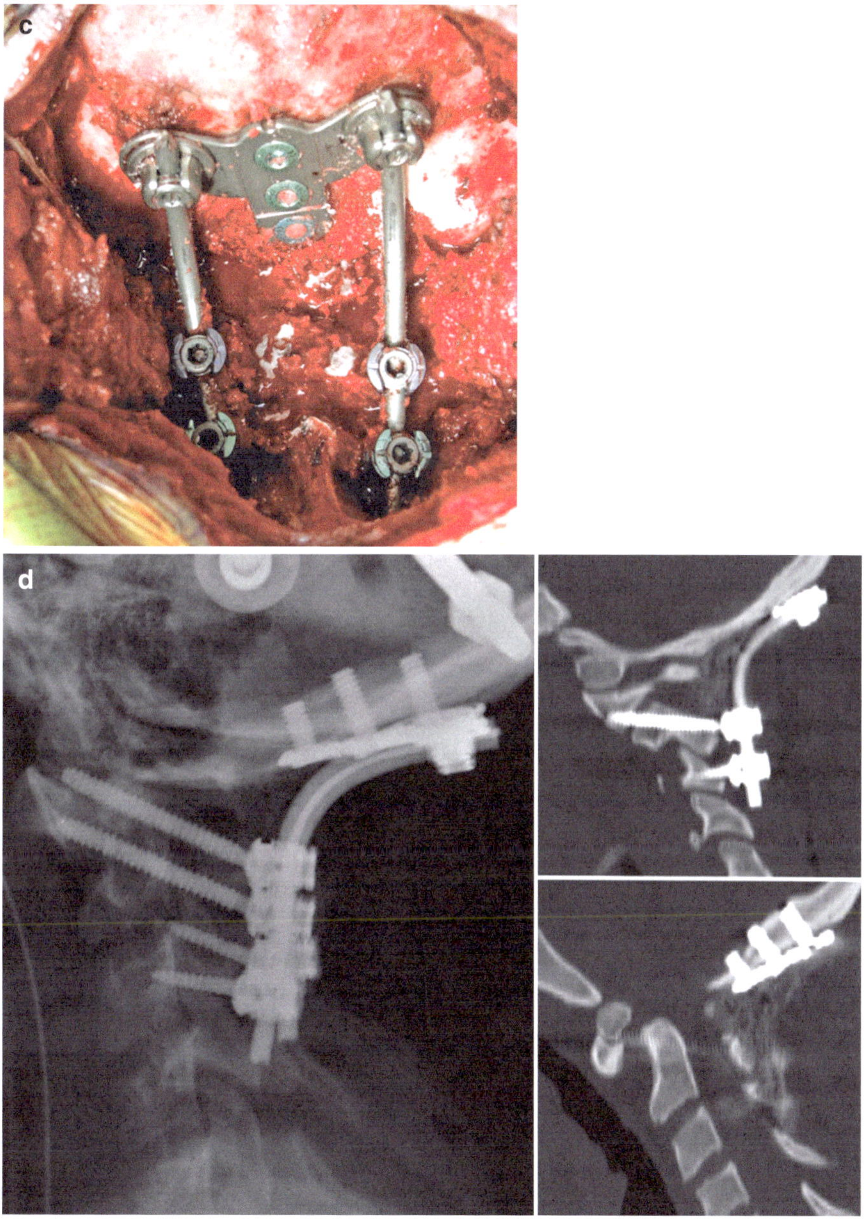

Fig. 31 (continued)

negating the necessary cleavage, prevents descent and subsequent joining of the apical segment with the centrum of the first cervical sclerotome to complete the dental pivot. The reason for this failure is unknown, but since proatlas resegmentation normally occurs at the transitional zone between somites 4 and 5, a caudal shift of this transitional zone along the body axis may affect the resegmentation process. In transgenic mouse mutant in which *Hox a-7* is expressed earlier and more rostrally in its anterior domain, the last occipital somite (O_4) is homeotically transformed (posteriorly) to become the atlas, bearing a "proatlas" centrum that remains attached to the basioccipital. C_1 then becomes C_2 and acquires a complete centrum while C_2 is deleted of its normal dens [24]. This extra "proatlas" bone in the murine mutant very much resembles the os avis in the human malformation and suggests that a Hox gene mutation causing posterior homeotic transformation of segmental identity may indeed underlie the genesis of the os avis. Alternatively, illegitimate *Pax-1* repression at the critical juncture of severance within the proatlas will prevent cellular cleavage through the original resegmentation fronts between somites 4 and 5, and allow the apical dental centrum to remain connected to the basion.

Clinical Significance

An os avis tends to be associated with neurological deterioration. The two patients with os avis described by Wollin [100] amongst seven others with "loose" ossiculum terminale and os odontoideum are the only ones with symptoms, and both had a hypoplastic dental pivot. Both cases of os avis described by Menezes and Fenoy are symptomatic due to posterior dislocations of C_1 on C_2 [62]. Of the two cases in our series, one had a hypoplastic dens, and the atlantoaxial complex is extremely unstable on extension; the TAL is strapped against the os and therefore moves with the skull (Fig. 32). Our other case is associated with other CVJ anomalies such as multiple hyposegmentation of vertebral bodies, short clivus, basilar impression, and a stenotic foramen magnum, even though the dens pivot is tall and sustaining for the TAL. The patient does not have instability but develops compressive symptoms (Fig. 33). In Wollin's cases, associated anomalies include a large median (third) occipital condyle (see below) and a hyperplastic anterior C_1 arch.

Treatment of os avis depends on the other anomalies. Pure instability can be remedied with C_1–C_2 fusion. An absent posterior C_1 arch or an occipitalised atlas would mandate inclusion of the occiput into the fusion. Concomitant neural compression due to basilar impression or invagination of the opisthion may require simultaneous decompression.

Failure of Midline Integration of Basal Dental Segment: The Bifid Dens

Aetiology

A completely bifid dens is an extremely rare entity. It is different from the "dens bicornis" described by von Torklus and Gehle in which only the tip of the dens is bicornuate and the function of the otherwise well-formed dental pivot is unaffected

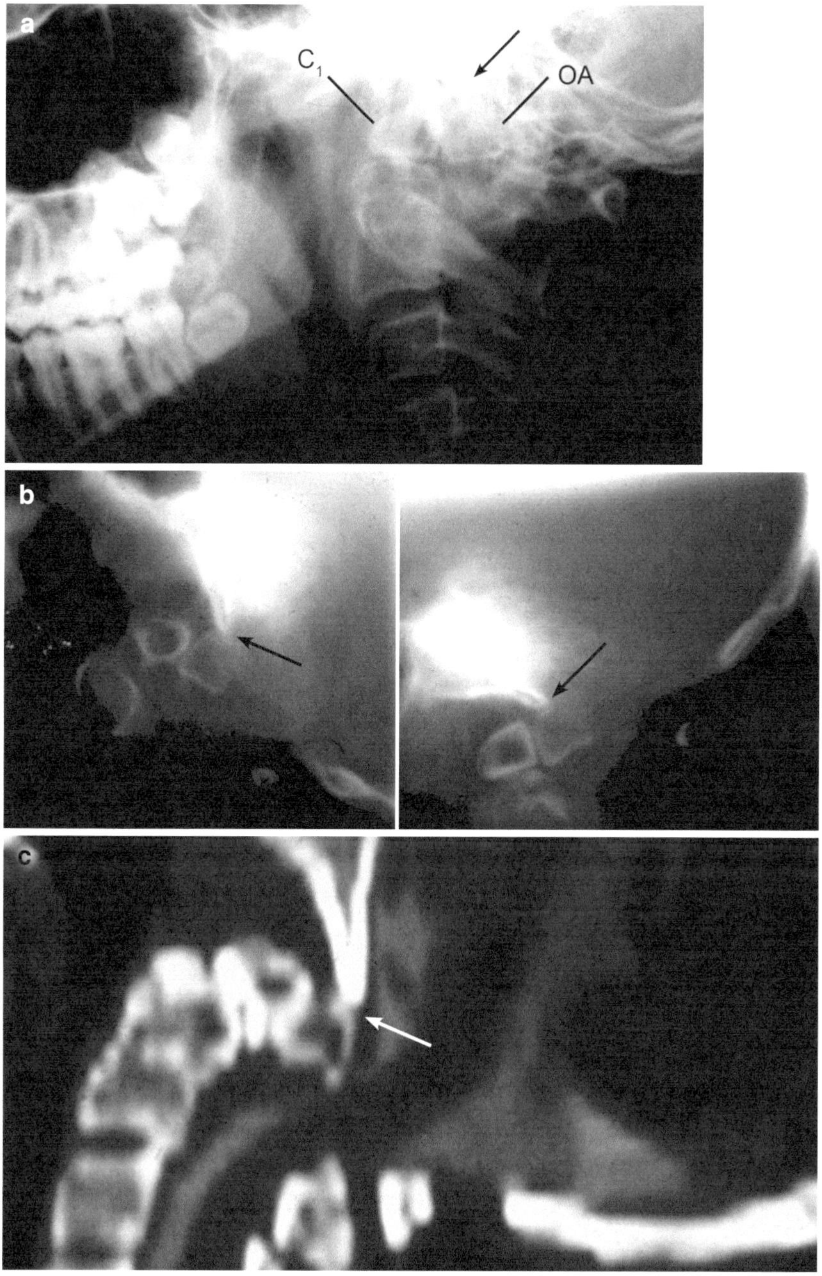

Fig. 32 Os avis with severe posterior subluxation of skull and C_1 on C_2 producing quadriparesis. (**a**) The bone directly above the dental pivot is in fact a posteriorly shifted C_1 anterior arch (*C_1*). The os avis (*OA*) is just behind the C_1 arch and is attached to the clivus marked by the *arrow*. Note posteriorly shifted posterior arch of C_1. (**b**) Flexion-extension polytomography shows relationship between C_1 arch, clivus, and os avis. Note attachment of the os with the clivus tip (*arrow*) and the unchanging (fixed) relationship with the clivus during flexion and extension. (**c**) CT myelogram shows spinal cord compression by the os avis during extension. *Arrow* marks attachment of os avis to clival tip

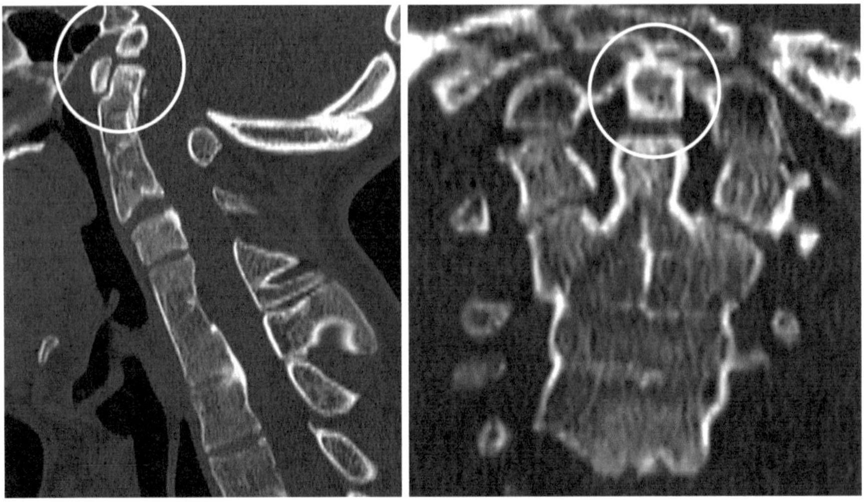

Fig. 33 Undescended apical dens still fused to the clivus (os avis). The dental pivot has a flat top but tall enough for the TAL and has no instability. Other anomalies such as multiple vertebral centra fusion, basilar invagination of the opisthion, and stenosis by C_1 posterior arch cause compressive myelopathy

[91]. Dens bicornis results from aberrant distal ossification late in development. In true dental bifidity, the partition in the basal dental segment goes full length of the process to the lower synchondrosis. In one example, the bifid dens is accompanied by a dislocated ossiculum terminale (Fig. 34). In two others, one half of the split dental base is unattached to the centrum of C_2 and is floating free, while the body of C_2 is fused with that of C_3, which is itself bifid. The anterior C_1 arch is also unfused in the midline (see Case 2). These examples suggest that the lack of midline integration occurs very early in development, probably in the mesenchymal prevertebral stage or during chondrification. The lack of midline integration in the primordium of the basal dental segment appears to interfere with fusion of the adjacent synchondrosis leading to a detached "hemi-os" in two patients and an ossiculum terminale in the other. Also, faulty midline integration in the second example given here is not confined to the basal dens but also extends to the primordium of the C_3 centrum and the hypochordal bow of the first cervical sclerotome, which forms the anterior C_1 arch. The multiplicity of primordial abnormalities occurring around resegmentation would make it unlikely for a truly bifid dens to be a result of anomalous ossification, which occurs much later.

Clinical Significance

Our entire experience of three cases suggests that the bifid dens is associated with atlantoaxial instability because the central pivot is hypoplastic when bifid. In our first case, the hypoplastic dens is aggravated by the dislocated ossiculum terminale, negating any possibility for TAL anchorage (Fig. 34b, c). In our second and third case, the hypermobile "hemi-os" pops backwards during flexion and accentuates the cord compression (see Case 2).

Stabilisation for case 1 had to include the occiput into the fusion because of an incomplete posterior arch of C_1. In the other two cases, occipital-cervical fusion is combined with a transoral resection of both halves of the dens to relieve the anterior compression.

Case 2

A 6-year-old boy presented with intermittent quadriplegia and somnolence whenever he flexed his neck to study. CT showed a bifid odontoid with the right half unfused to the axis body (Fig. 35a) so that on flexion this mobile "hemi-os" popped backwards against the lower brainstem. A previous occipital-cervical fusion failed to relieve neural compression from the anterior vector (Fig. 35b). Because the boy also had congenital microstomia and micrognathia, which prevented a conventional transoral approach to the odontoid, we split the mandible, tongue, mylohyoid muscle, and soft palate to access and resect the hemi-os and odontoid (Fig. 35c–g). The child recovered with complete abatement of symptoms (Fig. 35h).

Basioccipital Dysgeneses

Failure of Midline Integration of Basioccipital Primordium: Bifid Clivus

The rare entity of bifid clivus probably arises from failure of midline integration of the axial sclerotome of the proatlas, resulting in a split primordium of the basioccipital (Fig. 36). If the failure involves the other occipital sclerotomes, the bifidity may extend up to the sphenoclival synchondrosis (Fig. 36a, right).

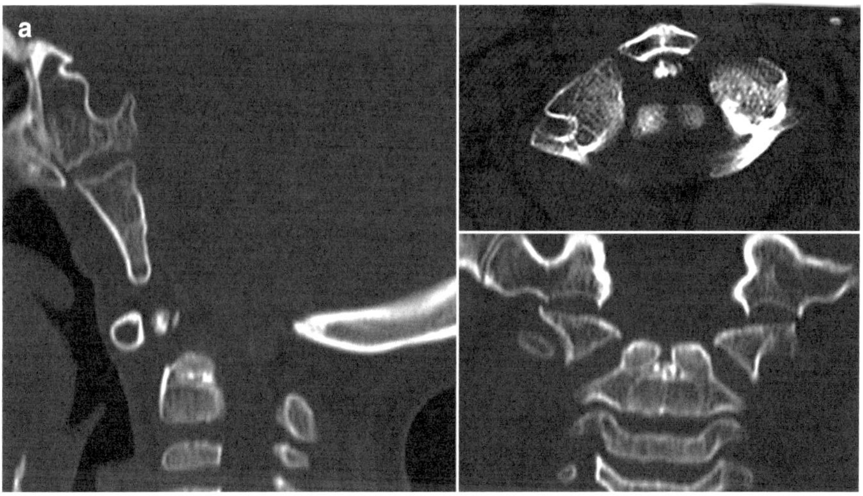

Fig. 34 Completely bifid dens. (**a**) Note complete lack of midline integration of basal dental segment down to lower dental synchondrosis, and an unfused and forward dislocated apical dens, suggesting midline integration abnormality interferes with growth and fusion of adjacent upper dental synchondrosis. (**b**) Flexion-extension CT shows C_1–C_2 instability. (**c**) Sagittal MR shows severe cord compression with flexion. *Arrow* points to small ossiculum

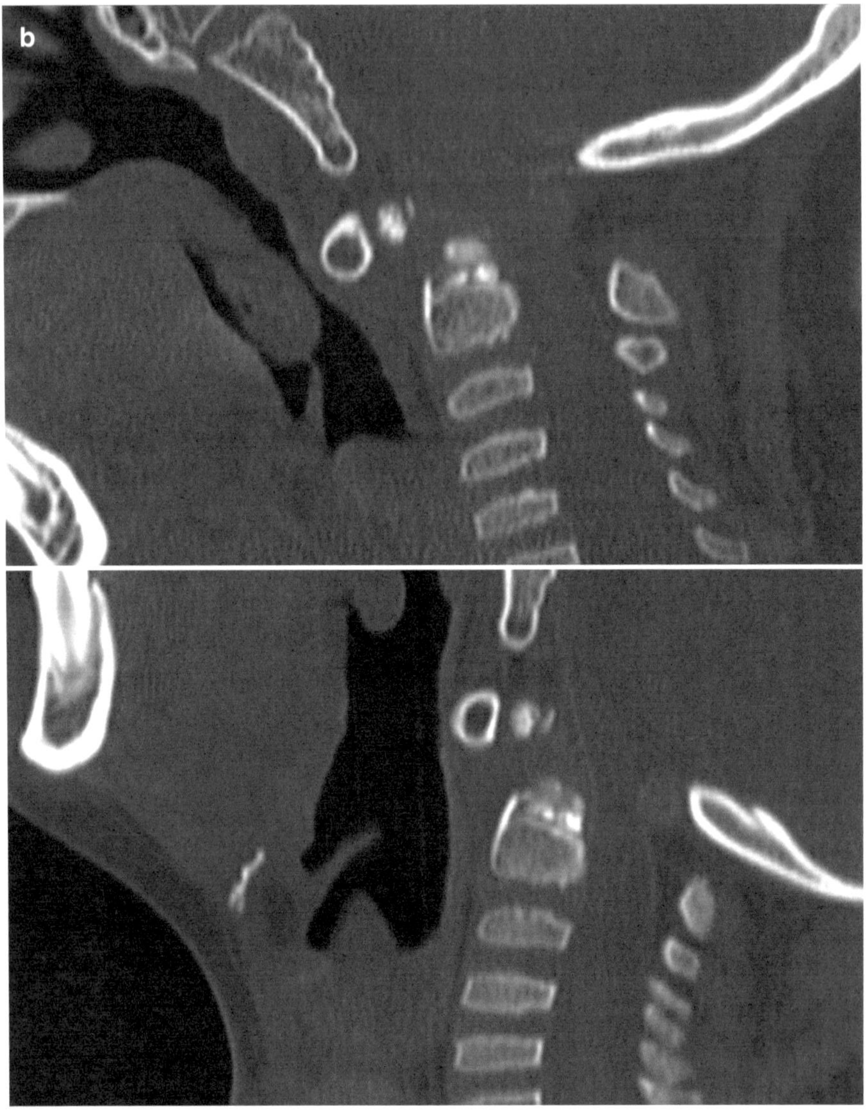

Fig. 34 (continued)

Fig. 34 (continued)

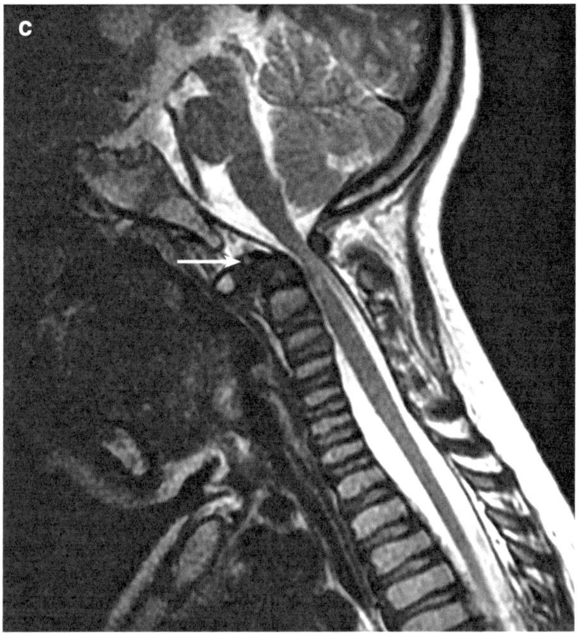

A widely split basioccipital may affect anchorage of the tectorial membrane, which normally straps the odontoid complex to the back of the clivus. The atlanto-occipital joint may become unstable, and the cervical spine may appear to have drifted away from the skull (Fig. 36a, right and b). Treatment depends on the degree of instability and consists of occipito-cervical fusion.

Basilar Impression, Platybasia, Retroflexed Dens, and Basilar Invagination

Basilar impression is present when the dens moves into the plane of the foramen magnum. In the pre-MRI era, basilar impression has been defined on plain x-ray by the relationship of the tip of the dens with anatomical lines: McGregor's line, the most reliable, is drawn between the hard palate and the lowest point of the occiput and should not be protruded by the dens for more than 5 mm. Likewise, Chamberlain's line between the hard palate and the opisthion should not be crossed by more than 2.5 mm, and McRae's line between the basion and opisthion not at all [57, 58] (Fig. 37). Today, the sagittal MRI is by far the best way to assess the clinical relevance of basilar impression.

Aetiology

Congenital basilar impression, which concerns us here, is less a result of active upward impingement of the dens against the brainstem, as the word "impression" implies, than a drop of the posterior fossa contents on to the unnaturally high-riding

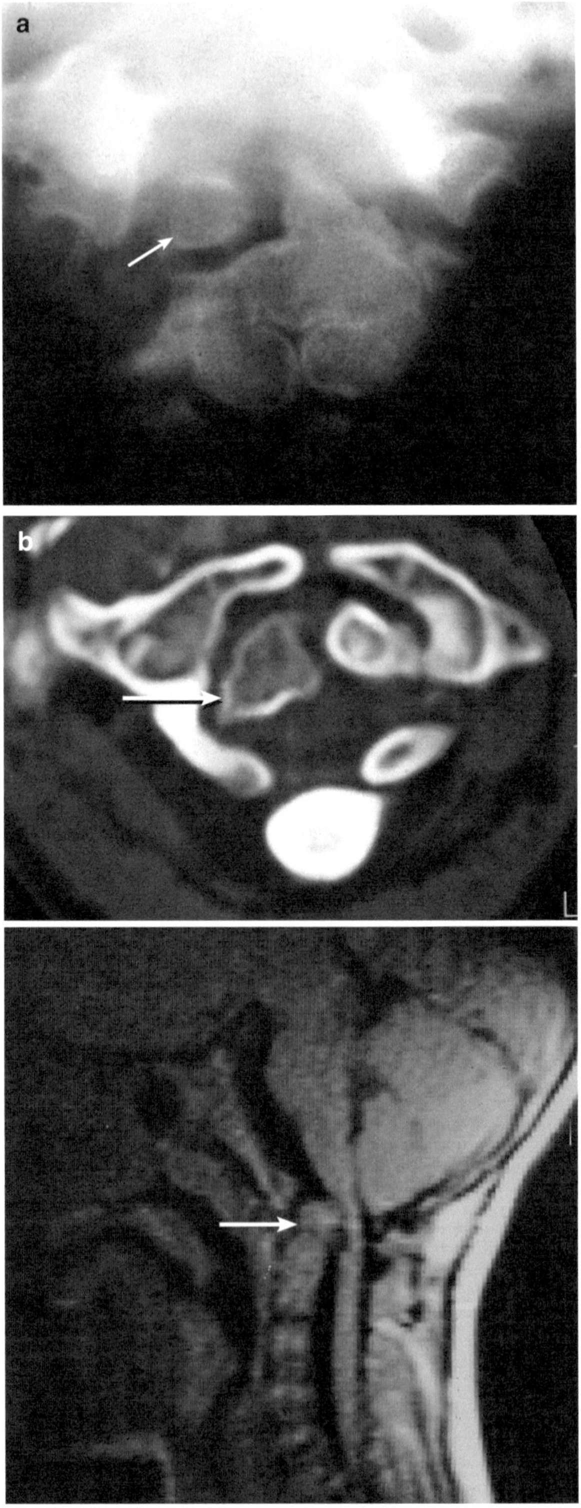

Fig. 35 Case 2: 6-year-old boy with absent midline integration of basal dental segment. (**a**) Non-fusion of right "hemi-os" (*arrow*) to the C_2 centrum suggests interference with adjacent dental synchondrosis fusion. Note bifid C_3 centrum and fusion of C_2 and C_3 centra. (**b**) Floating hemi-os (*arrow*) on the axial CT (*left*) and backward "popping" of the hemi-os with cord compression on MRI (*right*). (**c**) Incision for midline mandibulotomy. (**d**) Step-osteotomy of midline mandibulotomy for perfect reattachment. (**e**) *Left*: Difficulty in exposing the posterior pharynx even after mandibulotomy. *Right*: Both the tongue and part of the mylohyoid have to be split in the middle to expose the posterior pharynx. (**f**) *Left*: Exposure of the posterior pharynx after splitting the soft palate. *Right*: Exposure of the anterior C_1 arch after incising the pharyngeal mucosa. (**g**) Odontoid resection. *Left*: Subperiosteal exposure of the C_1 anterior arch. *Middle*: After drilling off the middle portion of the C_1 arch, the floating hemi-os is exposed. The fixed left hemi-os has been partially removed. *Right*: After removal of both the floating and fixed hemi-os, the transverse atlantal ligament (*TAL*) is exposed. (**h**) Post-operative axial CT showing complete removal of the mobile right hemi-os and most of the fixed hemi-os on the left

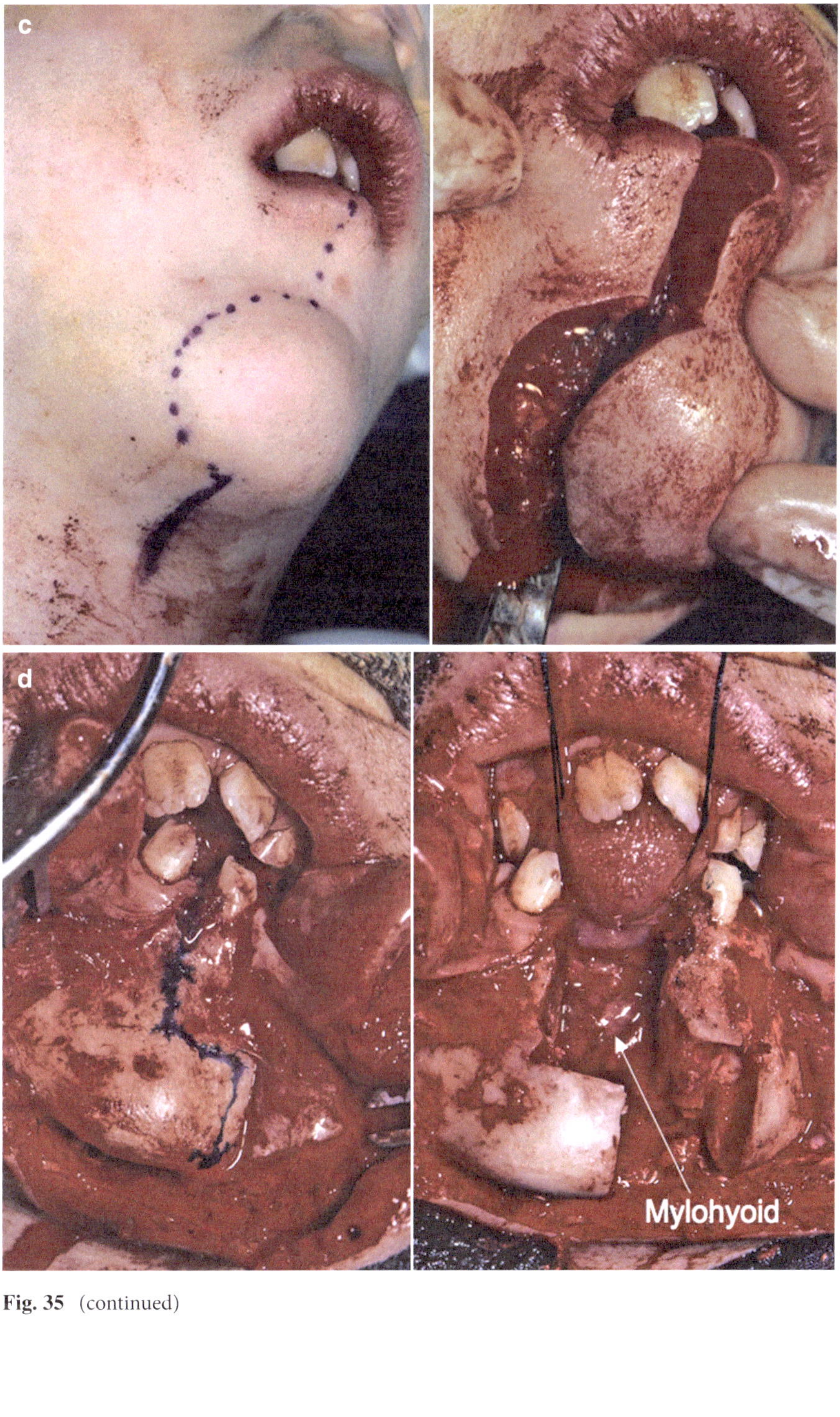

Fig. 35 (continued)

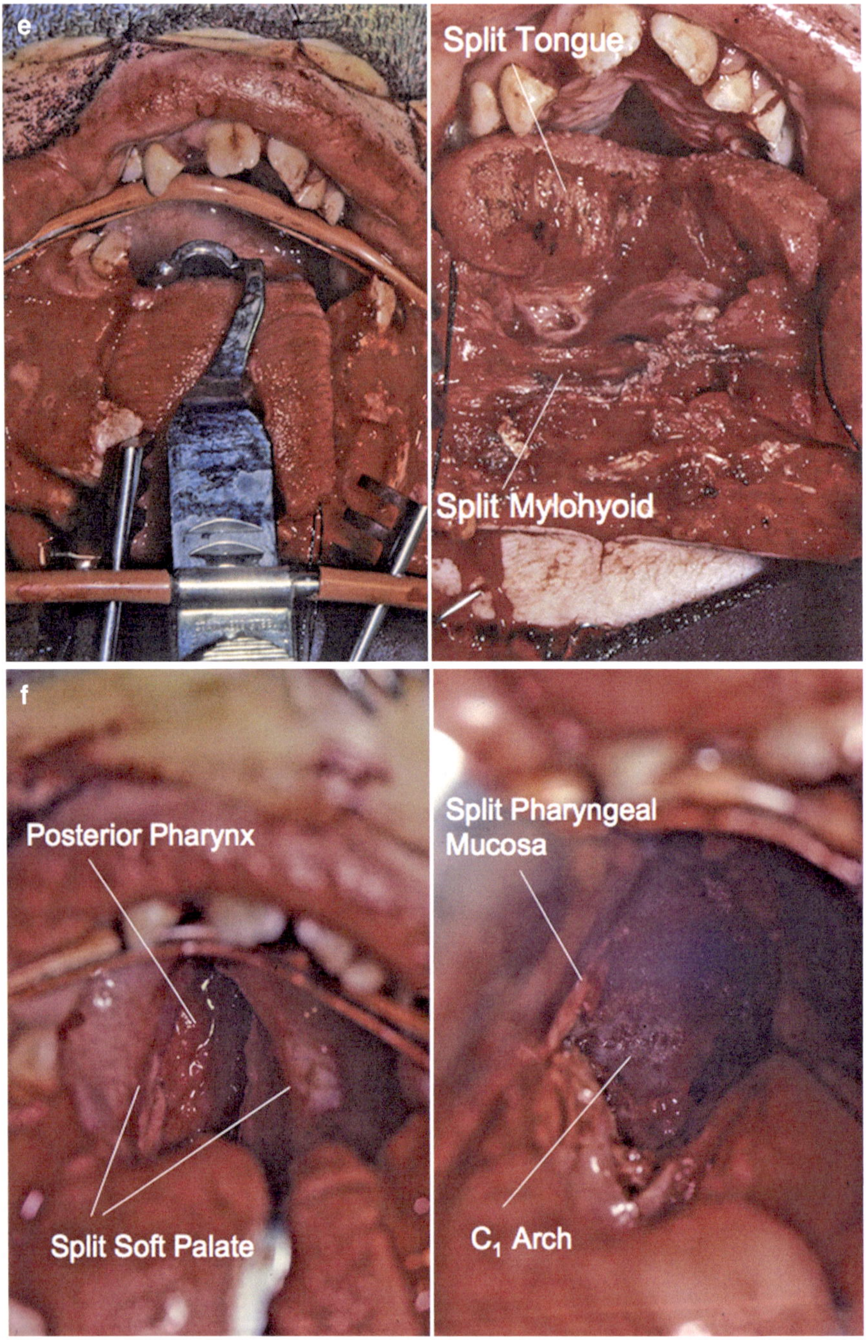

Fig. 35 (continued)

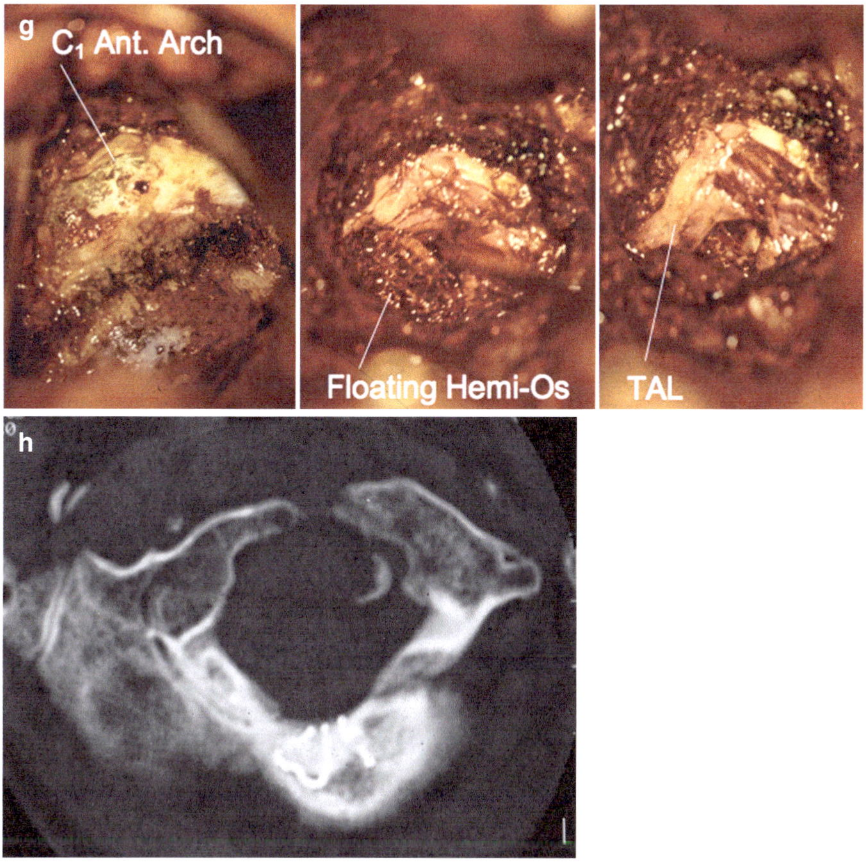

Fig. 35 (continued)

dens due to a shallow occipital "box" and flattened skull base. The causative occipital dysplasia is due to deformed growth of all three parts of the occipital primordium: the basioccipital (pars basilaris) and the exoccipital (pars lateralis including the condyles and the foramen magnum rim), which enlarge by endochondral ossification, are primarily hypoplastic; and the supraoccipital, the squama, which expands by membranous ossification and therefore depends on growth of the chondrocranial moulds of the other two parts, is obligatorily constricted.

Three etiological types of congenital basilar impression can be distinguished. Anterior basilar impression is caused by changes in the basioccipital complex, which derives from the four axial occipital sclerotomes. The most dramatic change is platybasia, when the nasion-tuberculum-basion angle (NTB angle of Welcker) is increased and the sphenoclival block appears severely flattened. Platybasia is often accompanied by a shortened basioccipital or clivus, which normally measures more than 3.2 cm from the sphenooccipital synchondrosis to the basion. The summated effect of a short and flattened clivus is that the basion, which normally lies below the nasion-opisthion

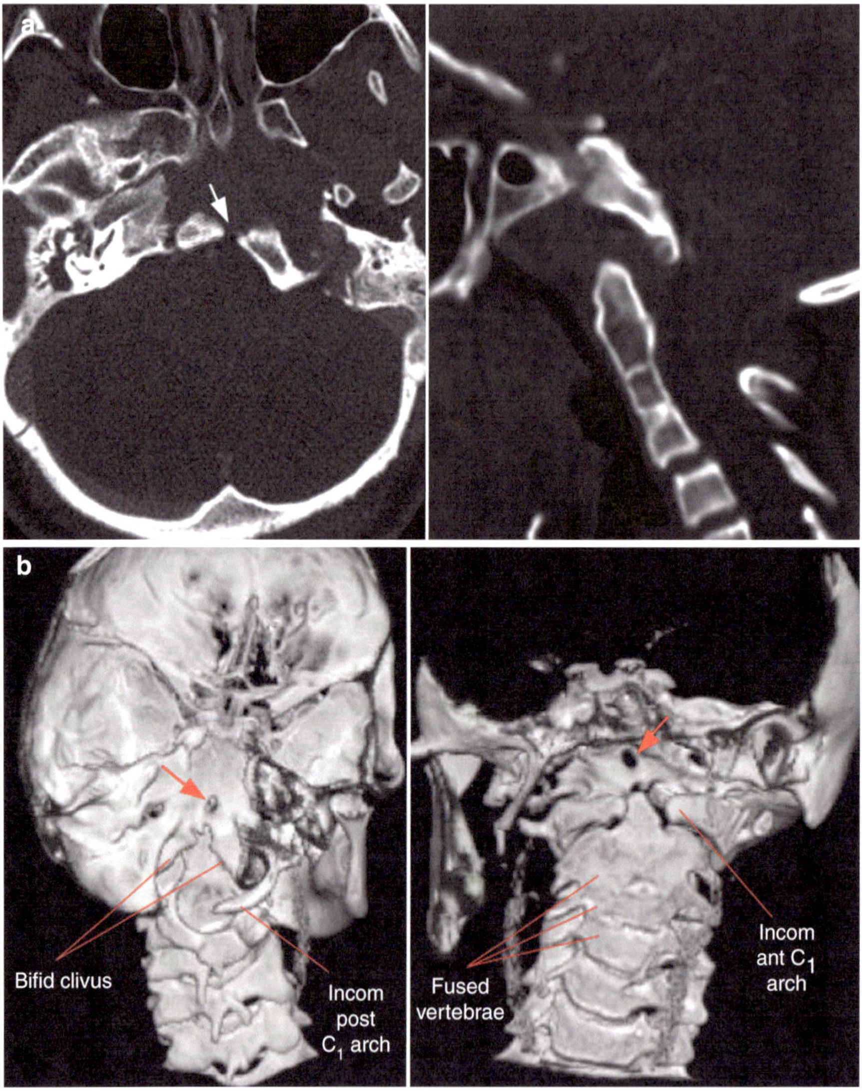

Fig. 36 Bifid clivus. (**a**) *Left*: Axial CT shows the gap in the lower clivus (*arrow*). *Right*: Sagittal CT shows the odontoid process is far anterior to its usual position below the clivus. Fusion of the C_2, C_3 and C_4 centra is also seen. (**b**) CT 3-D rendering of the skull base. *Left*: View from the back shows widely bifid basiocciput and an oval defect (*arrow*) higher in the clivus. The posterior C_1 arch is deficient. *Right*: View from the front shows the odontoid is far forward from the bifid clivus (mostly covered by the dens), and the anterior C_1 arch is also bifid. Note upper clival defect (*arrow*). *Incom post C_1 arch* Incomplete posterior C_1 arch, *Incom ant C_1 arch* Incomplete anterior C_1 arch

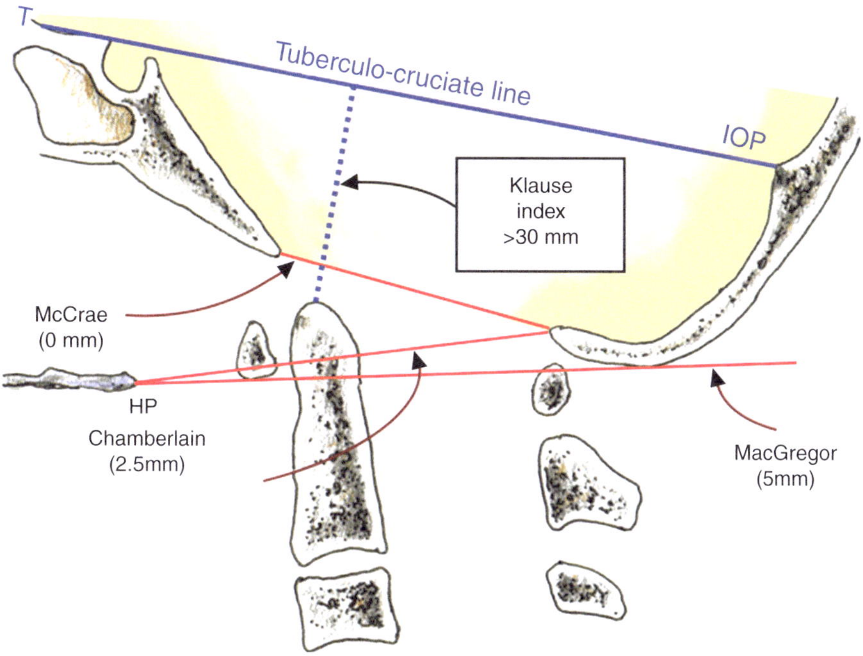

Fig. 37 Radiographic criteria for basilar impression. (1) McGregor's line between hard palate (*HP*) and the lowest point of occiput. Basilar impression is present if the dens protrudes >5 mm above this line. (2) Chamberlain's line between hard palate and opisthion. Positive diagnosis if dens protrudes >2.5 mm above line. (3) McRae's line between basion and opisthion should be above the dens. (4) Klaus index, distance between tip of dens and the tuberculum-cruciate line between tuberculum (*T*) and internal occipital protuberance (*IOP*). This measures depth of the posterior fossa and should be >30 mm

line (of Boogaard), is raised way above it and moves cranially (Fig. 38). This forces the plane of the foramen magnum to tilt upward in a lordotic angle, and with it the planes of the occipital condyles and of the condyle-atlas articulations (Fig. 39).

The fusion and chondrification of the basioccipital and the exoccipital sclerotomes occur slightly earlier than the resegmentation of the C_1–C_2 sclerotomes. A severely lordotic skull base angle consequently compels the emerging upper cervical sclerotomal column to rise up and bend backwards "in sympathy", whole hog but starting with the upper most centra complex that will ultimately form the dens-axis (Fig. 39). This explains why platybasia and short clivus are frequently associated with an elevated retroflexed and lordotic dens that, in severe cases, points sharply and wickedly backwards into the brainstem (Fig. 40). Clinical studies have indeed shown that patients with basilar impression have a significantly shorter clivus than control groups [69].

Case 3

A 10-year-old boy presented with long-standing painful scoliosis and a new onset of neurogenic dysphagia. Imaging studies show platybasia (NTB angle = 180°), a short clivus with a sphenoclival synchondrosis-basion length of

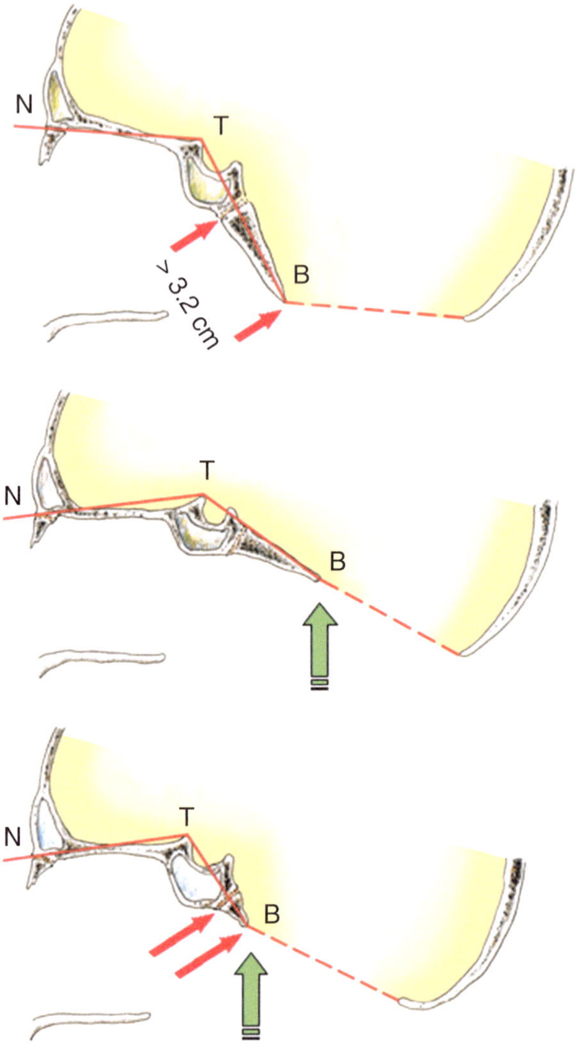

Fig. 38 Normal clival angle (*top*) measured by the NTB angle of Welcker joining the nasion (*N*), tuberculum (*T*), and basion (*B*). The angle should be less than 130°. Platybasia (*middle*) is marked by an NTB angle >130°. This raises the basion (*green arrow*) and forces the foramen magnum plane (*dotted line*) to tilt upward. The same upward tilt of this plane also occurs with a short clivus (*lower*). Clivus length is measured from the sphenoclival synchondrosis to the basion (B) (between *small arrows*). Normal clival length is >3.2 cm

1.8 cm, a retroflexed dens, and the anterior form of basilar impression (Fig. 41). There is also hindbrain herniation and syringomyelia. Both the clinical symptoms and syringomyelia improved following posterior bony decompression and occipital-C_2 fusion.

In the posterior form of basilar impression, the exoccipitals, derived from the lateral sclerotomes of the proatlas, rise up towards the foramen magnum, bringing with them the occipital condyles and opisthion. Alternatively, the exoccipital bones may be thin and the condyles flat and hypoplastic. In either case, the dens is secondarily elevated towards the cranial cavity without being lordotic or retroflexed. The opisthion, however, often invaginates into the cranial aperture (basilar invagination) (Fig. 42).

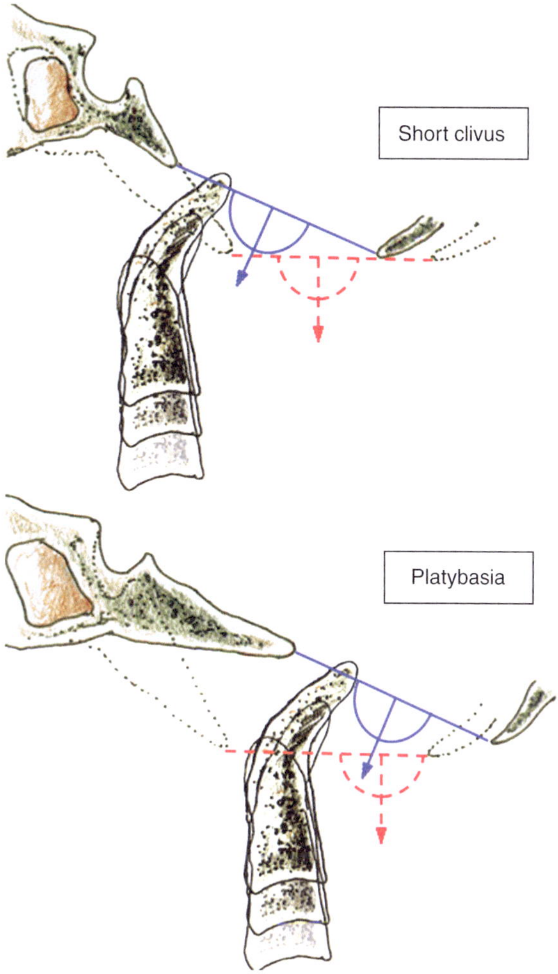

Fig. 39 Severe lordotic tilting of the plane of the occipital condyle in short clivus (*upper*) and platybasia (*lower*). Normal clivus and opisthion are represented by *dotted outlines*, and orientation and plane of the occipital condyle are represented by *arrow* and *semicircle*, respectively, *red* for normal and *blue* for abnormal. The overlapping images of the odontoid represent upward and backward tilting path of the prevertebra of the dens, induced by the lordotic tilt of the occipital-C_1 articulation

Case 4

A 12-year-old girl of normal intelligence presented with occipital headache, neurogenic dysphagia, nasal voice, and right arm and hand clumsiness. CT showed a steeply elevated occipital condyle (exoccipital), basilar (opisthion) invagination, and C_1 assimilation (Fig. 43a, left). There is no platybasia, and the dens, though migrated cranially into the foramen magnum, was not retroflexed (Fig. 43a, right). MR showed severe brainstem and upper cord compression mainly from the invaginating opisthion (Fig. 43b). At surgery, the posterior lip of the foramen was removed by careful drilling under microscopy (Fig. 43c). The thin occipital bone and the bizarre shapes of C_2 and C_3 precluded the use of regular occipital screw-plates and intra-axial cervical screws. We used instead the Inside-Outside Occipital Screw-plate system affixed to the C_2 and C_3 laminae with sublaminar cables (Fig. 43d–h). On-laid autogenous iliac crest grafts were put in place (Fig. 43i–k).

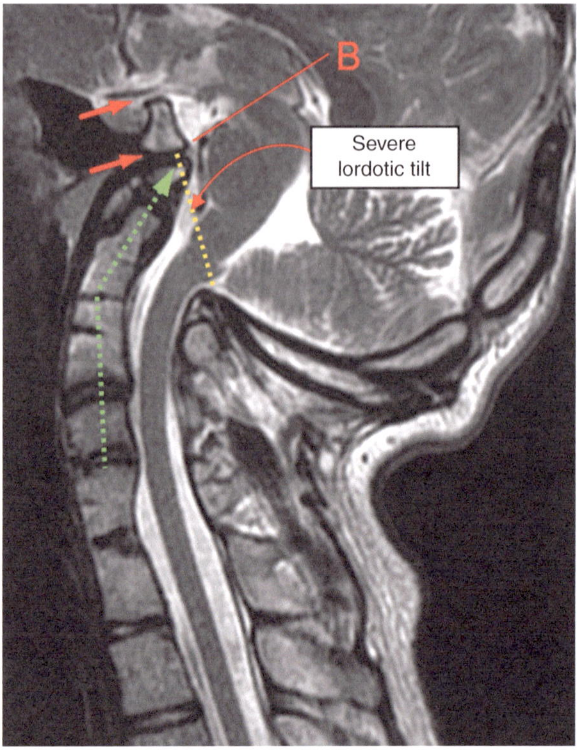

Fig. 40 Anterior form of basilar impression caused by an exceedingly short (<1 cm) and blunted clivus (*red arrows*) with severe lordotic tilt of the plane of the foramen magnum (*yellow dotted line*), leading to a "sympathetic" lordotic bend of the dental pivot (*green dotted arrow*) resulting in a retroflexed odontoid and basilar impression. *B* basion

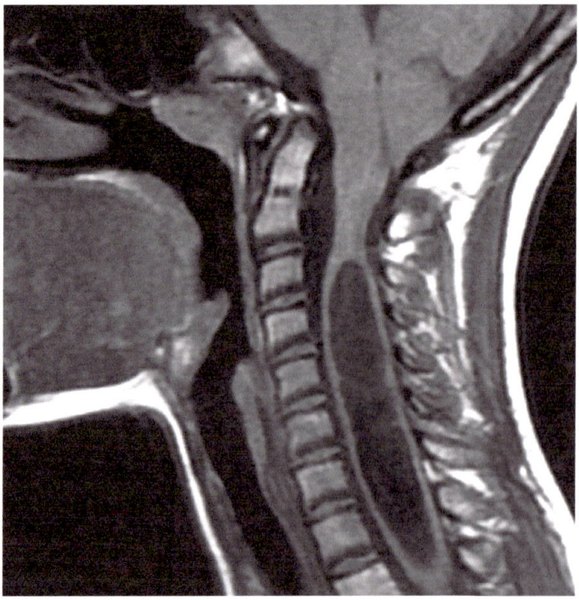

Fig. 41 Anterior basilar impression with severe platybasia, a short clivus (1.8 cm from sphenoclival synchondrosis to basion), and a retroflex and high-riding dens. The basioccipital dysplasia reduces the posterior fossa volume and leads to hindbrain herniation and secondary syringomyelia

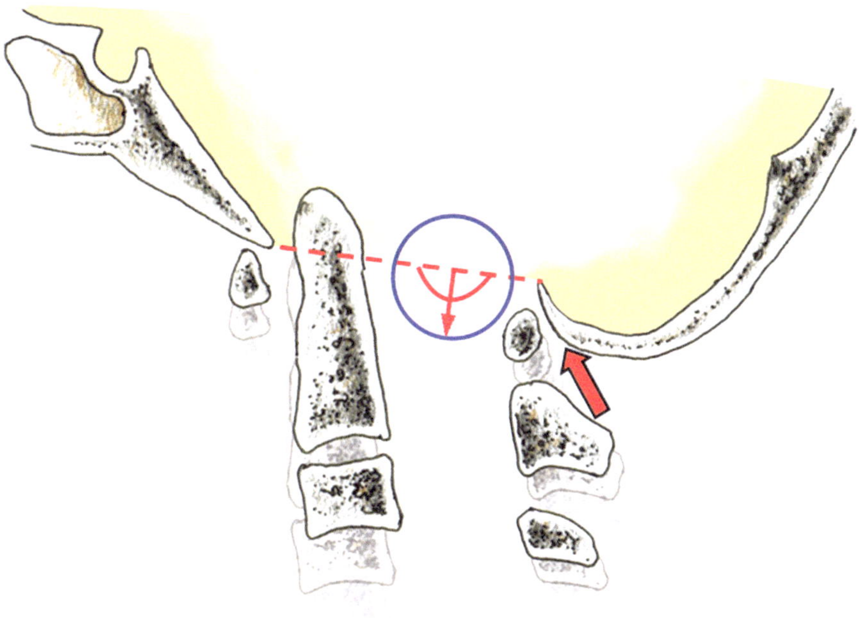

Fig. 42 Genesis of the posterior form of basilar impression. Elevation of the occipital condyle and invagination of the opisthion (*red arrow*) (basilar invagination) raise the occipital condyle-C_1 joint (*blue circle*) without much lordotic tilt, causing the odontoid process to rise up straight without backward tilt, resulting in basilar impression without a retroflex dens. Overlapping images of the odontoid represent its straight upward migration path

In the combined anterior and posterior form, severe basilar impression by a retroflexed dens is accompanied by posterior invagination of the opisthion, causing neural compression from both front and back.

Case 5

A 12-year-old girl presented with occipital headache, hemi-sensory loss, and tongue fasciculation. CT shows an essentially flat nasion-tuberculum-basion line and severe platybasia, an acute Wackenheim angle (basilar kyphosis), an elevated retroflexed dens, and severe basilar (opisthion) invagination (Fig. 44).

Hindbrain Herniation in Basioccipital Dysgenesis

The upward migration of the anterior and posterior occiput in severe basilar impression in essence reduces the posterior fossa volume, estimated by the index of Klaus, which measures the distance between the tip of the dens and the tuberculo-cruciate

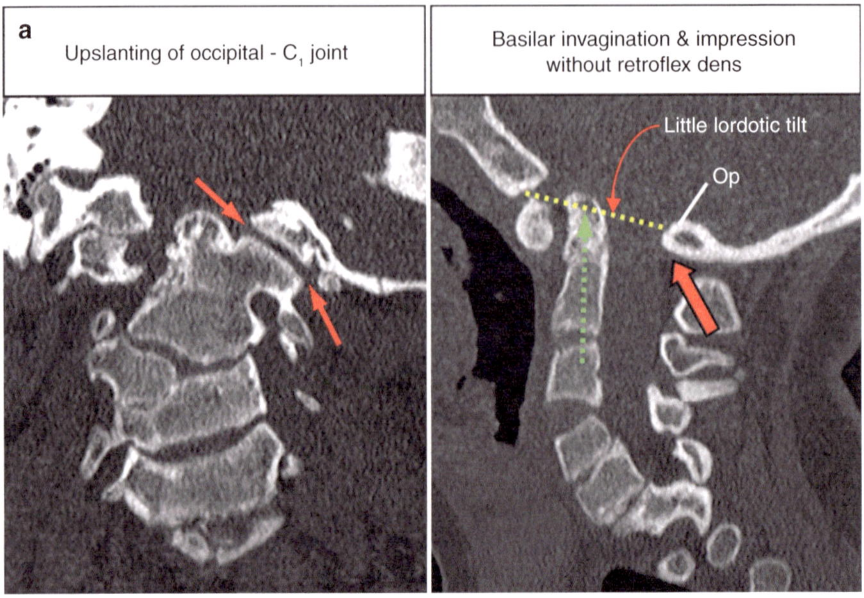

Fig. 43 Case 4 of the posterior form of basilar impression. Twelve-year-old girl with occipital headache, neurogenic dysphagia, and right hemiparesis. (**a**) CT of CVJ. *Left*: Coronal CT shows severely up-slanting and elevated left occipital condyle-C_1 joint (*arrows*). C_4 is a hemi-vertebra. *Right*: sagittal CT shows invagination of the opisthion (*Op*) (*red blocked arrow*) (basilar invagination) with elevation of the basion-opisthion plane (*dotted yellow line*) without much lordotic tilt. The posterior arch of C_1 is assimilated into the posterior rim of the foramen magnum. Note straight high-riding odontoid but absence of a retroflexed dens (*green dotted arrow*). (**b**)Sagittal and axial MRI shows compression of the medulla by the invaginating opisthion (*red blocked arrows*) and syringomyelia. Note elevated basion-opisthion plane (*dotted yellow line*) without lordotic tilt and straight indenting dens (*green dotted arrow*). (**c**) Intraoperative picture showing the invaginating opisthion and the rotated and knobbly spinous processes of C_2 and C_3. (**d**) The Inside-Outside screw plate with a slender sublaminar lower plate designed for sublaminar cable application for very young children. (**e**) Different Inside-Outside screws with different plate diameter (8–12 mm), screw-stem lengths (10–14 mm), and centre or off-set stems. The nut is shown with one of the screws. (**f**) Key holes in the occipital bone cut for insertion of the Inside-Outside screw. Note the invaginating opisthion lip has been removed. (**g**) Insertion of the Inside-Outside screw in holder. (**h**) Inside-Outside screw (I-O screw) and plates in place with sublaminar cable round the laminae of C_2 and C_3. (**i**) On-laid cortical and cancellous bone grafts (*G*) in place. (**j**) 3-D rendition of the fusion site at CVJ with the Inside-Outside screw (I-O screw) plates (I-O plate). *Right* picture and inset show subtracted CT 3-D images of the screw plates and sublaminar cables. (**k**) Post-operative CT. *Left* shows removal of the invaginating opisthion (*arrow*) and on-laid bone grafts (*G*). *Right upper* shows the Inside-Outside screw-plate assembly with the flat screw head pointing inwards and the screw stem (I-OS) outwards. *Right lower* shows axial CT of the decompressed foramen magnum

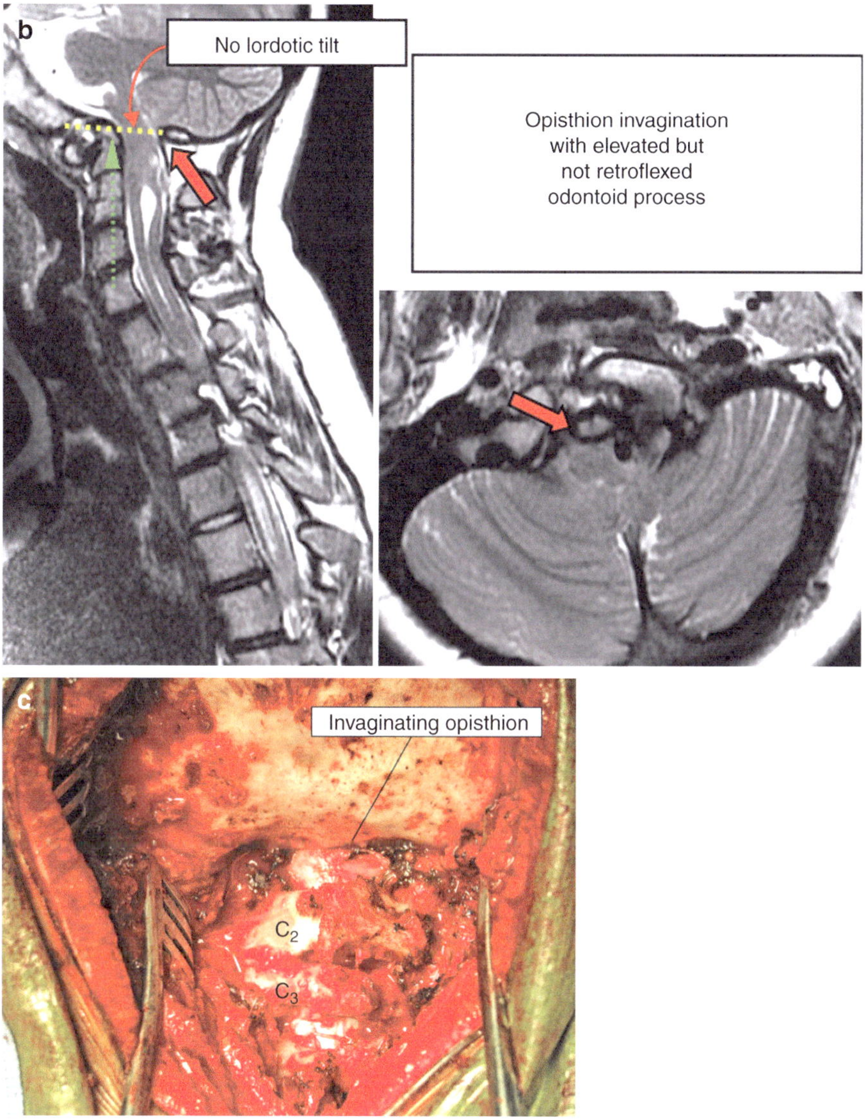

Fig. 43 (continued)

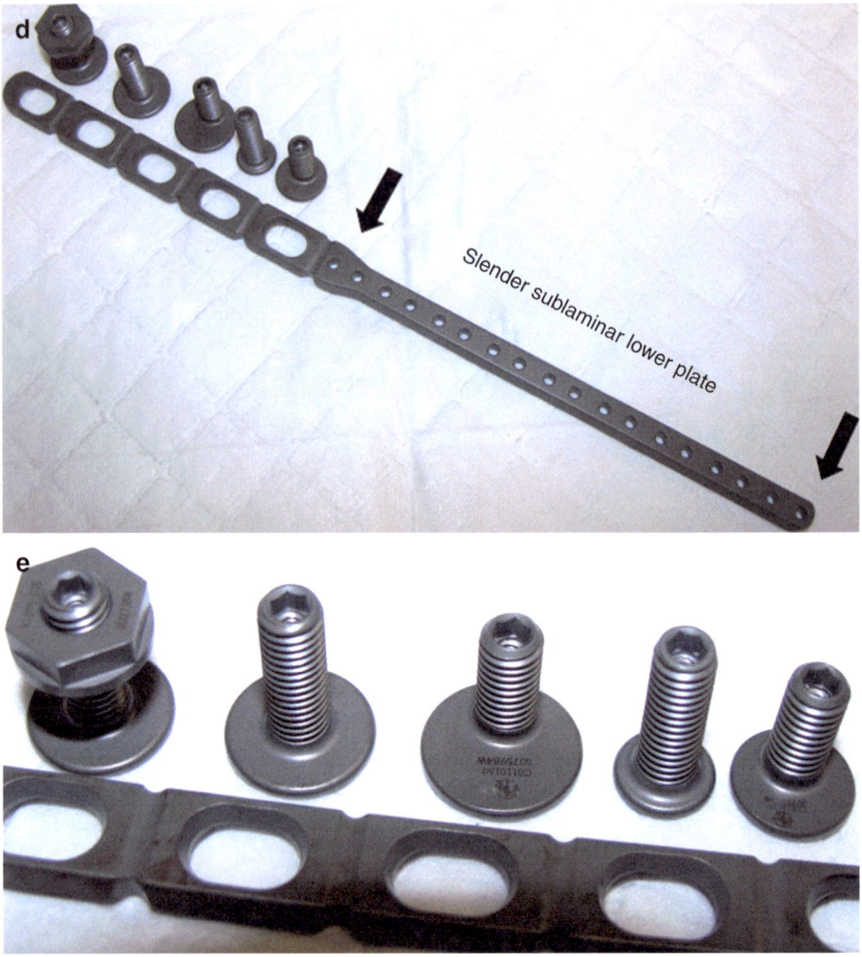

Fig. 43 (continued)

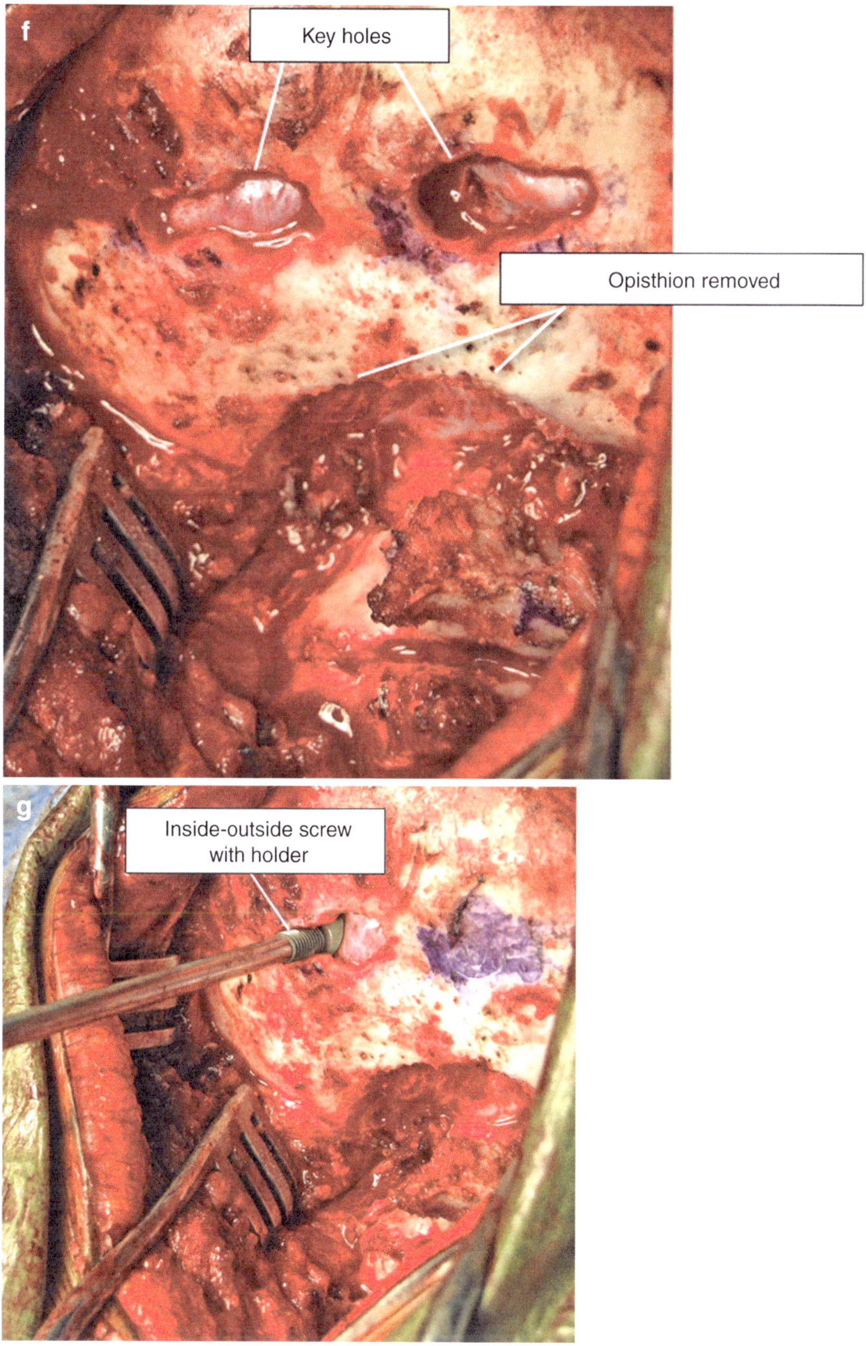

Fig. 43 (continued)

Fig. 43 (continued)

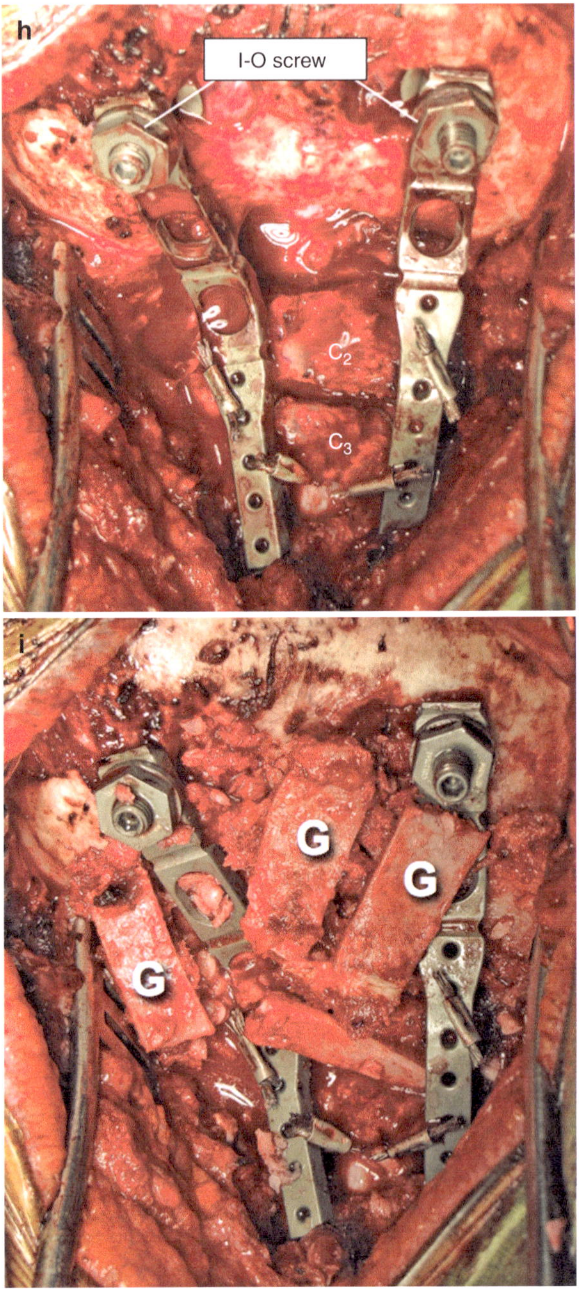

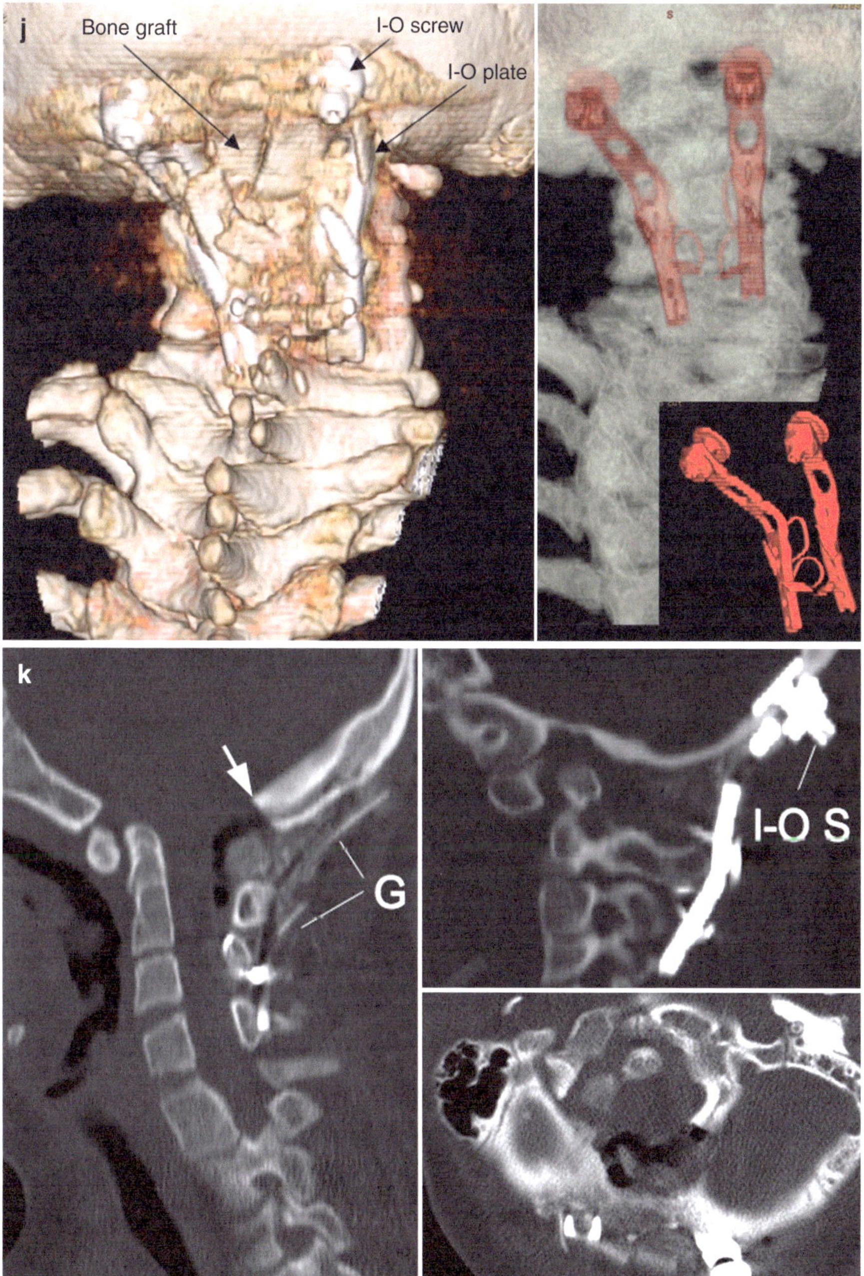

Fig. 43 (continued)

line (between the tuberculum sellae and the internal occipital protuberance) (Fig. 37). This line should exceed 30 mm [91]. With significant reduction to below 25 mm, the developing cerebellum and brainstem are desperately crowded and herniate downwards, accounting for the common association of ectopic cerebellar tonsils (Chiari I malformation) with severe basilar impression, platybasia, shortened clivus, and retroflexed dens (Fig. 45). Occasionally, the lower brainstem also lies well below the plane of the foramen magnum ("Chiari 1.5") [94]. It is our impression that the truly congenital form of Chiari I malformation often includes basioccipital dysplasia, and the much debated acquired Chiari I malformation (i.e., following lumboperitoneal shunting) consists only of ectopic cerebellar tonsils without skull base abnormality. Studies have shown that patients with hindbrain herniation and basilar impression have a higher brain to posterior fossa volume ratio than those with just hindbrain herniation, and both groups have higher ratios than controls [69, 89, 95].

Clinical Significance of Basilar Impression, Basilar Kyphosis, and Associated Chiari

Platybasia without basilar impression is asymptomatic (Fig. 46). Indentation of the anterior medulla by the dens, however, produces brainstem dysfunction and lower cranial neuropathies more frequently than "pure" cerebellar ectopia without an anterior compression vector. The brainstem deficits include neurogenic dysphagia [72, 73], nasal or hoarse voice due to paresis of the palatal levator and vocal cords, sleep apnea, and intermittent or progressive spastic quadriparesis. Tussive headaches, syncope, and gait discoordination are also common complaints.

Posterior decompression for Chiari I malformation with coexisting basilar impression carries a much higher late complication rate than for pure cerebellar ectopia. Even if the anterior vector is not initially symptomatic, the slightest amount of post-operative cranial settling after nullification of the dorsal tension band will deliver the brainstem straight on to the back-pointing dens to cause rapid onset of new brainstem signs [33]. In addition, platybasia and a decrease in the clivus-axis angle (of Wackenheim) (basilar kyphosis) accentuate the forward bending moment acting on the clivus-dens pivot point and accelerate the forward "folding" of the craniocervical hinge (see Case 6). It is our distinct impression that this type of post-operative instability occurs far more commonly in the associative type of Chiari I malformation. We therefore avoid removing the C_2 lamina during the decompression, if necessary at the expense of resecting the tips of the cerebellar tonsils.

If symptomatic post-decompression cranial settling does occur despite precautions, calipers skull traction with the neck in slight extension should be rendered under muscle relaxation and sedation for a few days, aiming at reversing the kyphotic deformity and telescoping effect at the foramen magnum. Occiput-C_1–C_2 fusion should be done after reduction. If brainstem indentation persists, transoral resection of the dens may be necessary.

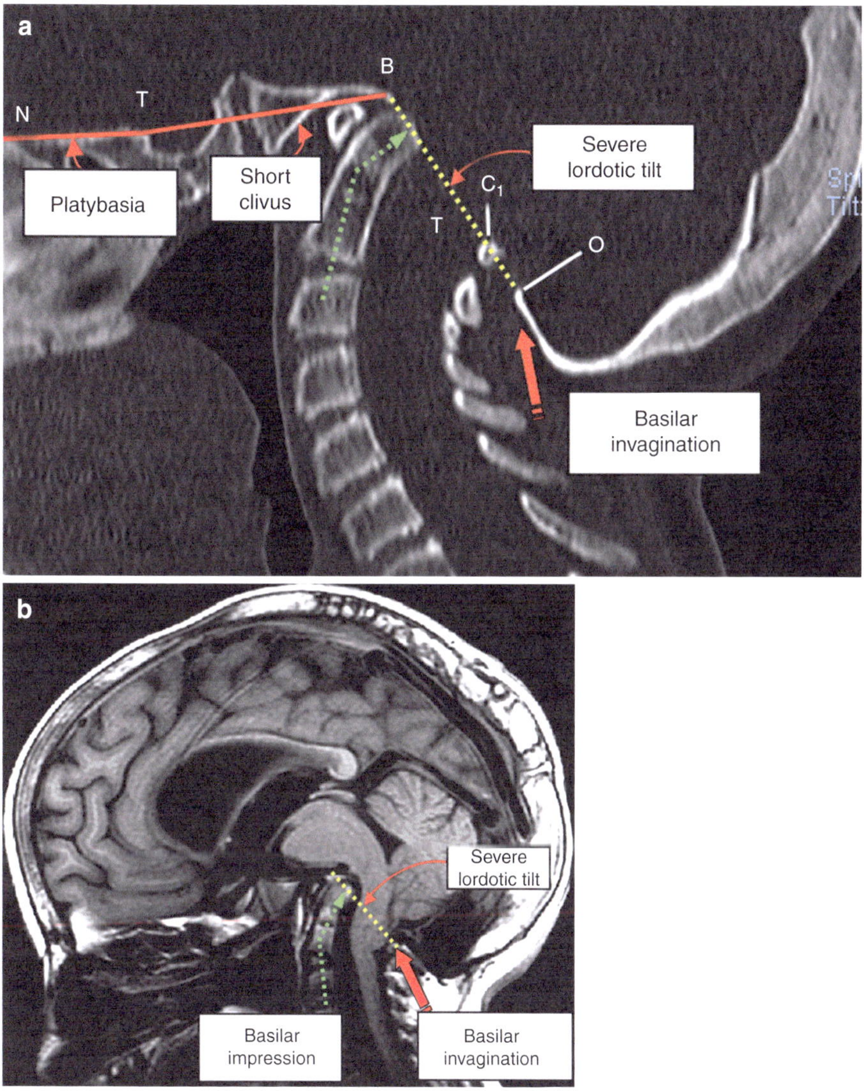

Fig. 44 Combined anterior-posterior form of basilar impression. (**a**) Sagittal CT shows extreme platybasia (NTB angle = 180°), short clivus (<1.5 cm), and forward folding of the clivus-axis angle of Wackenheim (80°), causing severe lordotic tilt of the foramen magnum plane and plane of the occipital condyles (*yellow dotted line*), resulting in a retroflexed dens and severe basilar impression (*green dotted arrow*). Note violation of McGregor's, Chamberlain's, and McRae's lines by the dens. Also, extreme invagination of the opisthion (*O*) and high posterior C_1 arch (C_1). (**b**) Sagittal MR shows distortion and compression of brainstem by both the dens (basilar impression) and the opisthion (basilar invagination)

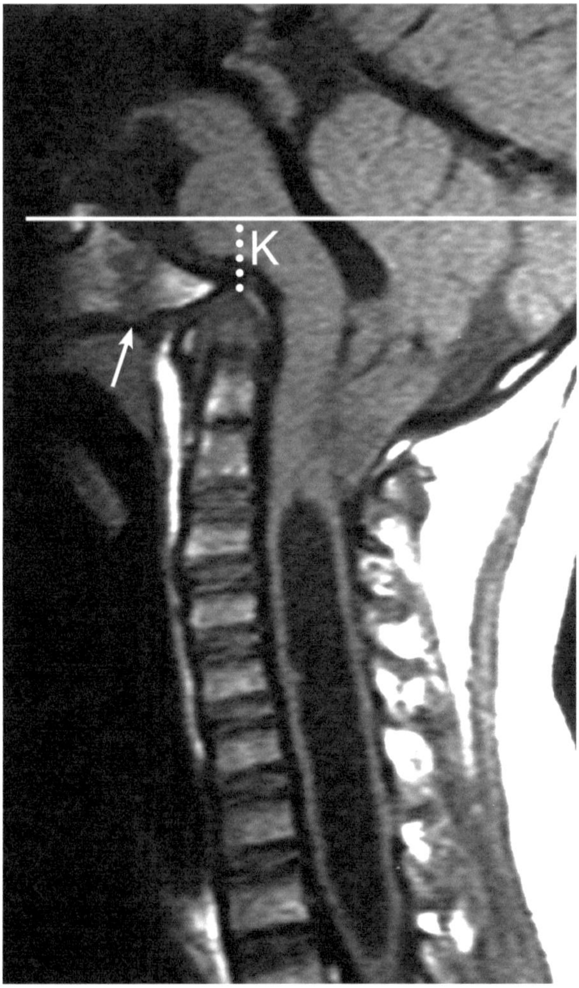

Fig. 45 Platybasia and short clivus (<1.5 cm; sphenoclival synchondrosis marked by *arrow*) causing severe basilar impression and mild retroflexed dens. This results in a shallow posterior fossa with a Klaus index (*K*) of less than 1.8 cm and ectopic cerebellar tonsils and cervical syringomyelia

Case 6

A 10-year-old girl presented with neck pain, diminished gag reflex, hand clumsiness, and poor truncal coordination. MRI and CT showed cerebellar ectopia, basilar impression, a retroflexed dens, and mild platybasia. The preoperative clival-axis angle was 130° (Fig. 47a). The child improved after suboccipital craniectomy and C_1–C_2 laminectomy. Six weeks after surgery, the child presented with rapid onset of nasal regurgitation, nasal voice, loss of gag reflex, and aspiration. MRI and CT showed cranial settling, extreme basilar kyphosis with the Wackenheim angle now reduced to 110°, and a shortened dens-basion interval (DBI) (Fig. 47b). Reduction with skull calipers traction and subsequent occipital C_1–C_2 fusion (Fig. 47c) promptly reversed her neurological defects. Post-fusion MRI and CT showed relief

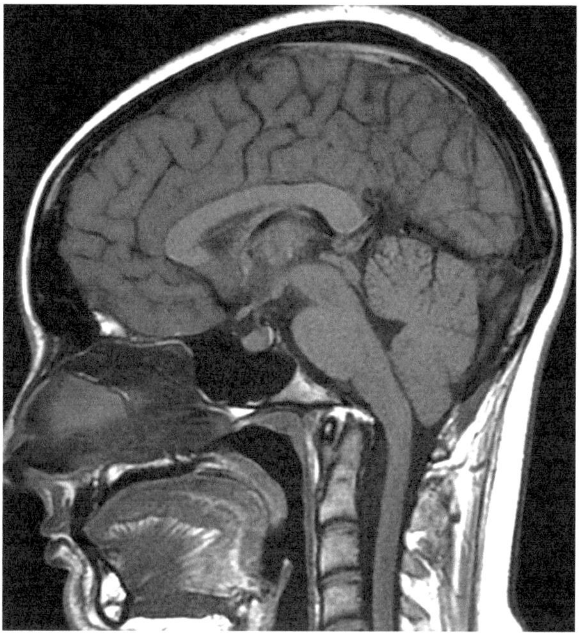

Fig. 46 Platybasia in a 9-year-old child with no symptoms. The clivus-axis angle (of Wackenheim) is about 100°. No CVJ compression is present

of the anterior basilar impression, straightening of Wackenheim's angle to 130°, and restoration of the initial DBI (Fig. 47d).

After repeatedly having to deal with similar post-decompression cranial settling as in Case 6, we have come to recognise a certain high-risk pattern of concomitant basioccipital kyphosis, anterior basilar impression, and hindbrain herniation that is best treated with pre emptive occipital-cervical fusion following posterior fossa decompression, to avoid the uncertain outcome of *post-factum* salvage of lost brainstem function. If there is already significant brainstem compression by an indenting odontoid process or a markedly small clival-axis angle, we take advantage of the "loosening effect" of posterior bony decompression by immediately placing the patient on weight-graded calipers traction for a few days before performing fusion, aiming to reduce the clival angulation and increase the dens-basion separation before fixation. The traction is rendered under strict monitoring and with muscle relaxation and sedation, and is terminated at the first sign of reversal of the kyphotic deformity and a more commodious foramen magnum on repeat CT. This new protocol creates new anterior as well as posterior space for the brainstem and significantly decreases the later need for transoral resection of the odontoid.

Case 7

A 7-year-old boy with a short neck presented with slowly progressive bilateral arm and hand weakness and worsening spastic gait. There was also chronic nuchal pain and spasm. CT showed anterior basilar impression and severe basilar kyphosis with

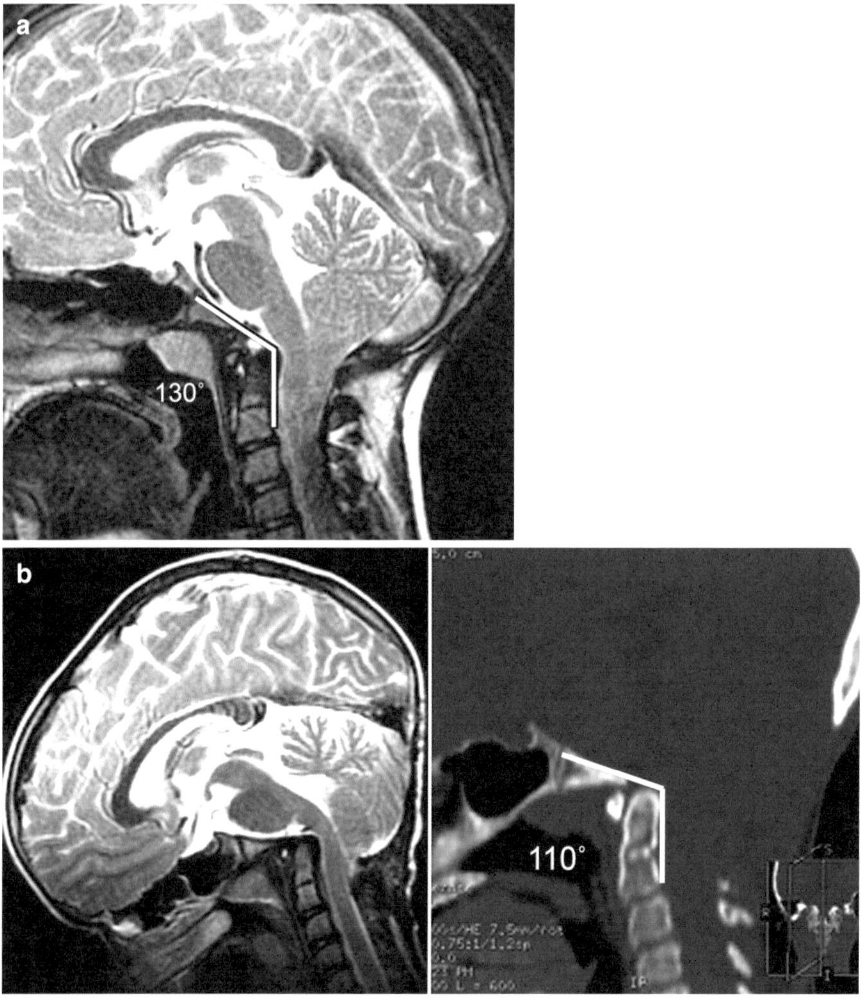

Fig. 47 Ten-year-old girl with retroflexed dens, mild basilar impression and Chiari I malformation. (**a**) Preoperative clivus-axis angle (of Wackenheim) of 130°. (**b**) Post-operative cranial settling causing forward folding of Wackenheim's angle to 110° and shortening of dens-basion interval (DBI). Note worsened anterior brainstem compression. (**c**) Caliper traction (*left*) for 4 days followed by C_1–C_2 Goel-Harm's screw-plate posterior fusion. (**d**) Post-fusion reversal of Wackenheim's angle to 138° and increase of DBI to 1.8 cm. Note relief of brainstem compression and symptoms

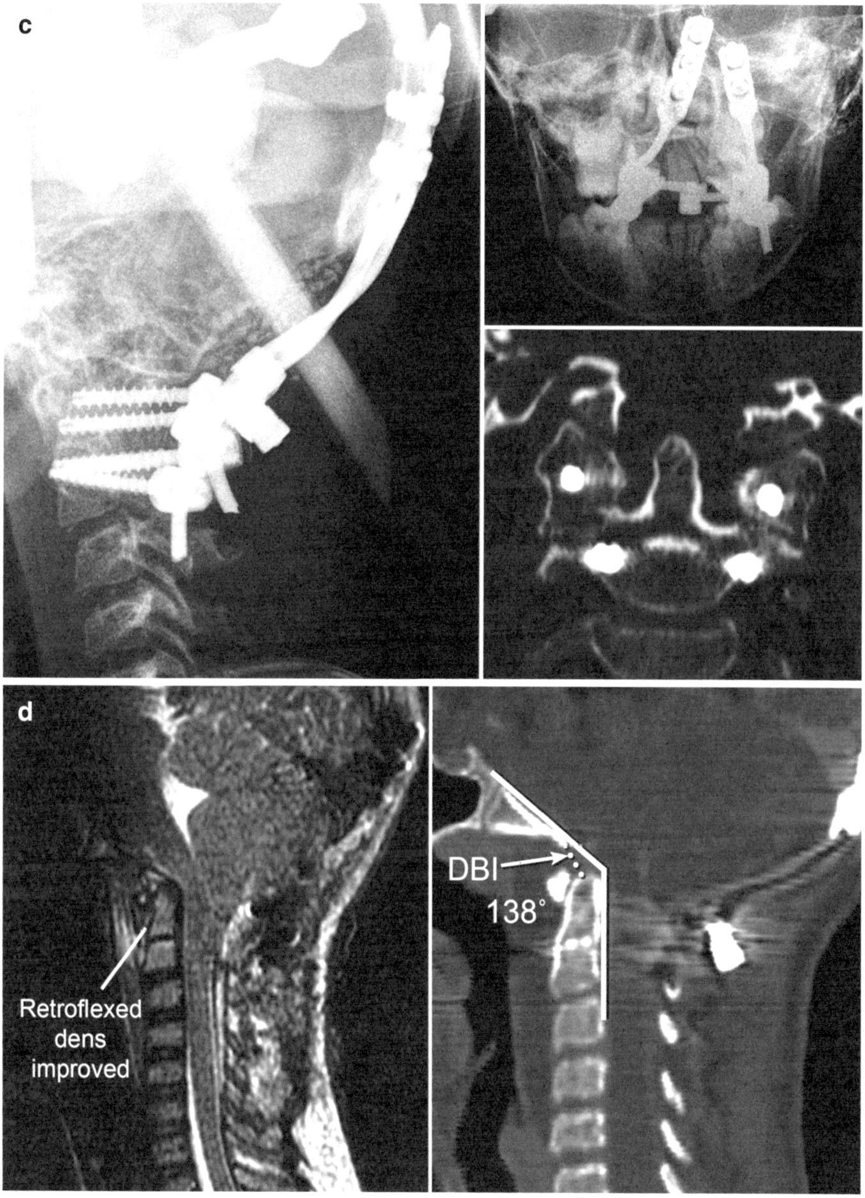

Fig. 47 (continued)

a clivus-axis angle of 95°; the blunt basion was anterior to and below the tip of the dens (Fig. 48a). MRI showed compression of the anterior medulla by the dens and impressive hindbrain herniation and syringomyelia (Fig. 48b). Following posterior bony decompression (sparing C_2), the child was put on cautious calipers traction using 3 lb. weight and kept in bed with adequate opiates and muscle relaxant for 1 week. The clival-axis angle increased to 120°, and the basion had risen to about 10 mm above the dens. Occipital-C_1–C_2 fusion was performed in this new clival-dental position using the Inside-Outside Screw-plate construct (Fig. 48c). The child showed dramatic improvement of extremity strength and gait coordination.

Disturbances of the Lateral Sclerotomes and Hypochordal Bows of Proatlas and C_1 Sclerotome: Anomalies of the Surrounding Ring Structures

These can be divided into anomalies of the proatlas and of the C_1 resegmented sclerotome.

Anomalies of Proatlas

Hyperplasia of the Proatlas Hypochordal Bow: Third Occipital Condyle

Embryogenesis

The hypochordal bow is an arcual strip of mesenchyme ventral to the axial sclerotome. In human, only the hypochordal bows of the proatlas and C_1 resegmented sclerotome persist [67]. The hypochordal bow of the proatlas normally forms a small midline osseus tubercle attached to the ventral surface of the basioccipital below the rim of the foramen magnum (Fig. 14). Rarely, it remains as a fully ossified structure distinct from the basioccipital bone. If the entire arc is preserved, it is called a pre-basioccipital arch, which looks like a U-shaped bony valance on the underside of the anterior rim of the foramen magnum [52, 76, 91] (Fig. 49). If only the paramedian arch persists, two parasagittal spikes project downwards from the clivus, called the basilar processes [52, 76, 91]. Neither of these bony excrescences encroach on the foramen magnum and are thus harmless. Occasionally, however, the median portion of the proatlas hypochordal bow becomes exuberantly hyperplastic and forms a prominent bone spur that juts obliquely backwards from the basioccipital tip that does cause neural compression. This median bony process is firmly attached to the basion, and, elongating it, frequently forms true synovial joints with the anterior arch of C_1 and the odontoid apex (Fig. 50) [52]; it is thus rather aptly termed a median or third occipital condyle

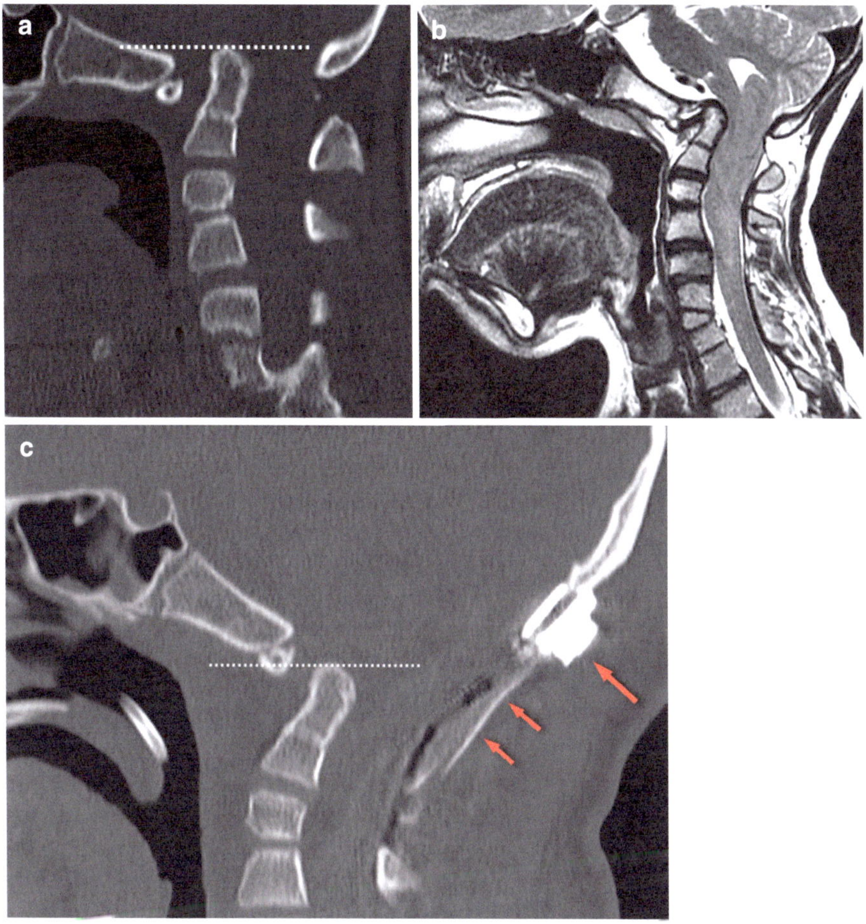

Fig. 48 Anterior basilar impression with severe hindbrain herniation. (**a**) Sagittal CT and (**b**) MRI show severe platybasia, retroflex dens, and a clivus that is below and anterior to the dens, which is retroflexed and high-riding causing anterior brainstem compression. There is also severe basilar kyphosis with a clivus-axis angle (of Wackenheim) of 95°. The *dotted horizontal white line* on the left is drawn tangential to the tip of the dens, to show its relative position to the blunt basion. (**c**) After 1 week of skull traction immediately following posterior bony decompression, the clivus has been raised significantly above the dens (above *dotted line* drawn tangential to the tip of the dens), and the clivus-axis angle has slightly improved. *Large arrow* points to Inside-Outside screw plate on the occiput, and *small arrows* show the on-laid bone grafts

(condylus tertius) [49, 52, 77, 79, 91]. These articulations, though bizarre, are not surprising if one remembers that the anterior arch of C_1 comes from the hypochordal bow of the first cervical sclerotome directly subjacent to the hypochordal bow of the proatlas, and the dental apex develops from the proatlas centrum; joint formation between corresponding components of adjacent sclerotomes is "normal" in the lower vertebral levels.

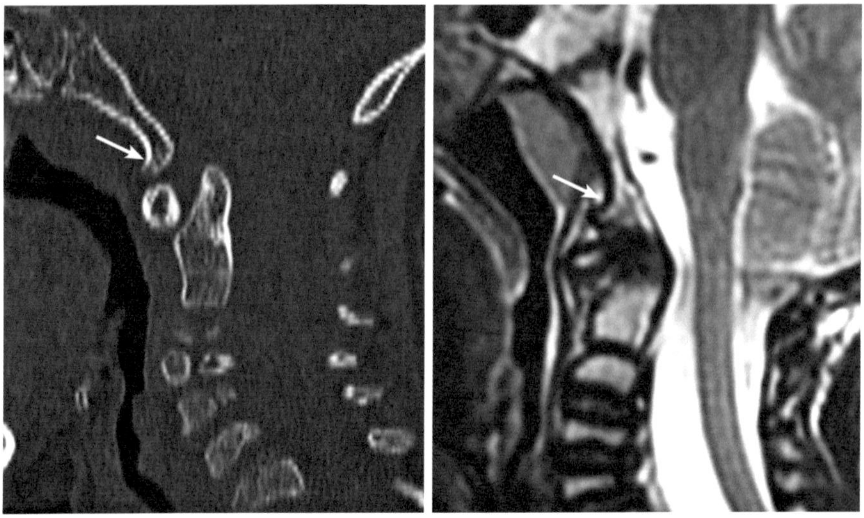

Fig. 49 Pre-basioccipital arch (*thin arrows*), a U-shaped bony valance on the ventral lip of the anterior foramen magnum rim. This results from complete preservation of the hypochordal bow of the proatlas

Clinical Significance

A third occipital condyle may be mistaken for an os avis on radiographs since both are osseous appendages of the clival tip. However, it is important to distinguish them because of their very different implications of stability. In os avis, the dental pivot has lost its top and becomes perilously hypoplastic, whereas the dental pivot in the case of the third occipital condyle has normal height and therefore remains solid anchor for the TAL; instability is unlikely. Although some third condyles are short and protrude along the contour of the clivus or even curl forward away from the brainstem (Fig. 51), others can be enormous backward pointing cantilevers [49, 62, 79, 91] producing serious neurological deficits. Because there is no instability, transoral, transclival resection of the third condyle is adequate treatment.

Hyperplasia of Exoccipital Sclerotome: Hypertrophic Occipital Condyle

Hyperplasia of the lateral sclerotome of the proatlas, precursor to the exoccipital bone, results in hypertrophy of the lateral and posterior rim of the foramen magnum and a massively gnarled occipital condyle. Bilateral condylar hypertrophy causes pincers-like cervicomedullary compression and early symptoms [62], but unilateral hypertrophy can also lead to severe lateral distortion of the lower brainstem and slow neurological deterioration. An uneven atlanto-occipital joint surface and chondromalacia may also produce chronic neck pain and stiffness. Treatment consists of resection of the occipital condyle, followed by occipito-cervical fusion for the expected O–C_1–C_2 instability.

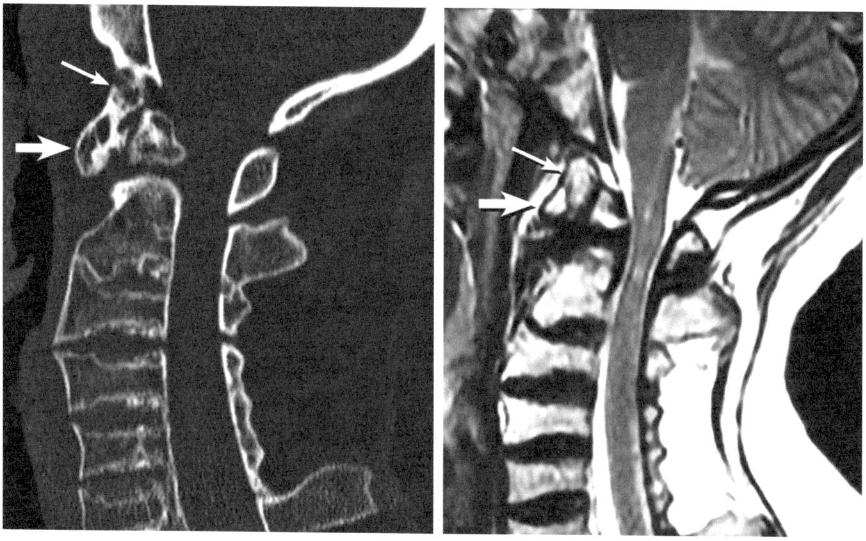

Fig. 50 Third occipital condyle or condylus tertius (*thin arrow*) attached to the ventral surface of the clival tip and fused to the anterior atlantal arch (*thick arrow*). On MRI, the condyle appears to form a synovial joint with an ossiculum terminale that is unfused to the basal dens. The third occipital condyle represents midline hyperplasia of the proatlas hypochordal bow

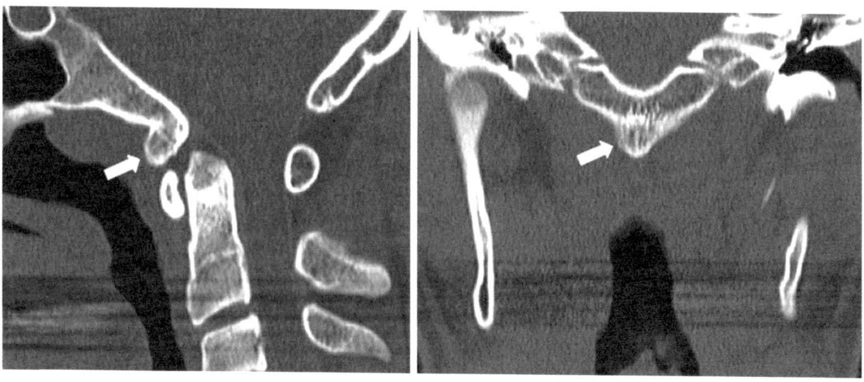

Fig. 51 Third occipital condyle (*arrow*) giving the clivus the shape of a boot with toes forward on sagittal CT (*left*). Coronal CT (*right*) shows the discrete midline nature of the bony condyle

Case 8

A 6-year-old boy was born with a fixed torticollis. At age 5, he began complaining of worsening neck pain and loss of rotation. He presented after a gentle fall on his back with right arm and leg weakness. CT and MRI showed a severe lateral tilt of the craniocervical junction, gnarly hypertrophy of the right occipital condyle, and compression and lateral distortion of the C_1 cord (Fig. 52). A right far-lateral approach was used to resect the condyle-C_1 joint followed by occiput-C_1–C_2 fusion.

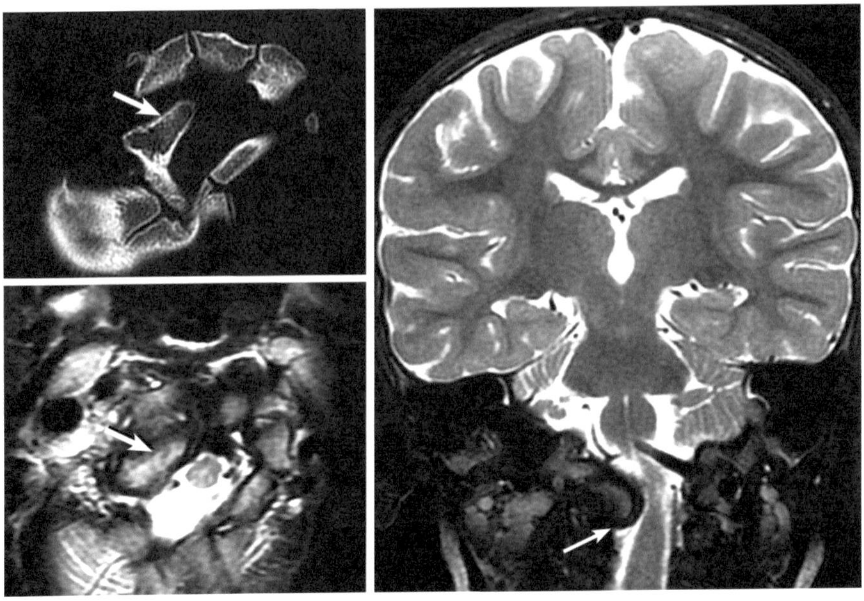

Fig. 52 Unilateral hyperplasia of the occipital condyle (*arrow*) with cervicomedullary distortion. This represents hyperplasia of the exoccipital (lateral) sclerotome of the proatlas

Assimilation of Atlas: Non-resegmentation of the Proatlas Sclerotome

Congenital fusion of the atlas with the occiput is one of the most common anomalies of the CVJ, with a prevalence rate from 0.08 to 2.8 % in the general population [5, 8, 54, 93]. Atlantal assimilation, or occipitalisation, ranges from complete incorporation of the atlas into the occiput to discrete osseous bridges between the two. Gholve et al. [31] identified three fusion zones. Zone 1 assimilation involves the anterior atlantal arch in front of the lateral masses (20 % in their series); zone 2 assimilation involves primarily the lateral masses (17 %); and zone 3 assimilation is fusion at the posterior atlantal arch (13 %) (Fig. 53). Combination of zones is seen in over 50 % of patients [31]. Thirty-seven percent of Gholve's patients also had associated basilar impression, 20 % had Klippel-Feil Syndrome, 17 % Chiari I malformation, and 37 % had cervical stenosis.

Embryogenesis

It has already been mentioned that inactivation of *Hox d-3* gene expression in mice results in anterior homeotic transformation at the CVJ such that the C_1 vertebra takes on an occipital identity and the head-neck transitional zone moves caudally to the C_1–C_2 junction (Fig. 21). All mutants have assimilation of C_1 to the basiocciput [13, 24]. It is therefore tempting to ascribe human cases of isolated C_1 assimilation to similar mutations of the human *Hox* gene homologues. However, in cases of

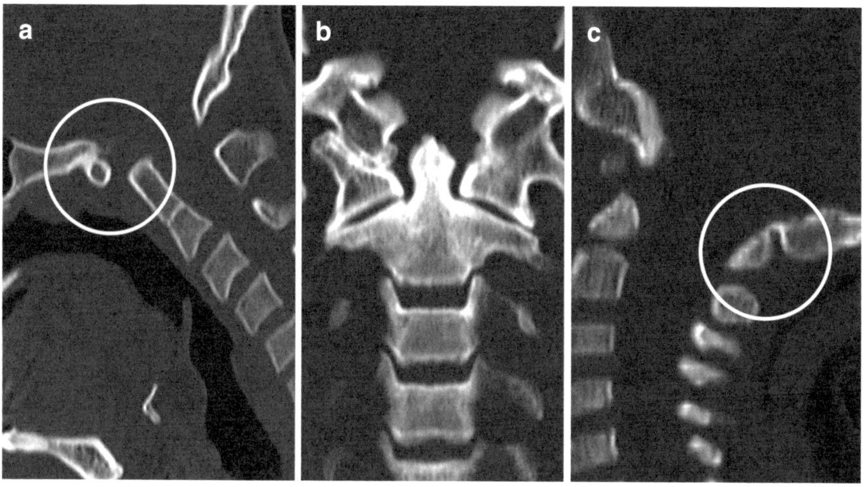

Fig. 53 C_1 assimilation or occipitalisation. (**a**) Assimilation of the anterior atlantal arch (Zone 1 assimilation). (**b**) Assimilation of the lateral masses (Zone 2 assimilation). (**c**) Posterior arch (Zone 3) assimilation

combined C_1 assimilation and Klippel-Feil syndrome in which multiple levels of cervical fusion are seen below C_2, the *Hox* gene theory will require multiple *Hox* mutations and alterations of multiple *Hox* codes, which is highly improbable. Since *Pax-1* expression is involved in resegmentation of all levels of the embryonic axis, inappropriate repression of *Pax-1* at the proatlas-C_1 sclerotome interphase and at other vertebral levels may be involved in cases of combined atlas assimilation and subaxial fusion.

Clinical Significance

Assimilation of the atlas to the occiput means that the first mobile segment between the skull and spine has been transferred to the C_1–C_2 junction, as are all the motion stresses including that of flexion-extension, normally of restricted range at this level and for which the local joint anatomy is ill-suited. This also means the supporting myoligamentous structures are more likely to suffer "over-stretch" failure. Almost 60 % of Gholve et al.'s patients with C_1 assimilation has C_1–C_2 instability defined as an atlantal-dens interval (ADI) greater than 4 mm in adults and 5 mm in children [31]. McRae and von Torklus and Gehle had similar findings [57–59, 92]. More than half of Gholve, et al.'s patients with instability also had C_2–C_3 fusion, which adds to the burden of stresses at C_1–C_2.

The symptoms of C_1–C_2 instability range from persistent neck pain and stiffness to frank myelopathy. Typically the neurological deficits begin in the third or fourth decade of life [57] and tend to worsen with age [58]. We have also seen concomitant hypertrophy of the posterior arch of C_2, which accentuates the neural compression. Management for symptomatic cases is stabilisation between occiput and C_2–C_3 in concert with treatment for the other associated malformations.

Unfused Occipital Condyle and Clivus: Posterior Homeotic Transformation

Unilateral or bilateral non-fusion of the occipital condyle with the skull base has been described [62]. The result is usually an unstable atlanto-occipital articulation and bony distortion around the joint that could indent the brainstem. Occasionally, only the clivus is unfused and the dens is fused to the anterior atlantal arch as if the atlas is acquiring its own centrum (Fig. 22). These phenotypes are reminiscent of the transgenic murine mutant with disturbance in *Hox d-4* expression and posterior homeotic transformation of the craniovertebral transitional zone, in which the exoccipital region contains unfused neural arch-like structures resembling the posterior arch of C_1, and C_1 acquires a centrum instead of an anterior arch (Fig. 22). Treatment of these rare entities consists of bony resection when necessary, followed by occipital-cervical fusion in case of instability.

Anomalies of the C_1 Resegmentated Sclerotome

Aplasia and Hypoplasia of the C_1 Hypochordal Bow: Anomalies of Anterior Atlantal Arch

Aplasia of the hypochordal bow of the C_1 sclerotome leads to complete absence of the anterior atlantal arch. This is an exceedingly rare anomaly; only a few postmortem cases can be found in the literature, in which the anterior arch was replaced by loose connective tissue [29, 50, 91]. Because the hypochondral bow may in fact be derived from the axial sclerotome, the centrum primordium of C_1, which gives rise to the principal bulk of the dens, is often simultaneously affected. In a representative case, the anterior C_1 arch is absent, and C_1 is unstable because the basal dental segment is unintegrated in the midline, and the two “hemi-os” are stunted (Fig. 54a). The insertion tubercles of the TAL are either greatly attenuated or nonexistent, and the TAL itself may also be absent since it is derived from mesenchyme adjacent to that of the hypochordal bow and centrum. It is not visualised on MRI (Fig. 54b). The result is severe anterior subluxation of C_1 on C_2 with cord compression (Fig. 54c).

In rare cases, the absence of the anterior arch may be due to delayed ossification of the cartilaginous mould and not true agenesis. We have encountered two children whose ossification centres of the anterior atlantal arch did not appear till 5–6 years of age (Fig. 55a). The TAL was present in both cases (Fig. 55b).

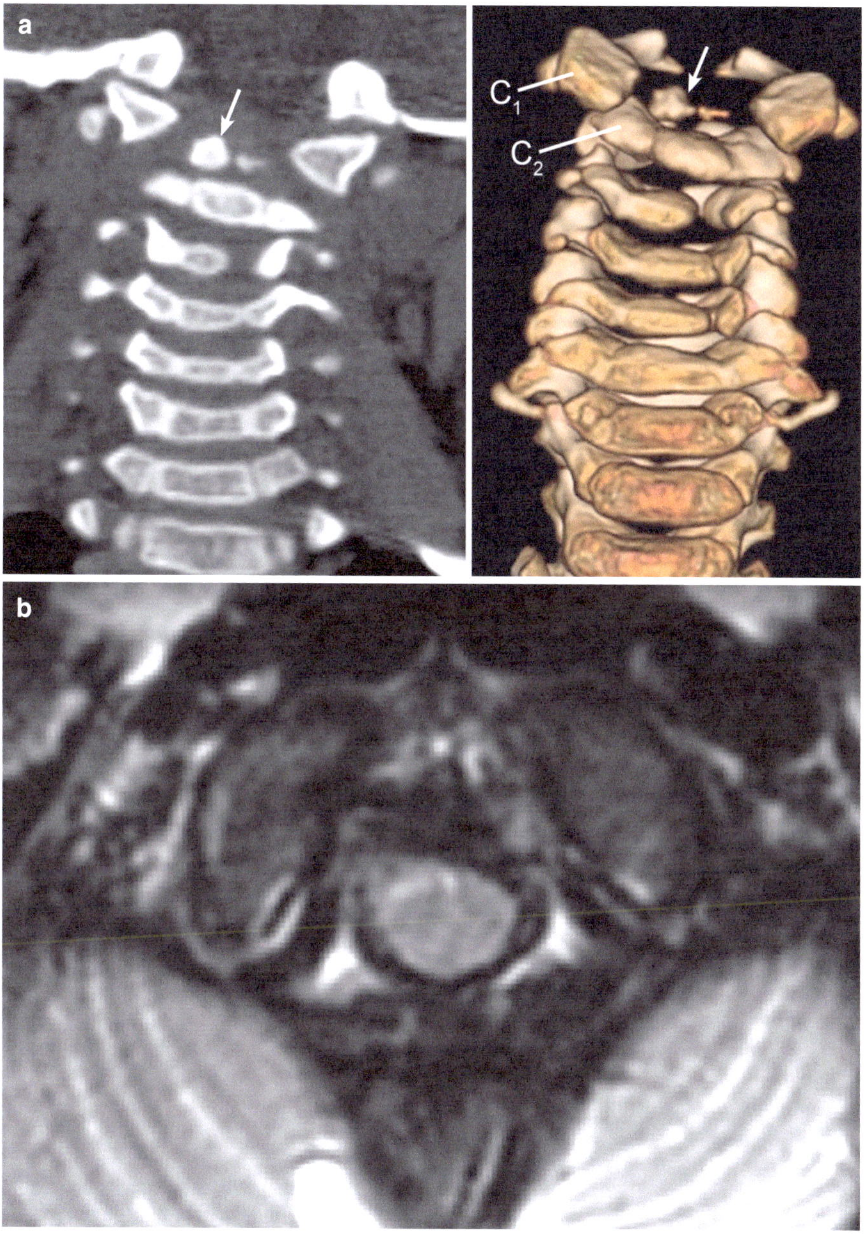

Fig. 54 Complete aplasia of C_1 hypochordal bow with complete agenesis of C_1 anterior arch. (**a**) CT and 3-D reconstruction shows no anterior atlantal arch or insertion tubercles for the TAL. The two stunted dental hemi-os (*arrow*) are unfused to the C_2 centrum. Posterior arch of C_1 is also unfused. (**b**) Axial T_2 MRI shows absence of the TAL behind the dens. (**c**) Extreme C_1–C_2 flexion instability and severe cord compression

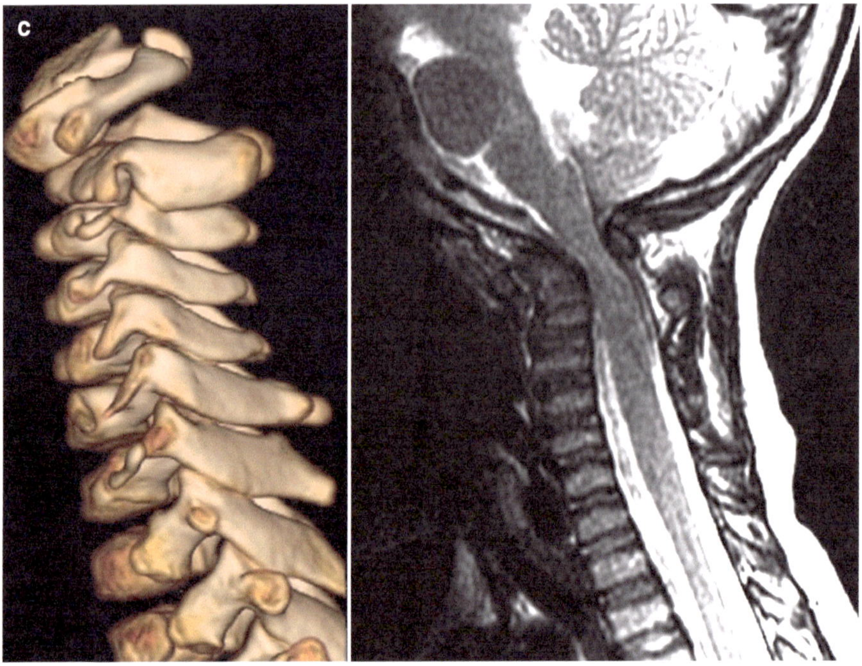

Fig. 54 (continued)

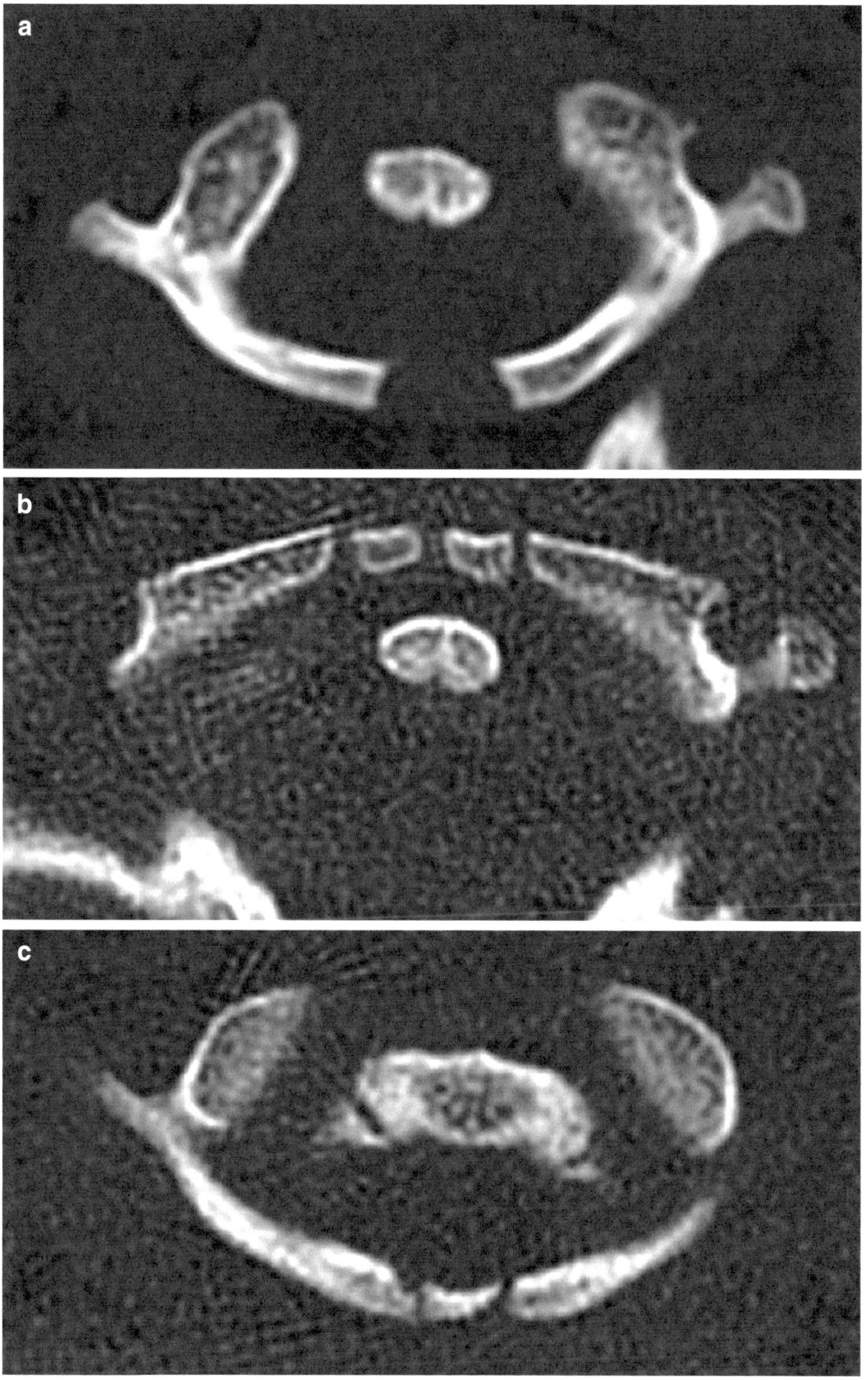

Fig. 55 Delayed ossification of the anterior and posterior C_1 arches presented at age 3 years as "absent" anterior arch and incomplete posterior arch (**a**). At 6 years of age, both anterior (**b**) and posterior (**c**) arches show ossification centres

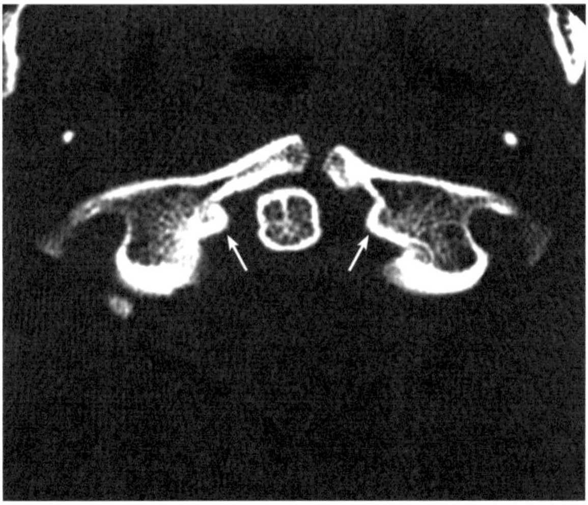

Fig. 56 Complete agenesis of posterior atlantal arch and bifid anterior atlantal arch. Normal TAL insertion tubercles (*arrows*). There is no C_1–C_2 instability

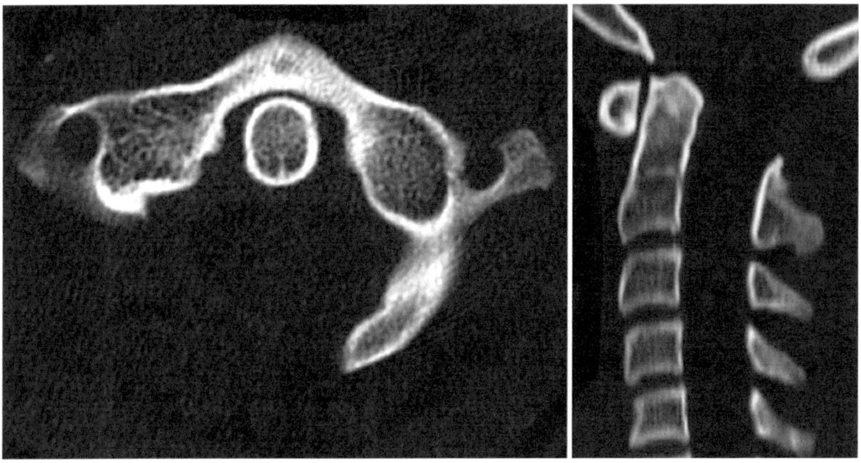

Fig. 57 Unilateral aplasia of the right posterior arch of C_1

Aplasia and Hypoplasia of the Lateral C_1 Sclerotome : Anomalies of Posterior Atlantal Arch

Varying degrees of aplasia of the lateral sclerotome of C_1 result in partial or complete agenesis of the posterior atlantal arch. Posterior atlantal arch deficiencies are ten times more common than anterior arch defects [22, 57, 58]. Von Torklus and Gehle [92] documented six subtypes, the rarest being total agenesis. The example of total agenesis given here has no bony arch posterior to the lateral masses, and the anterior arch is bifid (Fig. 56). Partial agenesis can be unilateral (Fig. 57), or

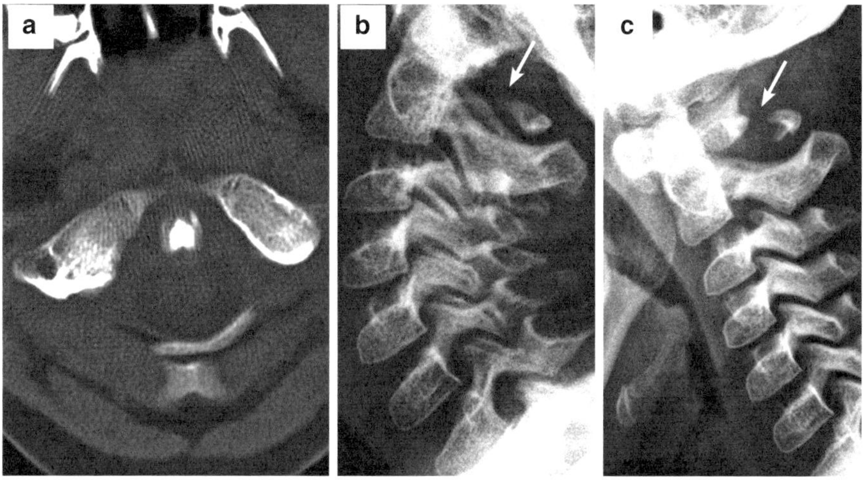

Fig. 58 Partial agenesis of posterior atlantal arch. (**a**) The posterior tubercle and arch remnant appear floating and unconnected to the lateral masses. (**b**, **c**) Flexion and extension shows ample tilting of the lateral masses away from the posterior tubercle (*arrows*), suggesting absence of a cartilaginous mould. In spite of this tilting, there is no translational instability

bilateral with preservation of all or portions of the posterior tubercle, which appears floating without bony attachment to the rest of the C_1 vertebra (Fig. 58a, b). MRI may suggest presence of cartilage in the scaffolding of the incomplete ring, but in our case, rather ample tilting of the lateral masses away from the remaining posterior tubercle during flexion (Fig. 58c) suggests that the cartilaginous mould was never formed, and the developmental error probably occurred at the mesenchymal (membranous) stage [9, 51, 83].

Stability of the C_1–C_2 Complex in C_1 Arch Dysplasia

As a general rule, the TAL, its anchorage to the medial tubercles of the C_1 lateral masses, and the structural integrity of the odontoid pivot jointly determine the translational stability between C_1 and C_2. Since the TAL, the base of the dens, and the anterior arch are all derived from the same primitive axial sclerotome (and its hypochordal bow), it follows that anterior C_1 arch agenesis tends much more often to be associated with instability than posterior arch defects. Even amongst the anterior arch defects, there are gradations of stability related to the soundness of the TAL-dens unit. Stability is usually maintained if the TAL and its sturdy anchorage are clearly seen on the MRI even if the two C_1 lateral masses are widely separated (Fig. 59). In the case of absent TAL or puny insertion tubercles, there is nothing restraining the excessive forward tilting movements of C_1 (Fig. 54b, c), and the cord is compressed by the intact posterior arch. Thus, axial T_2 MR imaging of the TAL is exceedingly important in predicting C_1–C_2 stability in C_1 arch defects.

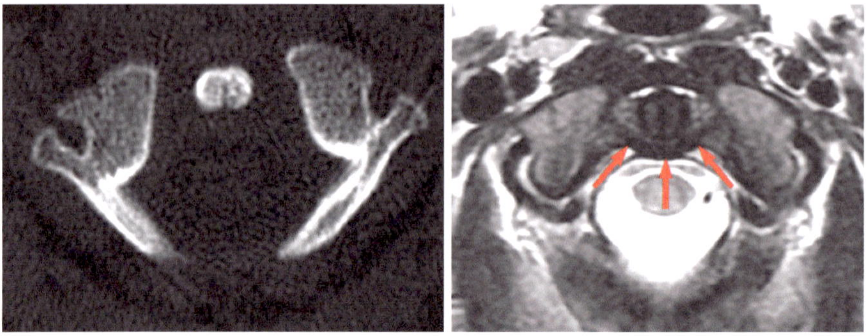

Fig. 59 Complete agenesis of the anterior C_1 arch with a normal TAL (*arrows*) shown on the axial T_2 MR image. Stability is maintained

When blighted development of the hypochordal bow is accompanied by complete aplasia of the primordium of the C_1 centrum, the instability is most extreme. Our example shows a match-head-sized remnant of the C_1 anterior arch in front of an axial body without any dental pivot (Fig. 60), and the TAL is either absent or greatly attenuated. The child presented with quadriparesis.

Because the atlas in these cases of unstable anterior arch defects is reduced, deformed, and feeble, posterior instrument fusion needs to incorporate the occiput and often has to be extended down to C_3 or C_4 to distribute the stresses on the upright plates. If the child is very young with a large head and puny nuchal musculature, post-operative halo is recommended.

Unlike anterior arch agenesis, posterior C1 arch defects are unaccompanied by dysplasia of the centrum sclerotome of C_1. The dental pivot and TAL anchorage are thus normal in both complete (Fig. 61) and incomplete (Fig. 62) posterior arch agenesis. The C_1–C_2 complex in patients with posterior arch defects is usually stable in spite of the intimidating appearance of the radiographs. None of our patients require fusion.

Aplasia and Hypoplasia of the Lateral C_1 Sclerotome: Anomaly of the C_1 Lateral Mass

Complete aplasia of one of the lateral masses of C_1 is due to disturbance or even absence of the transitional portion of the lateral sclerotome of C_1 that normally connects the posterior components to the hypochordal bow. There may thus be an associated absence or attenuation of the adjacent anterior atlantal arch (Fig. 63). The head is tilted towards the side of the aplasia and usually somewhat rotated to the opposite side due to the unusual orientation of the condyle-C_2 joint. In the 3-D rendering of the CT, the condyle appears to be floating in space a fair distance from the next available joint surface at the C_2 facet. The egregiously awkward articulation is unstable in limiting lateral sliding motion and rotation. Also, the inevitable loss of TAL anchorage due to absence of either the ligament or its insertion tubercle (normally on the medial aspect of the lateral mass) must also result in excessive translation of C_1 on C_2.

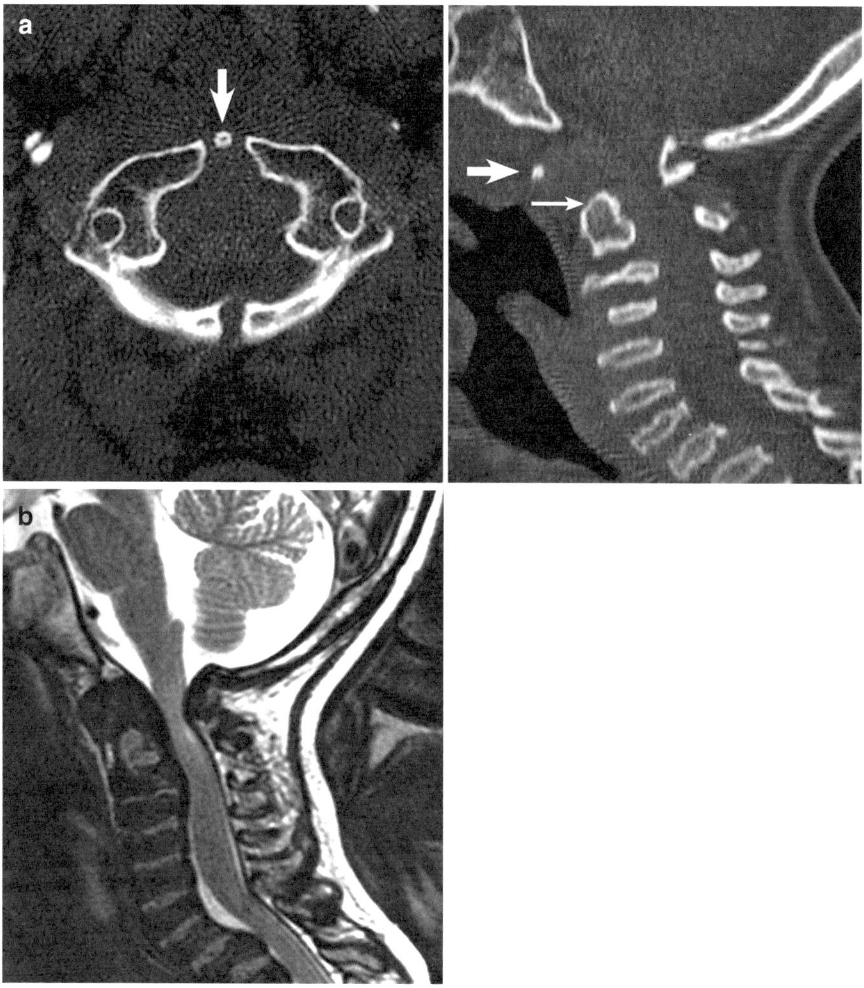

Fig. 60 Severe hypoplasia of C_1 hypochordal bow with minute anterior C_1 arch. (**a**) Match-head-sized anterior C_1 arch (*thick arrow*) associated with complete agenesis of the dens (*thin arrow*), a result of concomitant C_1 centrum aplasia. (**b**) Severe C_1–C_2 instability with cord compression

Combined Dysplasia of the Hypochordal Bow and Lateral Sclerotome of C_1-Combined Anterior and Posterior Atlantal Arch Defects

Simultaneous hypoplasia of the hypochordal bow and lateral sclerotome of C_1 leads to combined anterior and posterior atlantal defects. The anterior arcual defect is usually incomplete, and the insertion tubercles and TAL are mostly intact, thereby maintaining stability against translation. However, because the two lateral masses are essentially loose bones connected by soft tissues (Fig. 64), axial loading forces tend to split them apart similar to the mechanism of a Jefferson's fracture. The issue of stability in this situation is very different than in anterior arcual agenesis.

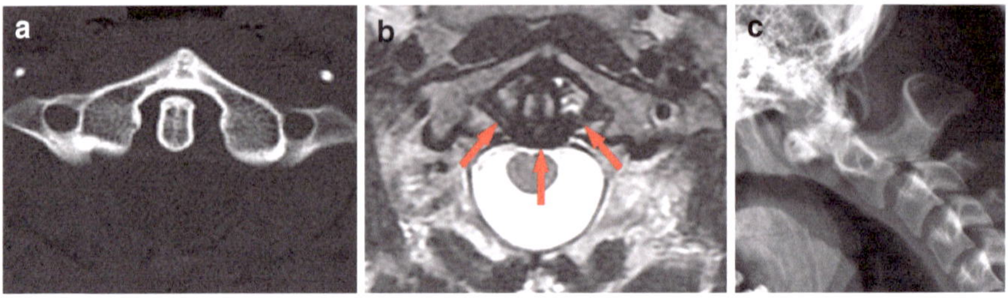

Fig. 61 Complete bilateral agenesis of the posterior C_1 arch (**a**). TAL is well shown on axial T_2 MR (*arrows*) (**b**), and there is no C_1–C_2 instability on flexion x-ray (**c**)

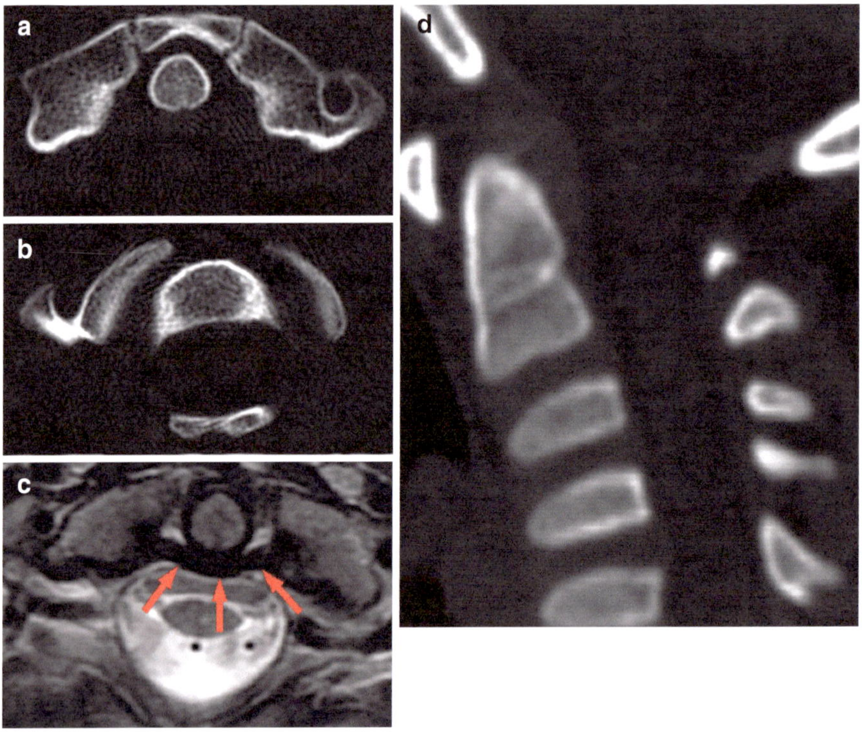

Fig. 62 Incomplete C_1 posterior arch agenesis. (**a**, **b**) Show preservation of the posterior tubercle. (**c**) TAL is well shown on axial T_2 MR (*arrows*). (**d**) No instability is seen on sagittal flexion CT

During axial loading, the vertical forces subjected to the upper and lower articular surfaces of the C_1 lateral mass are in effect translated into two force-vectors directed perpendicular to the upper and lower facet surfaces, respectively. Because the two articular surfaces of the occipital-C_1 joint and the C_1–C_2 facets are both slanted, these two perpendicular (to the joint surface) loading forces can each be resolved into two component vectors by the simple theory of parallelogram of

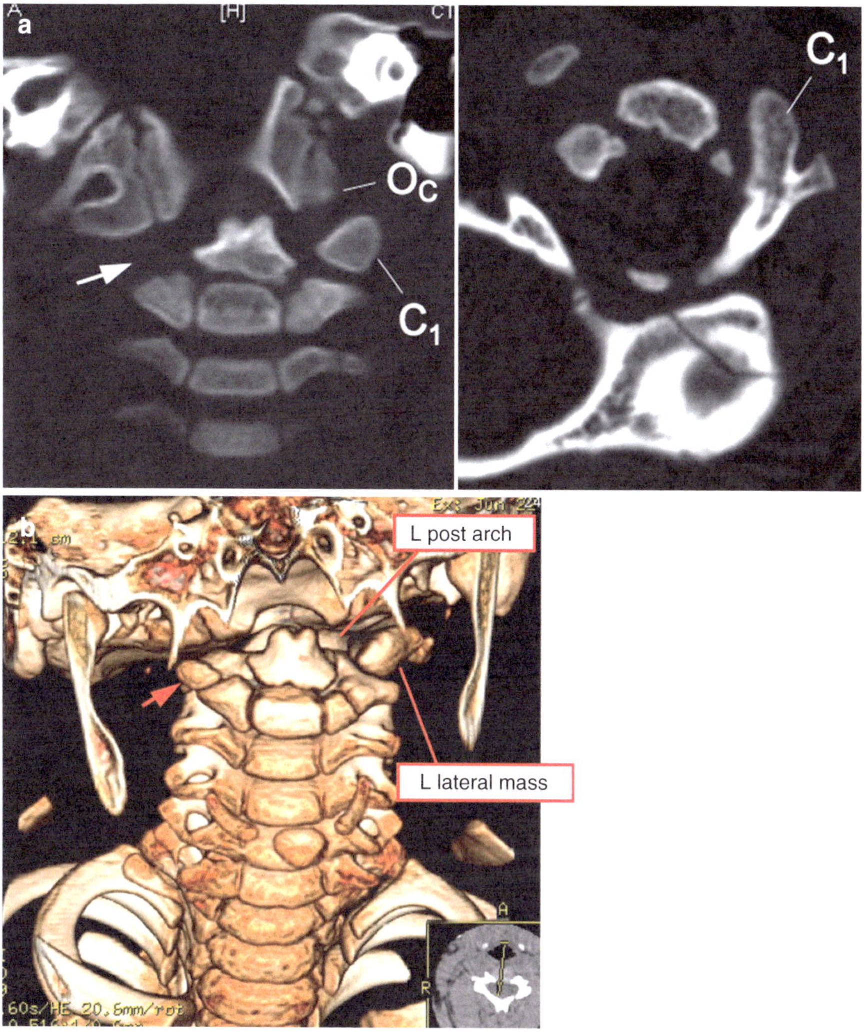

Fig. 63 Unilateral lateral mass aplasia in a 2-year-old with fixed right head tilt. (**a**) *Left*: Coronal CT shows aplasia of the right lateral mass. There is no real condyle-cervical articulation on the right side (*arrow*). Left Oc-C_1 joint is present. *Right*: Aplasia of right posterior arch and complete aplasia of the anterior arch. C_l left C_1 lateral mass, *Oc* occipital condyle. (**b**) 3-D rendering of the cervical spine from the front. Left lateral mass and left posterior arch of C_1 (*L. Post Arch*) are seen, but there is no equivalent structures on the right side except for a small ossified beadlike structure (*arrow*) lateral to the lateral mass of C_2. Note intact condyle-C_1 joint on the left but free-floating occipital condyle on the right. Anterior C_1 arch is also absent. (**c**) Sagittal CT reconstruction showing intact articulation between left occipital condyle (*Oc*) and C_1 lateral mass (C_l). Right condyle is free-floating

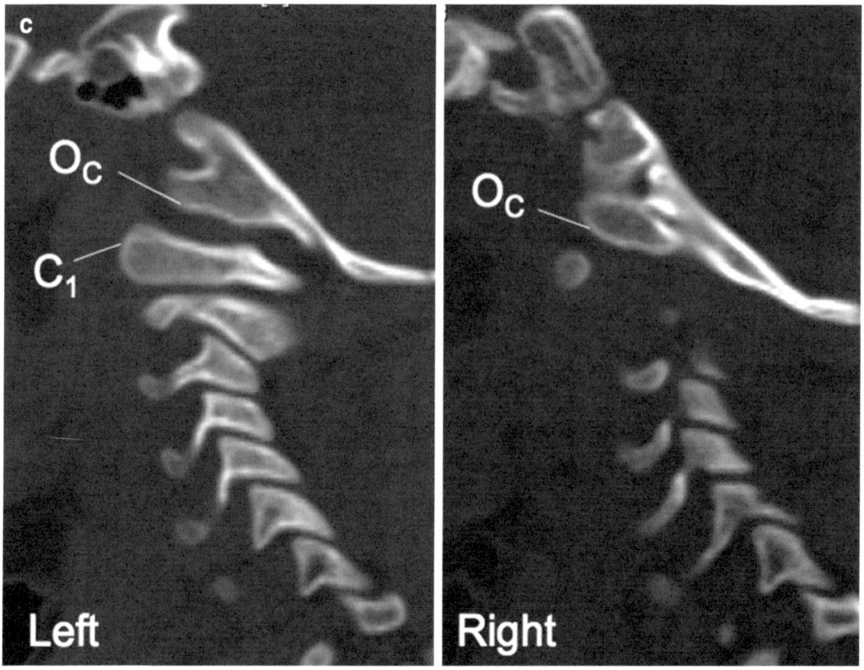

Fig. 63 (continued)

Fig. 64 Combined anterior and posterior atlantal arch defects

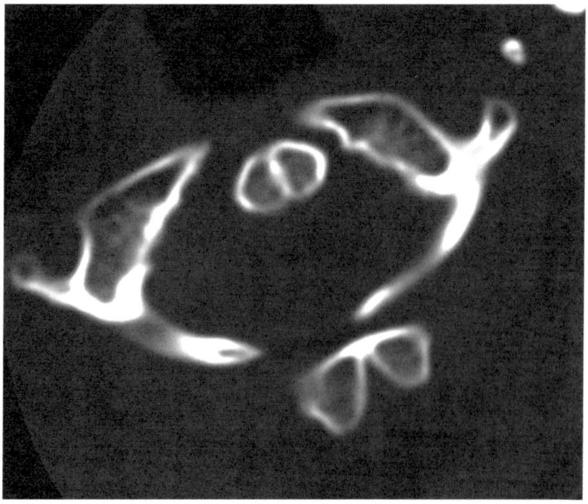

forces: a lateral vector pushing the lateral mass away from the central axis of the spine, the other a vertical vector crushing the lateral mass parallel to the spinal axis (Fig. 65). By elementary trigonometry, the larger the slanting angle of the joint to the horizontal, the larger will be the lateral vector because it is the product of the sine function of the angle, and the smaller will be the vertical vector because it is

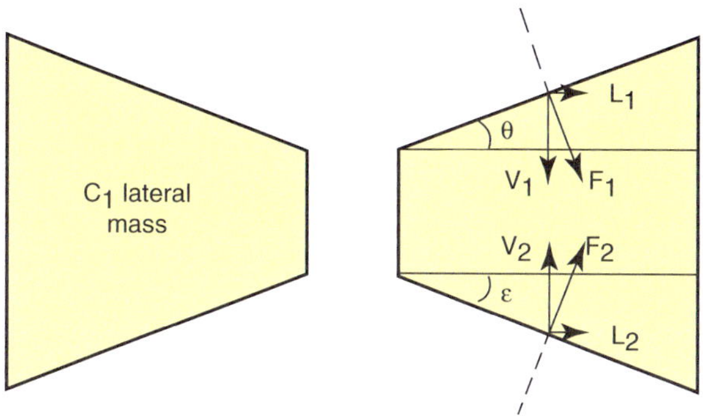

Fig. 65 Forces acting on the C_1 lateral mass during axial loading of the head. The lateral mass is wedge-shaped in the coronal plane, with an upper facet surface articulating with the occipital condyle, at a slanting angle of θ to the horizontal. The lower facet surface articulates with the C_2 facet and slants at an angle of ε to the horizontal. Axial loading stresses are translated into forces perpendicular to the facet surfaces, F_1 for the upper and F_2 for the lower facet. F_1 and F_2 are in turn resolved into a horizontal (lateral) and a vertical component vector, the former laterally displacing the lateral mass and the latter crushing it vertically. They are given by:
The larger θ and ε, the larger the centrifugal push on the lateral mass
For the upper articular surface:
Lateral vector $L_1 = F_1 \text{sine } \theta$
Vertical vector $V_1 = F_1 \text{cosine } \theta$
For the lower articular surface:
Lateral vector $L_2 = F_2 \text{sine } \varepsilon$
Vertical vector $V_2 = F_2 \text{cosine } \varepsilon$
Total centrifugal (lateral) force-vector pushing out lateral mass $= L_1 + L_2$
$= F_1 \text{ sine } \theta + F_2 \text{sine } \varepsilon$

the product of the cosine function of the same angle (Fig. 64). As the slanting angles of the upper and lower joints may differ in the same individual, as they do between individuals and certainly amongst patients with developmental anomalies of the atlas, the magnitudes of the lateral centrifugal forces due to any given axial loading also vary widely depending on the existing parameters, but are mathematically predictable.

In the case of a complete bony C_1 ring, the centrifugal forces tending to split apart the lateral masses are comfortably absorbed by the bony integrity of the anterior and posterior arches. In the classic Jefferson's fracture, both the anterior and posterior bony arches are abruptly broken on each side; the ring is cracked in four places, and the lateral forces push asunder the lateral masses (Fig. 66). In subjects with combined, congenitally incomplete (not absent) anterior and posterior atlantal arches, centrifugal migration of the lateral masses is seldom if ever seen, probably because whatever fibrous or fibrocartilaginous tissues bridging the unfused stumps of the arches of the front and back are inherently strong enough and together share the work of withstanding the continuous sundering stresses of normal vertical posture. One suspects the TAL also serves in this binding function.

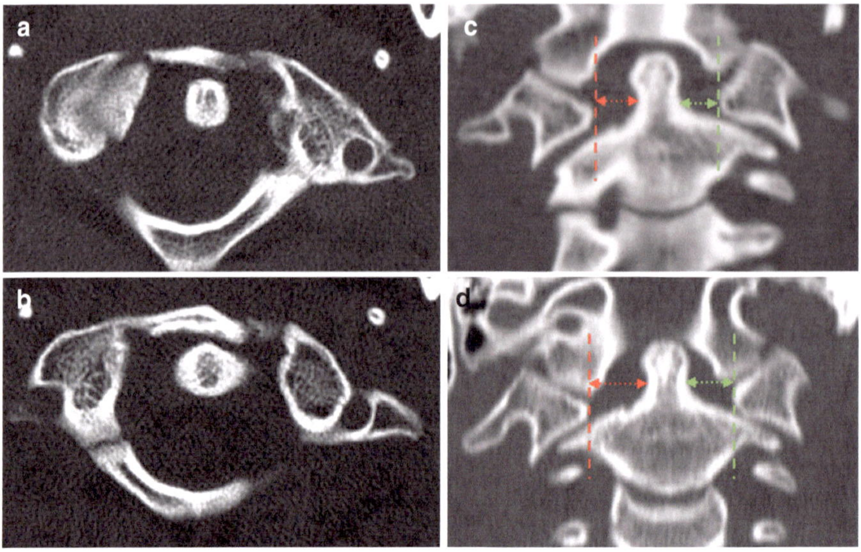

Fig. 66 Classic Jefferson fracture of C_1 with disruption of both the anterior and posterior arches on each side (**a**, **b**). The two lateral masses are thus disconnected from each other. Comparison of the coronal reformatted CT at injury (**c**), and after 4 weeks of treatment with cervical collar (**d**) shows lateral migration of both lateral masses, as seen in the lengthening of the distances between the medial aspect of the lateral masses and the sides of the dens (*double-headed arrows*, *red* for the right and *green* for the left) during the 4-week interval

In the unusual case of an anterior arch fracture in the presence of a developmental posterior arch defect, the sudden loss of continuity of the anterior ring shifts all centrifugal stresses abruptly upon the solitary posterior fibrous bridges, which consequently fails in preventing lateral migration of the lateral masses (Fig. 67). An equivalent situation may explain splaying of the lateral atlantal masses in a child with congenital anterior C_1 arch defect who had undergone C_1 posterior arch removal for foramen magnum stenosis (Fig. 68). Such scenarios are rare but are well worth monitoring with serial CT scans, particularly in patients with steep-slanting angles in their occipital-C_1 and C_1–C_2 joints. The coronal reformatted images are especially helpful in calibrating the "spread distance" between the medial edge of the lateral mass and the lateral surface of the dens (Fig. 67).

Bifid Ventral and Dorsal Atlantal Arches

Midline gaps in the dorsal atlantal tubercle are common incidental findings. Anterior bifid C_1 arch is less common but probably just as innocuous. Combined anterior and posterior C_1 bifidity is uncommon (Fig. 69). The examples we have seen are all stable entities, though the gaps never close with age. Rare cases with in-curling of the free ends of the unfused posterior arches have been known to compress the spinal cord [22] and require surgical decompression (Fig. 70).

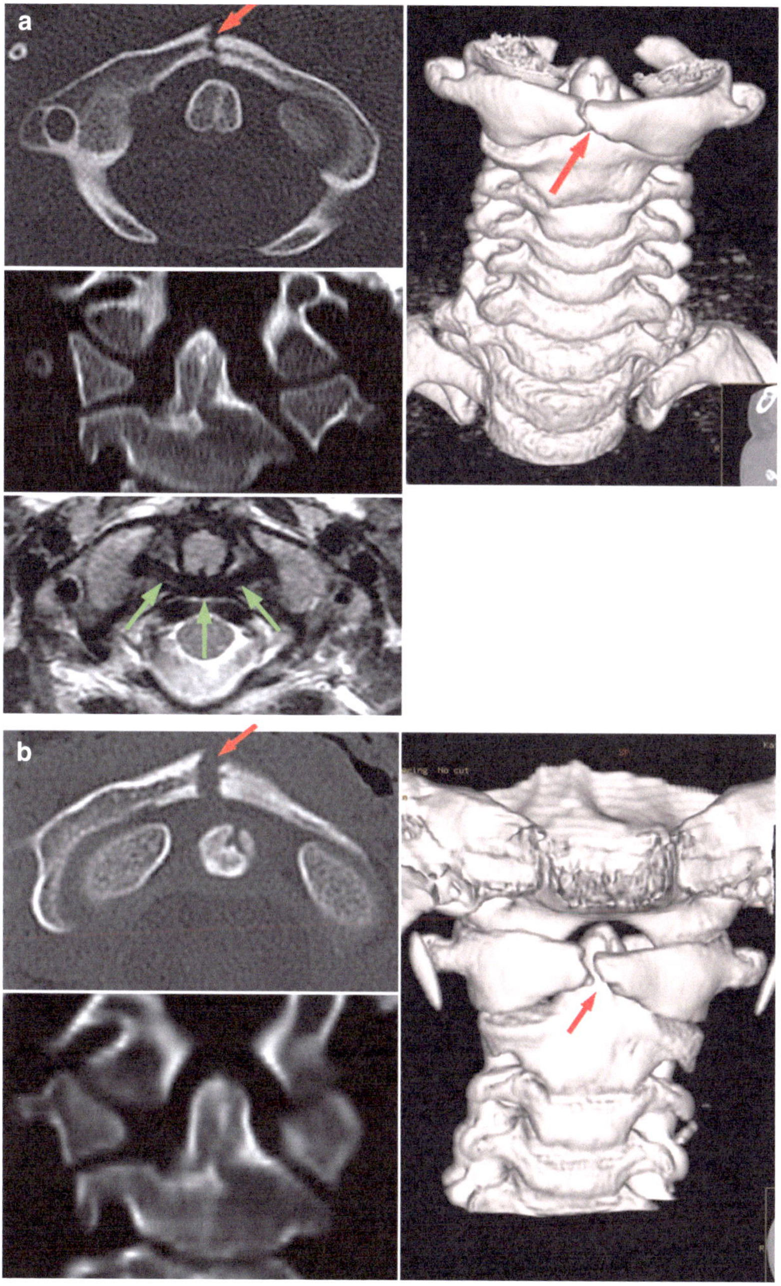

Fig. 67 Anterior C_1 arch fracture in a child with a congenital posterior arch defect. (**a**) Shows studies taken on day of injury. Fracture (*arrow*) and posterior arch defect are well shown on CT (*left upper*). Coronal CT (*left middle*) shows relationship of lateral masses with the dental pivot. TAL (*green arrows*) is present on axial MR (*left lower*). *Right side* shows 3-D rendering of the anterior arch fracture (*arrow*) and posterior arch defect. (**b**) Studies done 2 weeks after injury show widening of the anterior arch fracture (*arrow*) (*left upper* and *right side*) and lateral migration of the right lateral mass (*left lower*) similar to an unstable Jefferson fracture

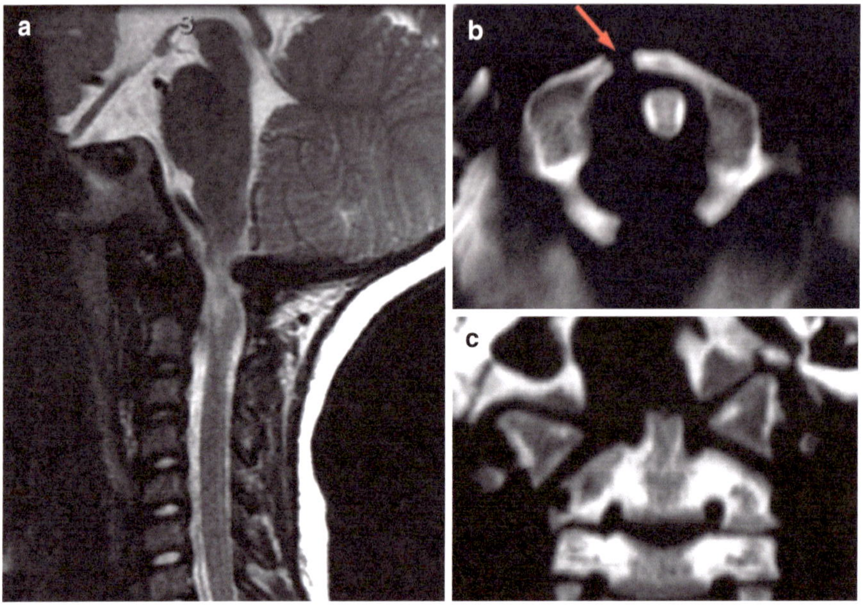

Fig. 68 Posterior C_1 arch resection in a child with congenital anterior C_1 arch defect. (**a**) Sagittal MRI shows severe foramen magnum stenosis with indentation of the cervicomedullary junction by the opisthion and posterior C_1 arch. (**b**) Axial CT shows iatrogenic posterior arch defect and the congenital anterior arch defect (*arrow*). (**c**) Four weeks after surgery, coronal CT shows lateral migration of the right C_1 lateral mass

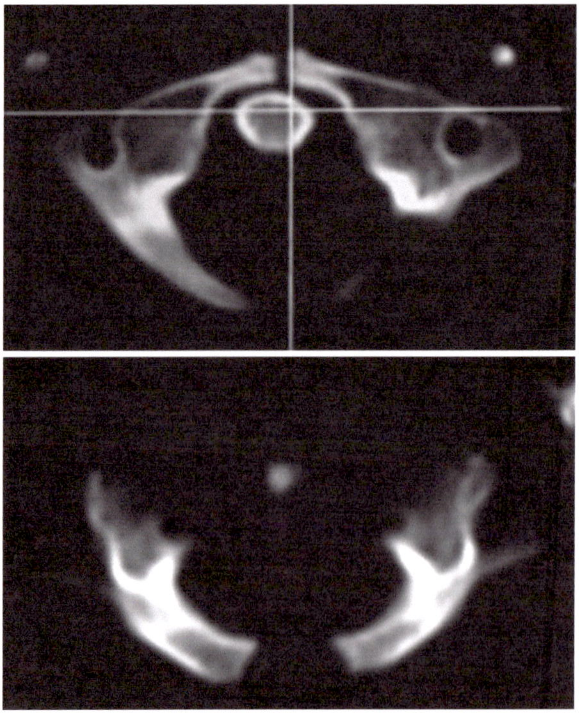

Fig. 69 Bifid anterior and posterior atlantal arches

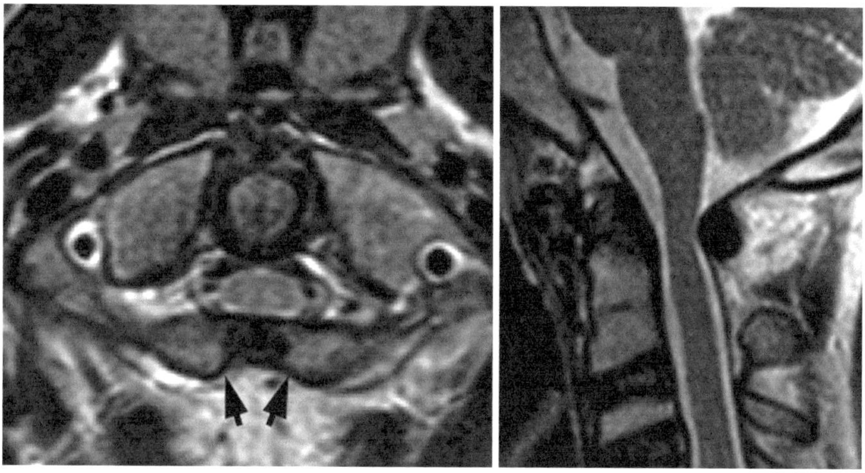

Fig. 70 Bifid posterior atlantal arch with hyperplasia and inward curling of the free ends (*arrows*) of the open arch. There is some narrowing of the spinal canal and slight indentation of the posterior surface of the cord

References

1. Aoyoma H, Asamoto K (1988) Determination of somite cells: independence of cell differentiation and morphogenesis. Development 104:15–28
2. Bagnall KM (1992) The migration and distribution of somite cells after labelling with the carbocyanine dye, DiI: the relationship of this distribution to segmentation in the vertebrate body. Anat Embryol (Berl) 185:317–324
3. Bagnall KM, Sander EJ (1989) The binding pattern of peanut lectin associated with sclerotome migration and the formation of the vertebral axis in the chick embryo. Anat Embryol (Berl) 180:505–513
4. Bellairs R (1980) The segmentation of somites in the chick embryo. Bolletino di Zoologia 47:245–252
5. Burwood RJ (1970) The cranio-cervical junction: anatomy. Thesis, University of Bristol
6. Cattell JS, Filtzer DL (1965) Pseudosubluxation and other normal variations in the cervical spine in children. J Bone Joint Surg Am 47A:1295–1309
7. Cave AJE (1938) The morphological constitution of the odontoid process. J Anat 72:621
8. Chevrel JP (1965) Occipitalization of the atlas. Arch Orthop Trauma Surg 13:104–108
9. Chigira M, Kaneko K, Mashio D, Watanabe H (1994) Congenital hypoplasia of the arch of the atlas with abnormal segmentation of the cervical spine. Arch Orthop Trauma Surg 113:110–112
10. Christ B, Jacob HJ, Jacob M (1978) On the formation of the myotomes in avian embryos. An experimental and scanning electron microscope study. Experentia 34:514–516
11. Christ B, Jacob HJ, Siefert R (1988) Über die Entwicklung der Zervikookzipitalen Übergangsregion. In: Hohmann D, Kügelgen B, Liebig K (eds) Neuroorthopädie, vol 4. Springer, Berlin/Heidelberg, pp 13–22
12. Christ B, Wilting J (1992) From somites to vertebral column. Ann Anat 174:23–32
13. Condie B, Capecchi MR (1993) Mice homozygous for a targeted disruption of *Hox d-3* (Hox-4.1) exhibit anterior transformations of the first and second cervical vertebrae, the atlas and axis. Development 119:579–595
14. Couly GF, Coltey PM, Le Douarin NM (1993) The triple origin of skull in higher vertebrates: a study in quail-chick chimeras. Development 117:409–429

15. Crockard H, Stevens M (1995) Craniovertebral junction anomalies in inherited disorder: part of the syndrome or caused by the disorder? Eur J Pediatr 154:504–512
16. Dalgleish AE (1985) A study of the development of thoracic vertebrae in the mouse assisted by autoradiography. Acta Anat (Basel) 122:91–98
17. David KM, Crockard A (2005) Congenital malformations of the base of the skull, atlas and dens. In: Benzel EC (ed) The cervical spine, 4th edn. Lippincott Williams and Wilkins, Philadelphia, pp 415–426
18. David KM, Thorogood P, Stevens JM, Crockard HA (1997) The one bone spine: a failure of notochord/sclerotome signaling? Clin Dysmorphol 6:303–314
19. David KM, Thorogood PV, Stevens JM, Crockard A (1999) The dysmorphic cervical spine in Klippel-Feil syndrome: interpretations from developmental biology. Neurosurg Focus 6(6):e1
20. Davis GK, Jaramillo CA, Patel NH (2001) Pax group III genes and the evolution of insect pair-rule patterning. Development 128:3445–3458
21. Davis GK, Patel NH (1999) The origin and evolution of segmentation. Trends Cell Biol 9:M68–M72
22. Devi BI, Shenoy SN, Panigrahi MK, Chandramouli BA, Das BS, Jayakumar PN (1997) Anomaly of arch of atlas – a rare cause of symptomatic canal stenosis in children. Pediatr Neurosurg 26:214–218
23. Dietrich S, Gruss P (1995) Undulated phenotypes suggest a role of *Pax-1* for the development of vertebral and extravertebral structures. Dev Biol 167:529–548
24. Dietrich S, Kessel M (1997) The vertebral column. In: Thorogood P (ed) Embryos, genes and birth defects. Wiley, Chichester, pp 281–302
25. Dietrich S, Schubert FR, Gruss P (1993) Altered Pax gene expression in notochord mutants of the mouse: the notochord is required for the dorsoventral patterning of the somite. Mech Dev 44:189–207
26. Dubrulle J, McGrew MJ, Pourquié O (2001) FGF signaling controls somite boundary position and regulates segmentation clock control of spatiotemporal Hox gene activation. Cell 106:219–232
27. von Ebner E (1888) Urwirbel und Neugliederung der Wirbelsäule. Sitzungsber Akad Wiss Wein III 97:194–206
28. Forsberg H, Crozet F, Brown NA (1998) Waves of mouse Lunatic fringe expression, in four-hour cycles at two=hour intervals, precede somite boundary formation. Curr Biol 8:1027–1030
29. Geipel P (1955) Zur Kenntnis der Spaltbildungen des Atlas und Epistropheus Teil IV. Zbl Path 94:19
30. George AW (1919) A method for more accurate study of injuries to the atlas and axis. N Engl J Med Surg 181:395–398
31. Gholve PA, Hosalker HS, Ricchetti ET, Pollock AN, Dormans JP, Drummond DS (2007) Occipitalization of the atlas in children, morphologic classification, associations, and clinical relevance. J Bone Joint Surg (Am) 89:571–578
32. Giacomini C (1886) Sull' esistenza dell' "osodontoideum: nell" uomo. Gior dr Accaddi med di Torino 49:24–28
33. Grabb PA, Mapstone TB, Oakes WJ (1999) Ventral brainstem compression in pediatric and young adult patients with Chiari I malformations. Neurosurgery 44:520–528
34. Haack H, Kessel M (1994) Homeobox genes and skeletal patterning. In: Hall BK (ed) Bone, vol 9. CRC Press, Boca Raton, pp 119–144
35. Hawkins RJ, Fielding JW, Thompson WJ (1976) Os odontoideum: congenital or acquired? J Bone Joint Surg (Am) 38:413–414
36. Hensinger RN (1986) Osseous anomalies of the craniovertebral junction. Spine 11:323–333
37. Hensinger RN, Fielding JW, Hawkins RJ (1978) Congenital anomalies of the odontoid process. Orthop Clin North Am 9:901–912

38. Huang R, Zhi Q, Ordahl CP, Christ B (1997) The fate of the first avian somite. Anat Embryol (Berl) 195:435–449
39. Jacob M, Christ B, Jacob HJ (1975) Über die regionale Determination des paraxialen Mesoderms junger Hühnerembryonen. Verh Anat Ges 69:263–269
40. Jenkins JFA (1969) The evolution and development of the dens of the mammalian axis. Anat Rec 164:173–184
41. Jones FS, Georges C, Guss P, Edelman GM (1991) Activation of the cytotactin promoter by the homeobox-containing gene *Evx-1*. Proc Nat Acad Sci USA 89:2091
42. Jones FS, Prediger EA, Dennis BA, DeRobertis EM, Edelman GM (1991) Cell adhesion molecules as targets for Hox genes: neural cell adhesion molecule promoter activity is modulated by cotransfection with *Hox 2.5* and *2.4*. Proc Nat Acad Sci USA 89:2091
43. Kessel M (1992) Respecification of vertebral identities by retinoic acid. Development 115:487–501
44. Kessel M, Gruss P (1991) Homeotic transformation of murine vertebrae and concomitant alteration of *Hox* codes induced by retinoic acid. Cell 67:1–20
45. Keynes RJ, Stern CD (1988) Mechanisms of vertebrate segmentation. Development 103:413–429
46. Kieny M, Mauger A, Sengel P (1972) Early regionalization of the somitic mesoderm as studied by the development of the axial skeleton of the chick embryo. Dev Biol 28:42–161
47. Kirlew KA, Hathout GM, Reiter SD, Gold RH (1993) Os odontoideum in identical twins: perspective on etiology. Skeletal Radiol 22:525–527
48. Koseki H, Wallin J, Wilting J et al (1993) A role for *Pax-1* as mediator of notochordal signals during the dorsoventral specification of vertebrae. Development 119:649–660
49. Kotil D, Kalayci M (2005) Ventral cervicomedullary junction compression secondary to condylus occipitalis (median occipital condyle), a rare entity. J Spinal Disord Tech 18(4):382–385
50. Le Double AF (1903) Traité des variations des os du crane de l'homme et de leur signification au point de vue de l'Anthropologie zoologique. Vigot Frères, Paris. 1912
51. Logan WW, Stuard ID (1973) Absence of posterior arch of the atlas. Am J Roentgenol 118:431–434
52. von Ludinghausen M, Schindler G, Kageyama I, Pomaroli A (2002) The third occipital condyle, a constituent part of a median occipito-atlanto-odontoid joint: a case report. Surg Radiol Anat 24:71–76
53. Lufkin T, Mark M, Hart CP, Dollé P, LeMeur M, Chambon P (1992) Homeotic transformation of the occipital bones of the skull by ectopic expression of a homeobox gene. Nature 359:835–841
54. Macalister A (1893) Notes on the development and variations of the atlas. J Anat Physiol 27:519–542
55. Markuske H (1978) Untersuchungen zur Static und Dynamik der kindlichen Halswirbelsäule: Der Aussagewert seitlicher Röntgenaufnahmen. In: Die Wirbelsäule in Forschung und Praxis, vol 50. Hippokrates, Stuttgart
56. McGrew MJ, Dale JK, Fraboulet S, Pourquié O (1998) The lunatic fringe gene is a target of the molecular clock linked to somite segmentation in avian embryos. Curr Biol 8:979–982
57. McRae DL (1953) Bony abnormalities in the region of the foramen magnum; correlation of the anatomic and neurologic findings. Acta Radiol 40:335–354
58. McRae DL (1960) The significance of abnormalities of the cervical spine. Am J Roentgenol 84:3–25
59. McRae DL, Barnum AS (1953) Occipitalization of the atlas. Am J Roentgenol Radium Ther Nucl Med 70:23–46
60. Menezes AH (1996) Congenital and acquired abnormalities of the craniovertebral junction. In: Youmans JR (ed) Neurological surgery, 4th edn. WB Saunders, Philadelphia, pp 1035–1089

61. Menezes AH (1998) Embryology, development, and classification of disorders of the craniovertebral junction. In: Dickman CA, Sonntag VKH, Spetzler RF (eds) Surgery of the craniovertebral junction. Thieme, New York, pp 3–12
62. Menezes AH, Fenoy KA (2009) Remnants of occipital vertebrae: proatlas segmentation abnormalities. Neurosurgery 64:945–953
63. Menezes AH, Ryken TC (1992) Craniovertebral abnormalities in Down's syndrome. Neurosurgery 18:24–33
64. Morgan MK, Onofrio BM, Bender CE (1989) Familial os odontoideum. Case report. J Neurosurg 70:636–639
65. Müller F, O'Rahilly R (1980) The human chondrocranium at the end of the embryonic period, proper, with particular reference to the nervous system. Am J Anat 159:33–58
66. Müller F, O'Rahilly R (1994) Occipitocervical segmentation in staged human embryos. J Anat 185:251–258
67. Müller F, O'Rahilly R (2003) Segmentation in staged human embryos: the occipitocervical region revisited. J Anat 203:251–258
68. Musil L, Goodenough D (1990) Gap junctional intercellular communication and the regulation of connexin expression and function. Curr Opin Cell Biol 2:875
69. Nishikawa M, Sakamoto H, Hakuba A, Nakanishi N, Inoue Y (1997) Pathogenesis of Chiari malformation: a morphometric study of the posterior cranial fossa. J Neurosurg 86:40–47
70. Palmeirim I, Henrique D, Ish-Horowicz D, Pourquié O (1997) Avian hairy gene expression identifies a molecular clock linked to vertebrate segmentation and somitogenesis. Cell 91:639–648
71. Pendergrass EP, Schaeffer JP, Hodes PJ (1956) The head and neck in Roentgen diagnosis, 2nd edn. Charles C. Thomas, Springfield, pp 1529–1530
72. Pollack I, Pang D, Albright LA, Krieger D (1992) Outcome following hind brain decompression of symptomatic Chiari malformations in children previously shunted with myelomeningoceles. J Neurosurg 77:881–888
73. Pollack I, Pang D, Kocoshis S, Putnam P (1992) Neurogenic dysphagia resulting from Chiari malformations. Neurosurgery 30:709–719
74. Pourquié O (2003) The segmentation clock: converting embryonic time into spatial pattern. Science 301:328–330
75. Pourquié O (2003) Vertebrate somitogenesis: a novel paradigm for animal segmentation? Int J Dev Biol 47:597–603
76. Prescher A (1997) The craniocervical junction in man, the osseous variations, their significance and differential diagnosis. Ann Anat 179:1–19
77. Prescher A (1990) The differential diagnosis of isolated ossicles in the region of the dens axis. Gegenbaurs Morphol Jahrb 136:139–154
78. Prescher A, Brors D, Adam G (1996) Anatomic and radiologic appearance of several variants of the craniocervical junction. Skull Base Surg 6:83–94
79. Rao P (2002) Median (third) occipital condyle. Clin Anat 15:148–151
80. Reiter A (1944) Die Frühentwicklung der menschlichen Wirbelsäule. II. Mitteilung: Die Entwicklung der Occipitalsegmente und der Halswirbelsäule. Z Anat Entwicklungsgesch 113:66–104
81. Remak R (1855) Untersuchungen über die Entwicklung der Wirbeltiere. Reimer, Berlin
82. Sawada A, Shinya M, Jiang YJ, Kawakami A, Kuroiwa A, Takeda H (2001) Fgf/MAPK signaling is a crucial positional cue in somite boundary formation. Development 128:4873–4880
83. Schulze P, Buurman R (1980) Absence of the posterior arch of the atlas. Am J Roentgenol 134:178–180
84. Sensenig EC (1957) The development of the occipital and cervical segments and their associated structures in human embryos. Contrib Embryol 36:152–161
85. Smith CA, Tuan RS (1994) Human PAX gene expression and development of the vertebral column. Clin Orthop 302:241–250

86. Stapleton P, Weith A, Urbanek P, Kozmik Z, Busslinger M (1993) Chromosomal localization of seven PAX genes and cloning of a novel family member, PAX-9. Nat Genet 3:292
87. Starck D (1979) Das Skelettsystem. In: Starck D (ed) Vergleichende Anatomie der Wirbeltiere, vol 2. Springer, Berlin/Heidelberg/New York, pp 44–95
88. Stern CD, Keynes RJ (1987) Interactions between somite cells; the formation and maintenance of segment boundaries in the chick embryo. Development 99:261–272
89. Stover LJ, Bergan U, Nilsen G, Sjaastad O (1993) Posterior cranial fossa dimensions in the Chiari I malformation: relation to pathogenesis and clinical presentation. Neuroradiology 35:113–118
90. von Torklus D, Gehle W (1975) Die Obere Halswirbelsäule, 2nd edn. Thieme, Stuttgart
91. von Torklus D, Gehle W (1972) Anomalies and malformations. In: von Torklus D, Gehle W (eds) The upper cervical spine. Thieme, Stuttgart, pp 14–53
92. von Torklus D, Gehle W (1969) Neue Perspektiven der Entwicklungsstörungen der oberen Halswirlbelsäule. Z Orthop 105:178
93. Tramontano-Guerritore G (1927) Die atlanto-occipital union. Anat Anz 64:173–184
94. Tubbs RS, Iskandar BJ, Bartolucci AA, Oakes WJ (2004) A critical analysis of the Chiari 1.5 malformation. J Neurosurg 101(2 Suppl):179–183
95. Vega A, Quintana F, Berciano J (1990) Basichondrocranium anomalies in adult Chiari type I malformation: a morphometric study. J Neurol Sci 99:137–145
96. Wadia NH (1967) Myelopathy complicating congenital atlantoaxial dislocation (a study of 28 cases). Brain 90:449–472
97. Wallin J, Mizutani Y, Imai K et al (1993) A new Pax gene, Pax-9, maps to mouse chromosome 12. Mamm Genome 4:354–358
98. Wallin J, Wilting J, Koseki H, Fritsch R, Christ B, Balling R (1994) The role of Pax-1 in axial skeleton development. Development 120:1109–1121
99. Wilting J, Ebensperger C, Müller TS, Koseki H, Wallin J, Christ B (1995) Pax-1 in the development of the cervico-occipital transitional zone. Anat Embryol (Berl) 192:221–227
100. Wollin DG (1963) The os odontoideum: separate odontoid process. J Bone Joint Surg Am 45:1459–1484

Extracranial Segments of the Vertebral Artery: Insight in the Developmental Changes up to the 21st Year of Life

Vasović Ljiljana, Jovanović Ivan, Ugrenović Slađana, Vlajković Slobodan, Jovanović Predrag, and Đorđević Gordana

Contents

V. Ljiljana (✉) • J. Ivan • U. Slađana • V. Slobodan
Faculty of Medicine, Department of Anatomy,
University of Niš, Blvd. Dr Zoran Đinđić 81, Niš 18000, Serbia
e-mail: likica@medfak.ni.ac.rs; ivanjov@junis.ni.ac.rs; sdugren@sbb.rs; sloti@ptt.rs

J. Predrag
Faculty of Medicine, Clinic of Ophthalmology,
University of Niš, Blvd. Dr Zoran Đinđić 81, Niš 18000, Serbia
e-mail: pedja.jovanovic64@gmail.com

Đ. Gordana, MD
Department of Pediatric, Health Center,
Street Vojvode Tankosića 15, Niš 18000, Serbia
e-mail: dr.goca@yahoo.com

C. Di Rocco, N. Akalan (eds.), *Pediatric Craniovertebral Junction Diseases*, Advances and Technical Standards in Neurosurgery 40,
DOI 10.1007/978-3-319-01065-6_3,

Abstract The vertebral artery (VA) bilaterally arises usually from the subclavian artery and courses within the bony canals of cervical vertebrae, and then it reverses directions on the first vertebra before piercing the dura to enter the cranium.

The aim was to follow (ab)normal developmental changes of extracranial VA from prenatal status to age 21. This chapter included a brief description of the arterial embryology and morphofunctional specificity of the VA in prevertebral, cervical, and atlantic parts, during prenatal and postnatal period.

The authors concluded that the subclavian origin of the VA was in most of fetal and adult cases. The incidences of variable VA origins and domination of one of the VAs were different from one series of human specimens to the second one. Although in most of cases, anomalous origin and/or variable course of the extracranial VA had little or did not result in clinical symptoms in infants and young adults, the true value of their discovery is in the diagnostic gain before vascular surgery of supra-aortic arteries.

Keywords Human vertebral artery • Prevertebral part • Cervical part • Atlantic part • Prenatal and postnatal status

Introduction

The vertebrobasilar system includes paired vertebral arteries (VAs) and unpaired basilar artery (BA) with their branches. The VA arises usually from the subclavian artery (SA) and courses within the bony canals of six cervical vertebrae, anterior to the cervical nerve roots, encircled by veins and nerve elements; then it reverses directions on the first cervical vertebra (atlas) before piercing the dura to enter the cranium [11]. The VA characterizes by a small diameter (0.5–5.5 mm) in relation to great length (5.0–35 cm), asymmetry, segmental branches, and convergent junction in the direction of forward flow [13]. The composition of the VA varies both among its layers and along its length, as a response to the different demands along its course [60].

The VA provides blood supply to the spinal cord, the rhombencephalon, the mesencephalon, the occipital lobe, and part of the temporal lobe of the telencephalon. The VA is a distributing artery and, as such, functions to transport blood between the SA and the small parenchymal arterioles of these brain parts [67].

The vertebrobasilar system distinguishes from the carotid system as follows: (1) the collateral circulation is more developed in the vertebrobasilar system, (2) the proportion of the vertebrobasilar circulation fed by small penetrating arteries is much higher, and (3) vascular anomalies are more common in the vertebrobasilar system [32]. Peculiarities in development of the vertebrobasilar system are responsible for the apparent greater tendency to arteriovenous malformations in the distribution of the vertebral vessels than in the carotid system [35]. Generally carotid artery wall of fetuses and newborns is more tensile and has greater strength and less rigidity than that of the VA [43]. The main findings of the study of Ganesan et al. [30] were

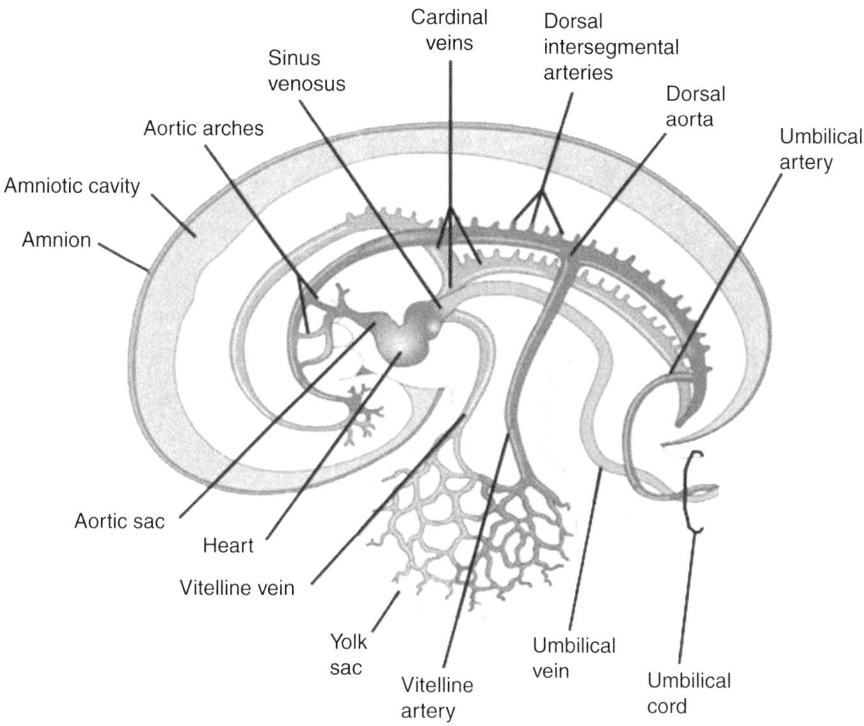

Fig. 1 Modified scheme [131] of the vasculature in the human embryo (right half) at week 4

that the majority of children with posterior circulation stroke are boys with vertebrobasilar abnormalities.

Embryology of Arteries

The cardiovascular system develops in the 3rd week of the human embryo. The heart begins to beat on 21st or 22nd day, and blood begins to circulate. Blood leaves the heart via the truncus arteriosus in this early stage. It is divided by the aorticopulmonary septum into the ventral aortas, which later become the aortic sac and the pulmonary trunk.

Due to the caudal movement of the heart relative to the pharynx, the six pairs of primitive aortic arches connect on each side the aortic sac with the corresponding dorsal aorta during 4th and 5th week (Fig. 1). During the 2nd month, the heart gradually migrates caudally with respect to the axial skeleton, progressively elongating the arteries which extend between the outlet of the heart and the cervical and upper thoracic levels. In addition to this alteration in the length and diameter of the arteries, there are changes in their relationships to one another [7].

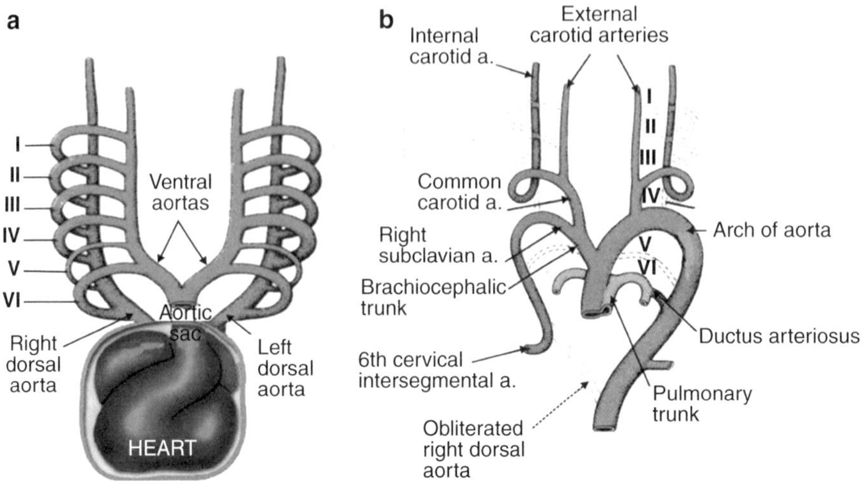

Fig. 2 (**a**, **b**) Modified scheme [131] of six (I–VI) primitive aortic arches during weeks 4–5 (**a**) and final arterial arrangement during weeks 6–8 of gestation (**b**)

Primitive aortic arches develop in regular order from cephalic to caudal. There are two distinct phases in the development of the aortic arches: (1) the branchial phase, in which the vessels approximate to the branchial pattern of lower vertebrates, and (2) the postbranchial phase, during which the branchial pattern is being replaced by the adult arterial arrangement. During the branchial phase, the blood stream from the heart to the dorsal aorta on each side makes use of the following arches in succession: (a) first arch; (b) first and second arches; (c) second and third arches; (d) third and fourth arches; and (e) third, fourth, and pulmonary arches. During weeks 6–8, the aortic-arch pattern is transformed to the final fetal arterial arrangement (Fig. 2). The conversion of the early embryonic circulatory system to the adult configuration involves the following steps: (1) degeneration of parts of some primitive vessels, (2) hypertrophy of some primitive vessels' parts, (c) anastomosis and/or fusion of some primitive vessels, (3) separation of one primitive vessel into two, (4) loss of connection between some primitive vessels, and (5) formation of new vessels [20].

The first primitive aortic arch largely disappears but the remaining parts form maxillary arteries and may also contribute to the formation of the external carotid arteries. The dorsal part of the second primitive aortic arch persists and forms the stem of the hyoid and stapedial arteries. Proximal parts of the third primitive aortic arch form the common carotid arteries; the distal part of the third pair of aortic arches joins with corresponding dorsal aorta to form the internal carotid arteries (ICAs). The left fourth aortic arch forms part of the arch of the aorta, whereas the right fourth aortic arch becomes the proximal part of the right SA [131]; the distal part of the right subclavian SA forms from the right dorsal aorta and right sixth cervical intersegmental artery (CIA). The left SA is formed from the left sixth CIA [83]. The primitive SA can first be recognized in embryos at the stage when the fourth arches are present but the pulmonary arches are not complete, yet [11].

Caudally to the aortic arches, the paired dorsal aortas merge to form a single descending aorta. Paired ventral aortas receive blood from the truncus arteriosus. It is worthy of note that no ventral aortas occur in the human embryo [11].

The aortic arch has a composite origin as it develops from the aortic sac, left fourth aortic arch, and part of the left dorsal aorta. The dorsal aorta degenerates between the third and fourth aortic arches. Failure of the normal caudal migration of the fourth aortic arch in the growing embryo from the occipital level in the thoracic cage at the 7th week of gestation has also been invoked as a cause of cervical ectopic of the aortic arch, as happened in a 3½-year-old boy and an adolescent [27].

Embryology of the Vertebrobasilar System

During the 4th week of gestation, 42 somites (4 occipital, 8 cervical, 12 thoracic, 5 lumbar, 5 sacral, and 8–10 coccygeal pairs) are formed. Each somite differentiates into an outer dermatome and inner myotome and a medial sclerotome. Each dorsal aorta gives off about 30 or more intersegmental arteries that pass dorsally between somites. Segmental arteries send ventral and dorsal branches to the trunk wall. The sclerotomes are ventral–medial in their location and will form the vertebral bodies. The first four sclerotomes essentially fuse to form the occipital bone and posterior portions of the foramen magnum [65].

The serial cervical parts in the human embryo are eight nerves (and somites), seven vertebrae, and six CIAs [83]. These CIAs extend from the corresponding dorsal aorta toward the anterolateral aspects of the developing vertebrae, where they give rise to dorsal branches that pass between the vertebral transverse processes toward posterior vertebral muscles. The tunica adventitia of the large arteries of the neck became more evident than at 15 weeks [68].

At the 7–12 mm (5th to 6th week), the VA is formed as a longitudinal canal dorsal to the costal elements, interconnecting the dorsal branches of the CIAs from the first to the seventh [52], i.e., between the PIA and proximal six CIAs [83]. The trunk of the VA develops from the three parts: (1) cervical vertebral artery (a longitudinal anastomosis extending from the brachiosegmental to the suboccipital artery), which is subdivided into prevertebral and transversal parts; (2) atlantic part is portion of a vessel including the transversal spinal branch and the suboccipital artery; and (3) subarachnoidal part—a metencephalic longitudinal anastomosis in the direction of the caudal branch of ICA [52].

It is well known that anomalous origins of the VA arise from aberrant anastomosis at any time during the embryonic development of the aortic arch and/or cervical intersegmental arteries [114, 115].

In the hindbrain area, paired, separate, longitudinal neural plexus, as a precursor of the basilar artery (BA), appears at the 5- to 6-mm crown–rump length of the embryo (29-day). At this stage, the caudal branch of the ICA communicates with the ipsilateral longitudinal neural artery, which later becomes the definitive posterior communicating artery. Blood reaches them from dorsal aortas and ICAs via some primitive vessels—the trigeminal (PTA), otic (POA), hypoglossal (PHA), and proatlantal intersegmental (PIA) arteries. Bilaterally, the longitudinal neural plexus is supplied cranially by the PTA and caudally by the PIA [119, 121]. The caudal supply is also supported by input from the POA at the level of the VIIIth cranial nerve and from the PHA at the level of the XIIth cranial nerve [118, 120]. The longitudinal neural arteries have begun to form prominent anastomoses across the midline of the hindbrain or, rarely, they can completely persist, as in a 3-year-old boy [38].

Aplasia of the Vertebral Artery

Unilateral or bilateral aplasia of the VA in fetal and/or postnatal period can cause by persistence of carotid-vertebrobasilar anastomosis or it can to be a "satellite" of some syndrome or disease.

Khodadad [47], in his study of persistent PHA (PPHA) based on 50 dissected fetal brains, described that in most of the specimens, one of the VAs was absent while the second one was hypoplastic or, rarely, normal. Absence of the both VAs in the presence of the left PPHA was showed in a 14-day-old male baby with Arnold–Chiari malformation [36]. There were descriptions of absence of the both VAs in the presence of bilateral persistent PIA (PPIA) in a 4-year-old girl [78] and in a 6-year-old girl [89]. There was the absence of the left VA in the presence of the ipsilateral PPIA in a 3-day-old male neonate and in a 14-month-old girl [89] and in a 6-year-old boy [1]. Left vertebral angiogram showing retrograde flow in the persistent PTA (PPTA) indicated the absence of the ipsilateral VA in a 17-year-old girl [79]. A rare case of a "segmental aplasia" of the VA, the termination of hypoplastic right VA at the atlas level in the presence of the left PPTA, was also reported [44].

It was reported an absence of the right VA in a 4-year-old girl with PHACES syndrome and moyamoya vasculopathy [37], as well as an agenesis of the vertebrobasilar system and the ICA on both sides in a possible PHACE syndrome of a 14-year-old girl [126]. Investigation with Doppler ultrasound followed by arch aortography proved absence of the left VA in a 14-year-old boy with Takayasu's disease [127].

Histology

The wall of the cerebral arteries of a 7-week-old embryo was composed of a single layer of endothelial cells. In a 9-week-old embryo, the walls consisted of an inner tunica intima, a central tunica media, and an outer tunica adventitia. At 12 weeks of gestation, two or three layers of smooth muscle cells had been added to the muscle coat of the media. In the embryos of more than 18 weeks old, the medial defect was not observed at the lateral angle of their branches; defects were observed at the lateral angle of the distal segments of these branches. The cerebral arteries of the embryos of more than 20 weeks old exhibited configurations similar to those of adult ones [29].

In addition to highlighting the striking difference between intracranial and extracranial arteries, data giving by Napoli et al. [71] indicated that brain arteries were

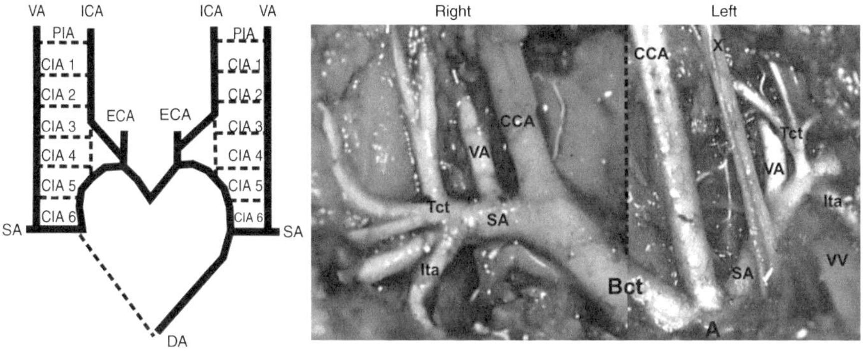

Fig. 3 Modified scheme and photo of the vertebral artery (*VA*) origin on both sides in the human fetus. *Scheme*: Normal embryonic origin of the VA from the sixth cervical intersegmental artery [56, 83]. *DA* dorsal aorta, *SA* subclavian artery, *CIA 1–6* six cervical intersegmental arteries, *PIA* primitive proatlantal intersegmental artery, *ICA* internal carotid artery, *ECA* external carotid artery. *Photo*: Origin of the VA from a superior wall of the SA, medially to the thyrocervical trunk on both sides [114]. *A* arch of the aorta, *CCA* common carotid artery, *Bct* brachiocephalic trunk, *Tct* thyrocervical trunk, *Ita* internal thoracic artery, *VV* vertebral vein, *X* vagus nerve

less susceptible to hypercholesterolemia than extracranial ones in human fetuses and prematurely newborns (6.2 months, in average).

Extracranial Parts of the Vertebral Artery

The VA, usually the first ascending branch of the SA, bilaterally courses through the neck (prevertebral, cervical, and atlantic parts) and through the foramen magnum and enters in the posterior cranial fossa (intracranial part), where it joins with the second one forming the BA. Incidence of an aortic origin of the left VA is on the second place among different patterns origin of the both VAs [4, 81, 114, 115].

Prevertebral Part

The prevertebral (V1) part of the VA extends from its origin to the point of entry into the foramen transversarium of the cervical vertebra, usually CVI.

Some authors stressed that an anomalous origin of the VA occurs mostly on one side, usually on the left [21]. In a study of 100 human fetuses [114], aged from 18 to 26 weeks of gestation and of both gender, the right and left VAs, as single vessels, originated directly from the superior or posterior wall of the SA in 94 and 83 % of cases, respectively (Figs. 3 and 4). In a study of 30 patients aged 19 years and older, the origin of the VAs was always from corresponding SA [21].

The VA orifice on the right SA was most frequently between 20 and 30 mm, at the junction of the posterior and superior surfaces of the SA in adults aged 20 years and older [4]. In relation to the thyrocervical trunk, the VA was usually located 5 mm

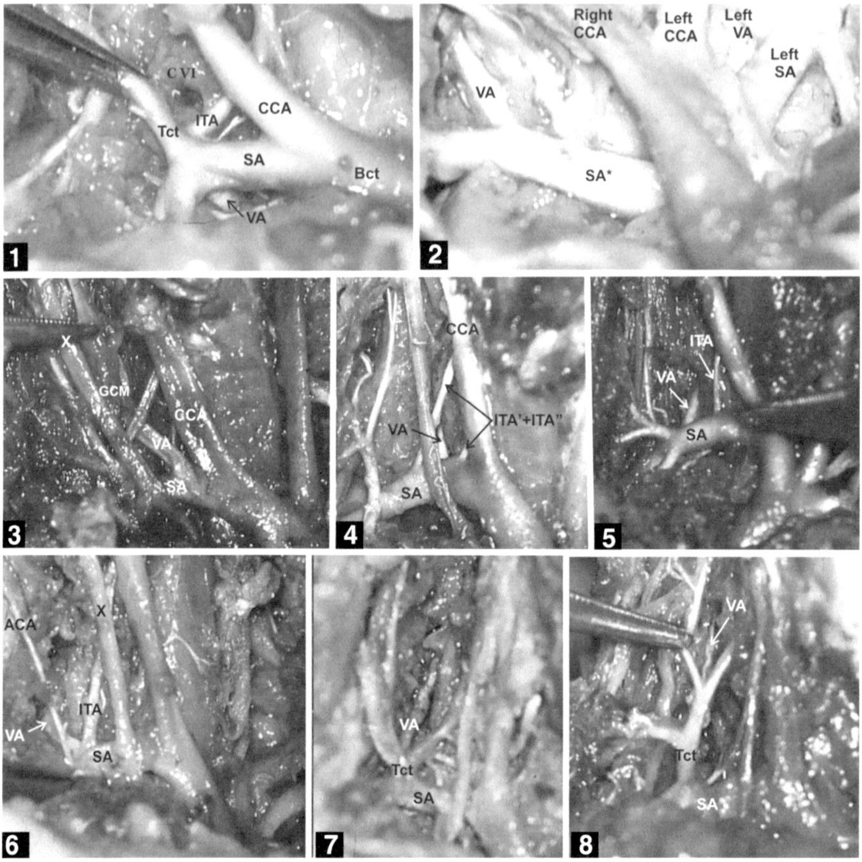

Fig. 4 Different modes of subclavian origin and relation of the right vertebral artery (*VA*) in human fetuses [114]. *Case 1*: Right VA originates from the posterior wall of the subclavian artery (*SA*) and penetrates CVII foramen transversarium. *Case 2*: Right VA originates from the superior wall of the arteria subclavia dextra lusoria (*SA**). *Case 3*: Right VA originates from the superior wall of the normal right SA, just laterally to the bifurcation of the brachiocephalic trunk, and courses through the middle cervical ganglion. *Case 4*: Right VA originates from the posterior wall of the ipsilateral SA and courses between the two inferior thyroid arteries. *Case 5*: Right VA originates from the posterior wall of the ipsilateral SA and courses between the inferior thyroid artery and a "cervical" trunk. *Case 6*: A common origin of the right VA and inferior thyroid artery, just medially to the ascending cervical artery. *Case 7*: Right VA of normal caliber originates from the thyrocervical trunk. *Case 8*: Right VA of extreme hypoplastic caliber originates from the thyrocervical trunk. *Bct* brachiocephalic trunk, *CCA* common carotid artery, *Ttc* thyrocervical trunk, *ITA* inferior thyroid artery, *ACA* ascending cervical artery, *X* vagus nerve

medially, as cited in the paper of Sartor et al. [92], or 10 mm before, sometimes at and less frequently immediately beyond the thyrocervical trunk, as noted Argenson et al. [4]. An origin of the VA at the level, or laterally from the thyrocervical trunk, Jung and Kehr [42] and Zlotnik and Gitkina [132] defined as a lateral displacement of the VA orifice, when scalene muscles can compress the VA. Incidences of 0.58 % was noted in the literature for a common stem of the VA and thyrocervical trunk originating from the

SA; the incidences of 0.64 and 0.13 % were noted for a common stem of the right and left VA and inferior thyroid artery, respectively [92].

On the tomographic image demonstrated by Borenstein et al. [9], it was evidenced that the normal right SA lies 3 mm above the level of the aortic arch and 14.8 mm above the level of the four-chamber view in the 20-week fetus. The values of an external diameter of the left SA ranged from 0.68 to 2.89 mm for the 4-month and 9-month fetuses, respectively [104]. Average external diameters of the right (left) SA were 3.6 (3.4), 4.8 (4.7), and 6.4 (5.9) mm of 19 mature newborn babies, infants, and children to the 4th year [59]. An average depth from the skin to the VAs in infants of about 20 months old was 15.1 ± 3.3 mm [111].

It is fact that VA is usually the branch of the SA; however, it is well known that SA could not be the branch of the brachiocephalic trunk on the right side and/or last branch of the aortic arch. There are a lot of these examples. One of these is the arteria subclavia dextra lusoria (ASDL)—a last branch of the aortic arch (beyond the left SA). It was founded in 1 of 100 human fetuses (see case 2 at Fig. 4) [114, 117], as well as in 1 of 103 human fetuses [31], and in 1.5 % of chromosomally normal fetuses [9]. However, it was found only in 1 of 173 fetuses [107]. The ASDL was also founded in a 7-week-old infant with a large facial hemangioma [106], as well as in an 8-year-old girl and in a 9-year-old boy with frequent respiratory infections, and in a 10-year-old boy with epilepsy [5]. With regard to the VA, it was the branch of the ASDL in previous fetal and infant cases, as well as in 84.3 % of patients with proved ASDL, aged from 2 to 16 years [109]. However Loukas et al. [57] found ASDL simultaneous with a common trunk of the right VA, and left thyroid ima artery arose from the aortic arch between the right and left CCAs during a medico-legal autopsy of a 12-year-old boy.

Two cases (a 6-month-old boy and 2-year-old girl) with tetralogy of Fallot and a right aortic arch were unusual because in each of them an atretic left SA arose from the left pulmonary artery; however, the SA was pulsate distally in both cases, where the vertebral, internal thoracic, and thyrocervical vessels arose [53].

Three infants (2-day-old boys and girl) with aortic arch anomalies had an origin of both SAs from descending aorta; however the beginning of the VA was from the corresponding SA [97].

An anomalous vessel of irregular shape, up to 10 mm in diameter and 4 cm in length, arising from the VA at the level of the CVI transverse process and terminating in the subclavian vein in a 4.5-year-old boy was defined as a rudimentary accessory SA [50].

The average diameter of the aortic arch ranged from 1.08 mm in 14–15 weeks' gestation [2] to 4.09 mm in 29–30 weeks' gestation [31] and 4.79 mm in 36–38 weeks' gestation [2]. In two studies of 100 and 200 human fetuses in Serbia, the left VA, as a single vessel, originated from the aortic arch in 11 of 100 [114] and in 18 of 200 cases [115]; a segmental V1 duplication was found in 4 and 2 % of fetal cases, respectively. The VA was localized on the aortic arch between the left CCA and SA in 17 of 18 cases (Figs. 5 and 6) and beyond to the left SA in one case (see case 5 at Fig. 6). In a study of Colombian fetuses, a variation of the arch with four branches—brachiocephalic trunk, left CCA, left VA, and left SA—was founded in 15.7 % of aortic arches [81]. Opposite to previous findings, the left VA sprang directly from the aortic arch between the left CCA and left SA in 7/103 (6.8 %) human fetuses aged from 14 to 30 weeks of gestation [31], as well as in 7 of 131

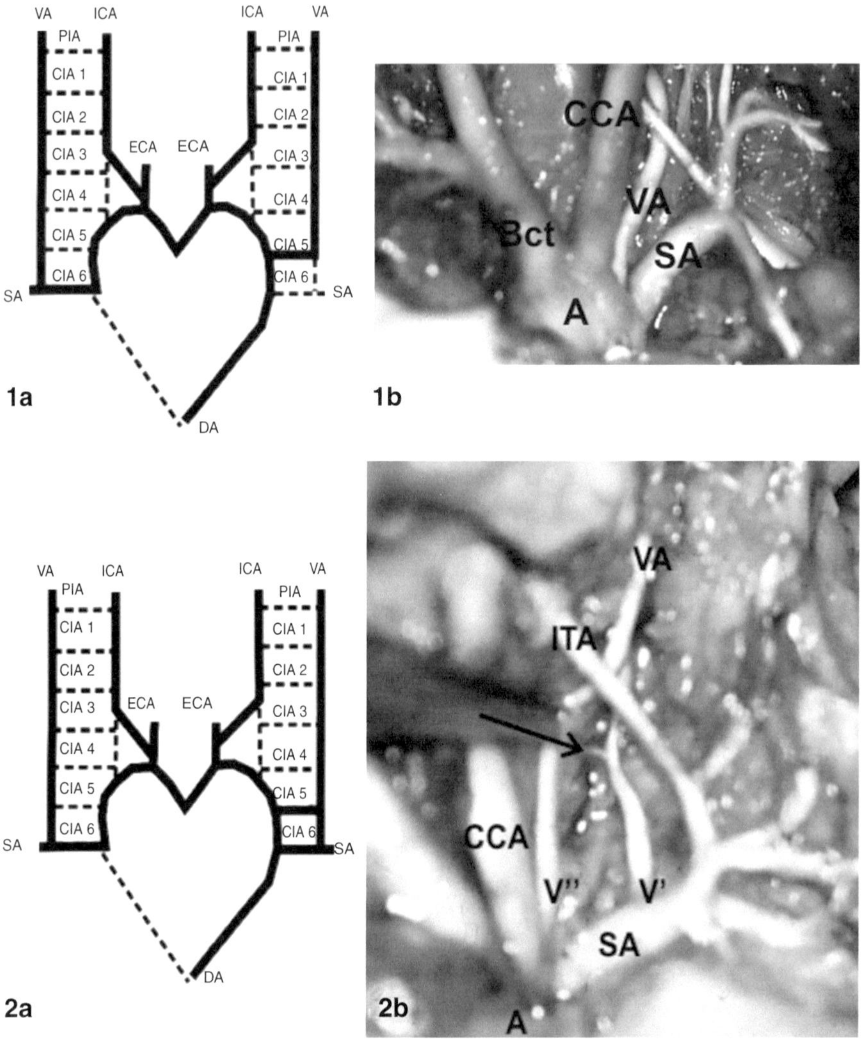

Fig. 5 Aortic origin of the left vertebral artery (*VA*) in two human fetuses [114, 115]. *Case 1a*: Modified scheme of embryonic origin of the VAs [56]. The left VA originating from the aortic arch is caused by a persistence of the 5th cervical intersegmental artery (CIA). *DA* dorsal aorta, *ICA* internal carotid artery, *ECA* external carotid artery, *PIA* primitive proatlantal intersegmental artery. *Case 1b*: Left VA, as a single vessel of aortic (*A*) origin (between left CCA, common carotid artery and left SA, subclavian artery). *Bct* brachiocephalic trunk. *Case 2a*: Modified scheme of embryonic origin of the VAs [56]. Segmental duplication of the left VA is caused by a persistence of the 5th and 6th cervical intersegmental arteries (CIAs). *Case 2b*: Dual vessels of aortic (V″) and subclavian (V′) origin; these vessels course through V1 part behind the ipsilateral inferior thyroid artery (*ITA*). A collateral branch (→) from V′ vessel is presented

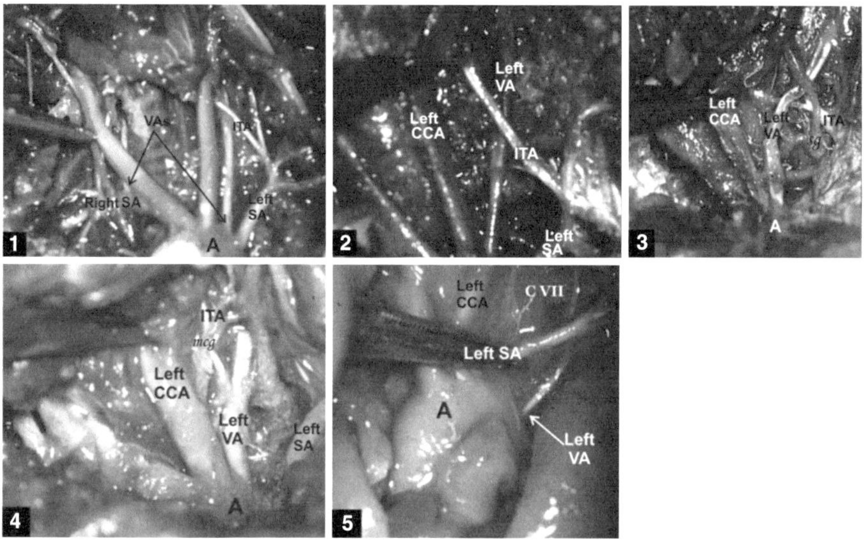

Fig. 6 Five cases of the aortic origin of the left vertebral artery (*VA*) in human fetuses [114, 115]. *Cases 1–2*: Left VAs of aortic (*A*) origin (between the left CCA, common carotid artery, and the left SA, subclavian artery) pass behind the left inferior thyroid artery (*ITA*) in both cases. *Case 3*: Left VA of aortic origin (between the left CCA and left SA) crosses anterior wall of the ipsilateral ITA at the level of the stellate ganglion (*sg*). *Case 4*: Left VA of aortic origin (between the left CCA and left SA) is vascular source of the left ITA; it passes through the middle cervical ganglion (*mcg*). *Case 5*: Left VA of aortic origin (behind to the left SA) passes in front of the CVII vertebra to the CVI foramen transversarium [115]

(5.34 %) human fetuses aged from 15 to 34 weeks [103]. Similar incidence is proved in adults; a beginning of the left VA from the aortic arch arose between the origins of the left CCA, and SA was noted in 6/104 subjects (54 Black African and 50 European subjects) aged 20 years and older, respectively [4]. Eighty-six (4.2 %) in series of 2,033 patients (between 3 months and 94 years) had a left VA originating directly from the aortic arch proximal to the left SA, except the one case where it was distal to the left SA [70]. However, digital subtraction angiographies belonged to 447 male and 186 female Greek patients aged 19 years and older revealed the left VA on the aortic arch between the left CCA and left SA in 0.79 % of cases [72].

Literature case reports showed an aortic origin of the left VA (between the left CCA and left SA) simultaneous with the ipsilateral aplasia of ICA in a 21-year-old male with subdural hematoma [128], as well as the beginning of the left VA from the aortic arch beyond the left SA in a 6-year-old boy with small perimembranous ventricular septal defect [102].

Oppido et al. [80] disclosed a right aortic arch with four separate branches—right CCA, right VA, right SA, and aberrant left SA—in a newborn girl with tetralogy of Fallot and DiGeorge syndrome. Felsont and Strife [27] presented an unusual literature case of the left VA origin from the cervical aortic arch (between the left CCA and left SA) in a 3.5-year-old boy.

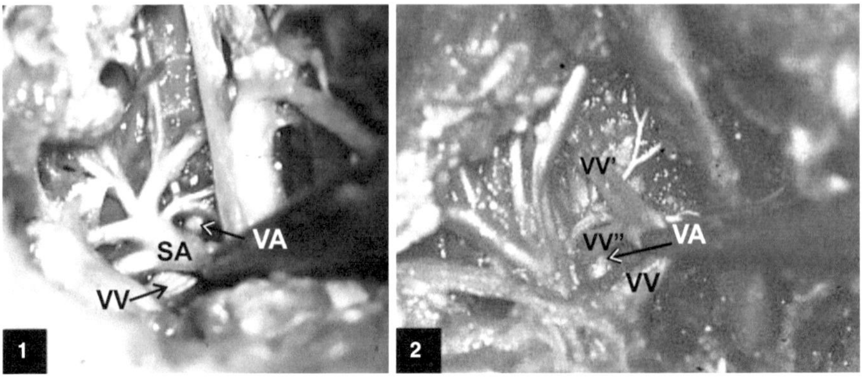

Fig. 7 Single (*case 1*) and dual (*case 2*) right vertebral veins (*VV*) at the exit from the transversal canal and their relation with the ipsilateral vertebral artery (*VA*) of the subclavian (*SA*) origin in human fetuses [114]

Both VAs originated separately from the aortic arch, which was narrow from the brachiocephalic trunk to the origin of the patent ductus arteriosus in a 6-day-old male infant [62]. Both VAs showed an anomalous origin in a 13-year-old female patient with ASDL: the right VA arose from the right CCA, whereas the left VA arose from the aortic arch [109]. The aortic origin of both VAs beyond the left SA origin was also shown in a 20-year-old male patient with a spondyloepiphyseal dysplasia [33]. Multidetector CT angiography performed by Oguz et al. [76] in a 7-year-old boy with symptoms of gastroesophageal reflux identified the left VA with two separate origins, from the left CCA and aberrant left SA (beginning from right-sided aortic arch). Segmental duplication of the right VA originating from the ipsilateral SA was proved in one human fetus [114, 116], as well as in an 18-year-old epileptic female [6].

The V1 part of the VA is surrounded by the cervical sympathetic plexus and by two vertebral veins [113]. The diameter of the vertebral vein in adults is variable but usually three times smaller than the VA [4]; however, this difference was not showed at V1 part of fetuses (Fig. 7) [114]. It was noted that 20 % of the cranial outflow of 16 normal babies normally passed down the vertebral veins [18]. In some instances an arteriovenous fistula could be found just below the transverse process of the CVI vertebra, as in a 20-year-old man [98].

Of the vessels examined, 60 % of VAs followed a relatively straight course from their origin to their entry into the foramen transversarium [21]. A tortuosity of the VA in fetal status was found only in one case of its origin from the left SA beginning on the aortic arch, whereas of 42 infants aging from 2.5 to 14 years, 15 infants had tortuosity of the extracranial VA, while 5 infants had bilateral asymmetric underdevelopment of the VA with tortuosity on the right side [125]. The tortuosity and/or compression of the VA can be congenital, muscular (due to compression by the longus colli and scalene), or because of advancing years [113]. So, Jung and Kehr [42] performed a section of the right scalene in a 16-year-old girl with vertigo symptoms in the aim of the VA decompression in the transversal canal from CVI to CIV vertebrae.

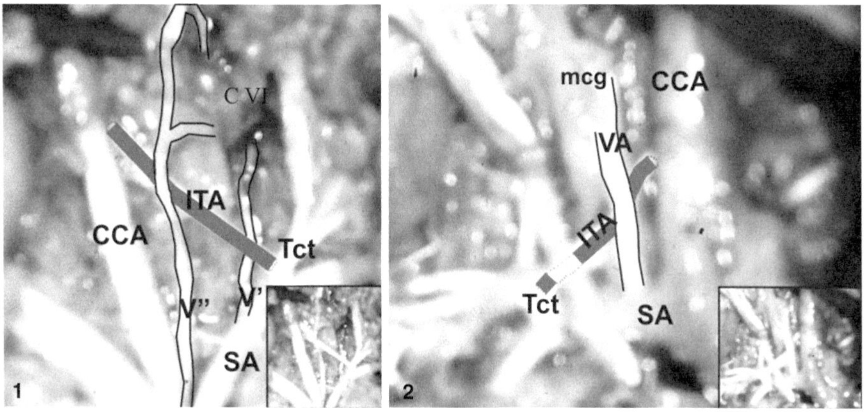

Fig. 8 Relationships between the vertebral (*VA*) and inferior thyroid (*ITA*) arteries [114]. *Case 1*: Vertebral vessel (*V''*) of aortic origin courses in front of the ipsilateral ITA; vertebral vessel (*V'*) of subclavian origin courses behind the ITA. *Insert*: original photo. *CCA* common carotid artery, *SA* subclavian artery, *Tct* thyrocervical trunk, *CVI* sixth cervical vertebra. *Case 2*: Right VA originating from the superior wall of the SA courses in front of the ipsilateral ITA, and through the middle cervical ganglion (*mcg*). *Insert*: original photo

From its origin from the SA, the VA traverses the subclavian triangle, lateral to the longus colli muscle and medial to the scalenus anterior muscle to penetrate the foramen transversarium of CVI vertebra. An anomalous vessel of irregular shape, up to 10 mm in diameter and 4 cm in length, arising from the VA at the level of the CVI transverse process and terminating in the subclavian vein, in a 4.5-year-old boy was defined as a rudimentary accessory SA [50]. Two vertebral vessels from the left CCA and aberrant left SA in a 7-year-old boy united at CVI vertebral level to continue as the single VA and entered the foramen transversarium at the same level [76].

The VA is vulnerable at the V1 part, where it is traversed by fascial bands and skeletal muscles [30]. In relation to the inferior thyroid artery (ITA), the fetal VA was located behind (see Figs. 3 and 5; case 3 at Fig. 4; cases 1–2 at Fig. 5) or in front of it (Fig. 8); however, a rule was not found [114].

Incidences of VA penetration of the foramen transversarium of cervical vertebrae at different levels in prenatal and postnatal status are presented at Fig. 9. Literature data indicated that in slightly over 10 % of subjects, the VA does not enter the foramen transversarium at CVI but at other levels, from CVII to CII, as well as that the entrance is symmetrical in 85 % of cases and asymmetrical in 15 % [32]. Some authors noted that VA penetration of the foramen transversarium at high cervical level was in relation with aortic origin of the VA. However, the left VA, as the last branch of the aortic arch in one fetus, penetrated the foramen transversarium of the ipsilateral CVI vertebra (see case 5 at Fig. 6). In addition, the right VA, as a last branch of the aortic arch distal to the origin of the left VA, coursed behind the trachea and the esophagus and entered the ipsilateral foramen transversarium of the CVII vertebra [33].

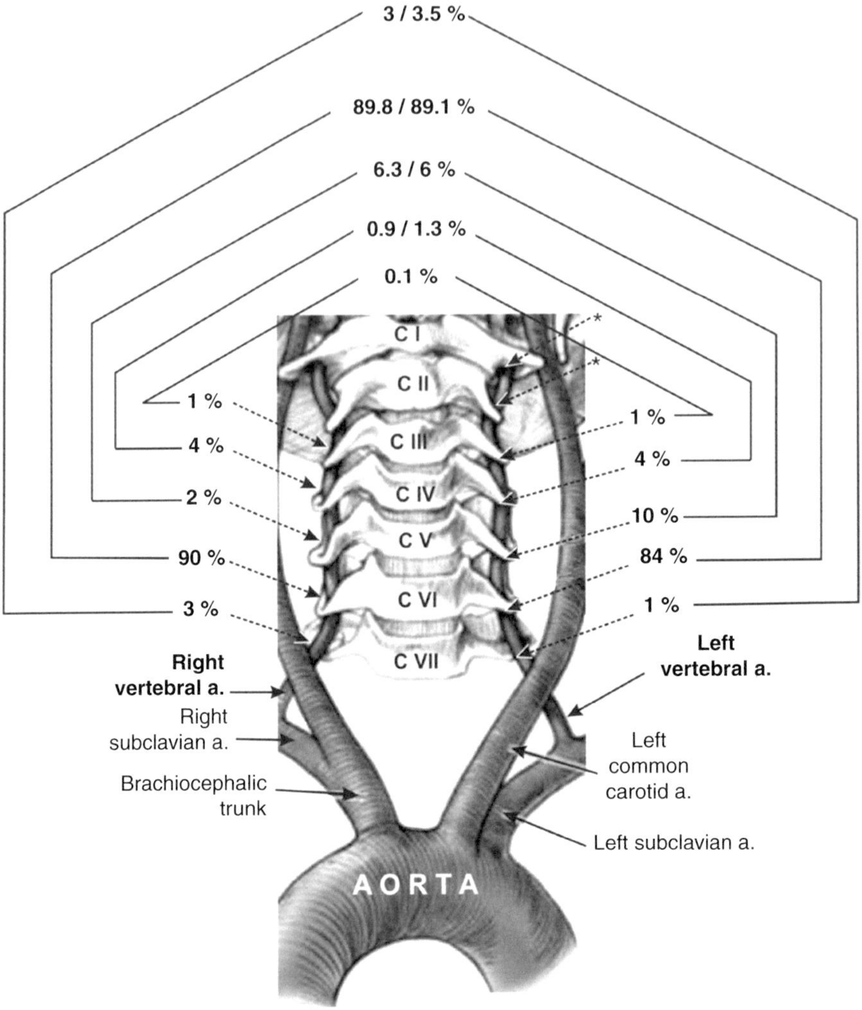

Fig. 9 Possible levels of the entrance in transversal foramina of fetal and adult cervical vertebrae by the vertebral artery (*VA*). Percentiles to the *arrows* relate to the fetal cases [114]; percentiles above the diagram relate to the adult ones [4, 32], respectively

Histology

The wall of the VA, like all human blood vessels, consists of three layers: tunica intima, tunica media, and tunica adventitia; it is a muscular (distributing) artery [43, 67].

The tunica intima of the VA in the newborn is thin, plane, whereas the internal elastic lamina is thicken and uneven. The tunica media consists of single elastic fibers, which are embedded between muscle fibers; its thickness is about 70 μm. The tunica adventitia consists of collagen and single elastic fibers; its thickness is about 100 μm. There is an increase of elastic fibers in the tunica media and adventitia in a 5-month-old infant; the thickness of the media and adventitia is about 100 and 200 μm, respectively. The number of elastic and collagen fibers increases in tunica media until the 15th year of life. The thickness of the tunica media and adventitia is 220 and 200 μm in the 16th year [48].

The adventitia of the VA is fixed at the transverse process of the CVI vertebra, and consequently this anatomical feature prevents injury to the VA from various neck movements [77].

Cervical Part

The cervical (V2) part comprises the segment of the VA that usually extends from the CVI to the CII foramen transversarium.

During the fetal–neonatal period, the cervical vertebrae (CIII–CVI) consist of three independent osseous components: a centrum and two neural arches which are joined to each other by a hyaline cartilage. The CII vertebra (axis) consists of four osseous components: a centrum, two neural arches, and dens. The CVII vertebra may be described as a transitional one; superior articular facets are seen to extend transversely to the top of the transverse processes [14]. The posterior aspect of the foramen transversarium is formed from the neural process; the anterior portion is formed by a vestigial costal element that fuses to the vertebral body, encasing the VA within the foramen [75]. Since a longitudinal anastomosis runs ventral to the 7th costal element in the human embryo, the VA usually does not pass through the foramen transversarium in the CVII vertebra [7]. The VAs ran vertically in the vertebral grooves (later foramina) in four human embryos (45, 50, 53, and 58 days) and in a 77-day-old fetus [19]. At 8 weeks of gestation, the cervical nerves and ventral branches of C2 to C6 lay laterally to the VA; the C4 to C7 nerves give twigs to the VA [75].

If the vascular system is a factor of the canal form through transverse processes of cervical vertebrae during embryonic development, vascular system tolerates an opposite effect and secondary changes caused by deformation of canal walls [22]. Since the CIA is instrumental in the formation of the definitive vertebral body during the stage of resegmentation, any abnormal distribution of the CIAs may induce malformation [108]. In addition, abnormalities in the fusion of CIAs can also contribute to some tortuosity of the VA [21, 113]. Tortuous VAs may have an eccentric position in an enlarged foramen transversarium; the area of this foramen occupied markedly in some patients aged 7 years and older was with a range of 8–85 % [91]. A straight course of the VA is found in 94 % of cadaveric specimens aged 16 years and older [45]. A dolicho left VA running in a short loop toward the midline was visible at angiographic film of an 18-year-old girl [6]. A fenestration of the left VA at the level of CV vertebra in a 19-year-old male was also discovered [49].

The posterior placement of the vertebral foramina in relation to the body of the vertebra increases vulnerability to VA compression by the subluxation of the apophyseal articulation [11]. The distance between the medial borders of the transversal foramina is the greatest at the level of C VI vertebra; it narrows as the VA ascends, and is the narrowest at the level of C III vertebra [82]. In the upper cervical spine, the VA is most vulnerable to compression and stretching, as well as forced lateral flexion, during head rotation. Veleanu (1974) has stressed that the transverse processes of the axis are not ossified in fetuses and newborns, and for this reason during a forced rotation or lateral flexion or extension of head and neck there is the possibility for the compression of the VA. James et al. [39], Pamphlett and Murray [84], and Mitchell [66] also supported the fact that an extreme extension or rotation of the head can occlude one or both VAs. One case involved a 7-year-old boy who sustained a left VA occlusion at the axis level after a chiropractic adjustment, whereas the second one involved a 21-month-old girl who suffered a thalamic stroke due to VA compression as a result of head turning [87]. A significant decrease in the VA blood flow velocities was found with both ipsilateral and contralateral rotation of the cervical spine in healthy adults aged 20 years and older; this significant difference was maintained in the male subjects but with contralateral rotation, only, in the female subjects [66].

An extraspinal system is highly developed in the cervical region, where the VA and the deep cervical and ascending cervical arteries form the most effective longitudinal anastomoses [17]. These anastomoses are proved in fetal cases (Fig. 10), too [114]. Anterior and posterior ascending arteries of the VA originating at the level of CIII vertebra ascend to the dens and meet superiorly to form an apical arcade [101]. This posterior branch of the VA in reality is the anterior meningeal artery or so-called C_3 artery; it anastomoses with ascending pharyngeal collaterals laterally or with occipital or deep cervical artery posterior [55].

Infant pattern of vascularization of the cervical spine is as follows: The cervical arterial anastomoses are built by the segmental arteries of the VAs; the thyrocervical and the costocervical trunks are an additional blood supply especially to the ventral anastomoses. Some decades of nutrient arteries come in the vertebral body from all sides, but only two up to four anterior central branches and two posterior central branches join in the middle of the vertebral body [63]. Generally, anastomoses between intraosseous arteries of the (cervical) vertebrae are widespread in infants and small children; they are less profuse by age 7 years, and atrophy by age 15 years, when the peripheral periostal arteries develop [64].

In fetuses with a crown–rump length of 70 mm, blood vessels can first be demonstrated between the lamellae of the annulus fibrosus; however, these vessels never reach the nucleus pulposus, and following the second year of life, these blood vessels degenerate [88]. At the vertebral margins of intervertebral discs, the capillary network is denser in children. Several vessels penetrate deeply into intervertebral discs of infants, while in adolescence and adult period no such vessels are found.

The VA by its pulsations interferes with the cerebrospinal fluid and the venous blood flow at cervical level. The cervical venous sinuses (epidural, periradicular, periarterial) are very obvious in the fetus and the newborn [123]. MRI of the cervical spine demonstrated the vascular abnormality extended from the CIV to CV level, whereas cerebral panangiography evidenced a direct arteriovenous fistula

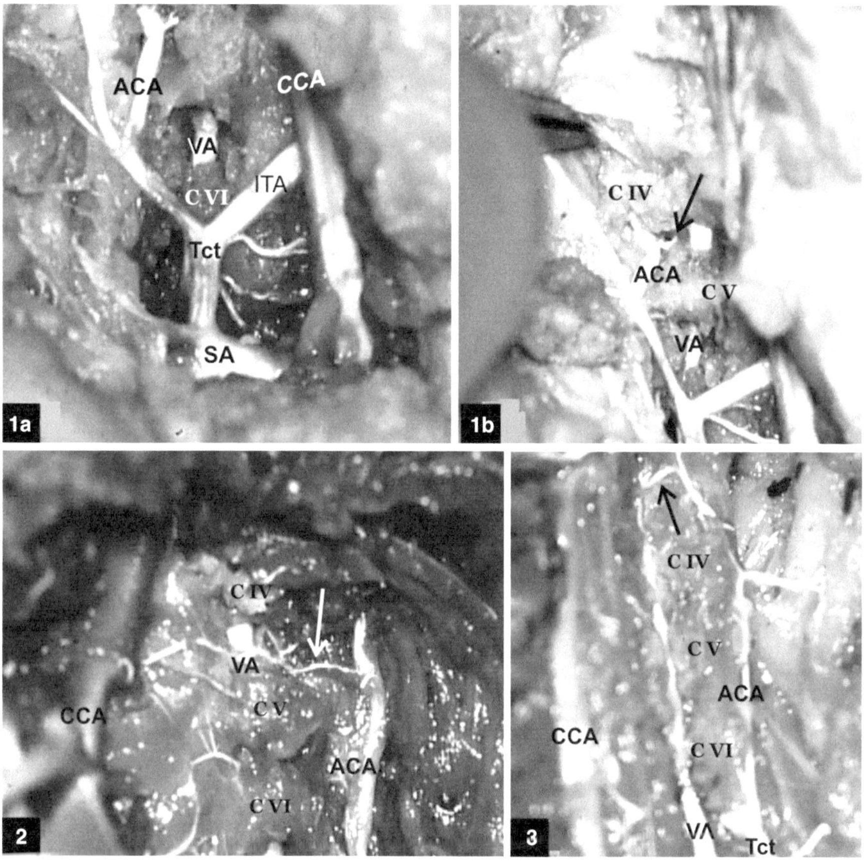

Fig. 10 Levels of anastomoses of branches of the vertebral (*VA*) and ascending cervical (*ACA*) arteries in cervical part (V2) of VAs of human fetuses [114]. *Case 1a*: Right VA, originating from the subclavian artery (*SA*) at the level of the thyrocervical trunk (*Tct*), traverses the CVI foramen transversarium and courses through the V2 part. It anastomoses (*black arrow*) with a branch of the ascending cervical artery (*ACA*) at the level of CIV foramen transversarium (*1b*). *CCA* common carotid artery. *Cases 2–3*: Anastomoses (*white* and *black arrows*) between branches of the left VA and ipsilateral ACA at the level of CV and CIV transversal foramina, respectively

between a radiculomedullary branch of the left VA and the posterior juxtamedullary venous system in a 9-month-old female infant [74].

Histology

A section of extracranial VA from a 9-month-old child shows early intimal thickening and obvious breaks in the internal elastic lamina. Mild degrees of fragmentation were almost universal from the age of 4 years and extent by the age of 20 years [41].

An increase of tensile strength of the VA between the 28th and 40th week is caused by enlarging of the elastin and decrease of the collagen; there are single elastic fibers in the tunica media, as well as collagen fibers of wavy course in the adventitia of newborn [43]. The thickness of the media and adventitia of the VA in 5-month- and 16-month-old children are 80 and 120 and 170 and 180 μ, respectively [48].

Spontaneous dissection of the right VA at the level of CII vertebra was found in a 9-year-old male patient [12].

Atlantic Part

The atlantic part (V3) comprises the segment of the VA that extends from the axis' foramen transversarium to the point of dural penetration at the foramen magnum.

The five curves of the VA were arc-shaped, which were discovered on CT angiographies of patients older than 16 years: the first curve was going through the transversal foramen of the axis, the second was up beside the atlantoaxial joint, the third was going through the transversal foramen of the atlas, the fourth was on the posterior arch of the atlas, and the fifth was going forward to the foramen magnum [23].

During the fetal–neonatal period, the atlas has ossification centers only in the lateral masses and the posterior arch, whereas the anterior arch is completely cartilaginous [14]. In the 3rd month of gestation, the cartilaginous ring of the posterior arch of the atlas is large. A relatively large vessel traverses the cartilage at the level where the arch merges into the lateral mass. The bony nucleus extends from the base of the pedicle beneath the VA (whose lumen is easily seen) and forms a considerable element of the lamina. In the middle of the 5th month, ossification extends outward into the cartilage of the transverse process, in front of which the VA ascends. In the 7th month more than three-fourths of the posterior arch is ossified, and the bony growth in the lateral mass extends in front of the VA [58].

At 27 mm embryo, the ventral branch of the C1 nerve is at first below the VA and then crossed the vessel medially [75]. On the posterior arch of the atlas, the VA lies superior to the suboccipital nerve [113].

A bony ring on the posterior arch or arcuate foramen is observed in atlases of two children's skeletons aged 2 and 4 years, respectively, and also in the x-ray of the cervical spine of a 13-year-old boy [51]. Tubbs et al. [110] noted that the arcuate foramen has been reported with an incidence of 1.14–37 % and that it has been documented in children as young as 2 years old. Paraskevas et al. [85] found that the incidence of incomplete canal for VA is higher in the age of 5–24 years than in older adults. The CVA will be thicker and wider on the left side due to the left VA dominance [90].

Generally, the most vulnerable location for intimal injury of the cervical VA is the point at which the artery exits from the CII foramen transversarium before piercing the atlantooccipital membrane [30, 39, 85]. It is known that in children, the atlantoaxial joints are horizontal and shallow and the ligaments and joint capsules have sufficient elasticity to give increased mobility without disruptions [34]. The cervical muscular tonus of infants, and especially premature infants, is physiologically reduced, which results in poor control of head posture with the possibility of a greater degree of cervical rotation [124]. It was noted that during head rotation or extension conductance in one VA was less than half that of the contralateral artery in 41 % of infants [84]. However, Vanhatalo et al. [112] could not identify any child among 27 infants whose brain stem circulation would be significantly compromised during head turning.

Angiographic images proved that anomalies of the vertebral vessels occur even in cases of malformation of the occipitocervical joint [8] or cervical spine [95]. Four from five patients showing marks of torticollis from infant period had VA anomalies (double vessels that were smaller than normal, multiple loops, and an abnormal route between the atlas and axis) on the side of the hemi-aplasia or hypoplasia of the atlas [24]. Computed tomography angiography performed in a 16-year-old woman with trisomy 21 and abnormalities at the craniovertebral junction (hypoplastic odontoid and ossiculum terminale) showed that right VA bifurcated after exiting the CII foramen transversarium with one branch passing through the CI foramen transversarium, whereas the other turned posteromedially and entered the vertebral canal between the atlas and axis [129]. Similar abnormalities at the level of CII–CIII vertebrae are proved in an 18-year-old girl [24]. The right and left VAs terminated in the posterior inferior cerebellar arteries (PICAs) without filling of the BA in a 6-year-old boy with a history of vertebrobasilar transitory ischemic attacks [28]. A proximal origin of the right PICA from both C_1 and C_2 roots was documented in a 15-year-old boy, as well as a single PICA from the VA at the atlas level in a 20-year-old woman [100].

Kowada et al. [49] revealed fenestration of the left VA at the level of the foramen magnum in a 7-year-old girl, as well as the right VA fenestration at the level of the atlantoaxial junction in a 17-year-old boy.

The fetal VA distributes spinal and muscular branches in the suboccipital region (Fig. 11), as in adults. The precise site of the vertebral–occipital anastomosis is usually considered as a muscular anastomotic channel [54]. There were descriptions of a vertebral–occipital anastomosis on the right side in one fetus [119], as well as 8 bilateral and 20 single (10 on the left and 10 on the right) vertebral–occipital anastomoses with corresponding veins in 15 newborns and a 4-month-old infant [61]. Lateral projection of the right common carotid angiogram showed filling of the VA (and BA) via prominent vertebral–occipital anastomosis in a 6-year-old girl and boy with histiocytoma of the right orbit and brain stem glioma, respectively [96]. An artery located next to the atlas was observed; this was thin-walled aneurysmatic PPIA with a diameter of 8–10 mm and a length of 5–6 mm, extending from the right VA to the occipital artery in a 9-year-old child with a history of vomiting and ataxia [105]. In addition, an anastomosis between prevertebral branches of the ascending pharyngeal artery and muscular branches of the VA occurred inferior to the level of the vertebral–occipital anastomosis in a 12-year-old boy with a small tumor in the pineal region [96].

The VA and its venous plexus in fetuses and newborns have been demonstrated to go in the nearest vicinity to the atlanto-occipital joint; the veins are adhered to the joint, and the common fascial vascular sheath entwines in the fasciae of the oblique muscles, periosteum, and joint capsule [113]. The superior oblique and inferior oblique and rectus capitis posterior major muscles can press vertebral vessels to the joint [130]. The vertebral veins at the suboccipital level deserve mention because of its complexity. Vertebral venous channels receive tributaries from the suboccipital venous plexus,

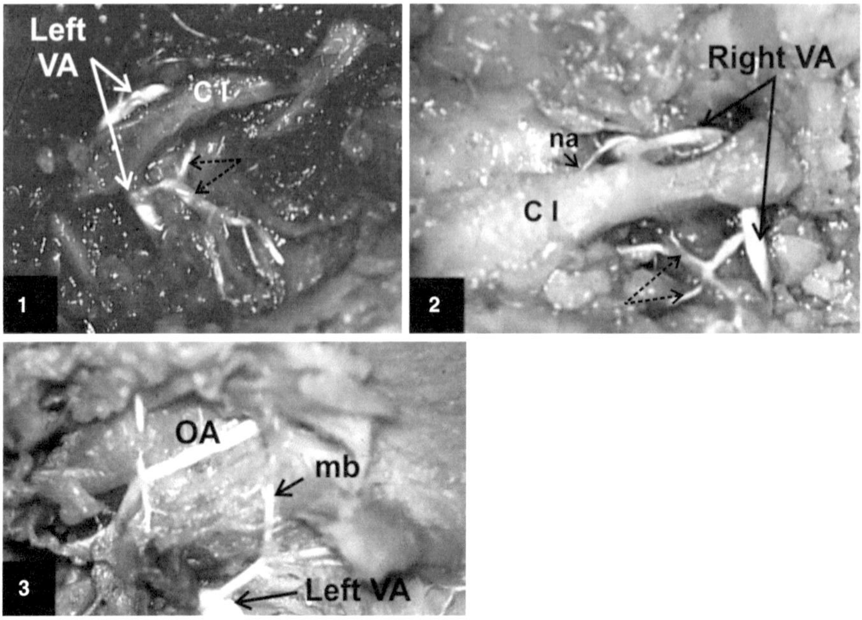

Fig. 11 Atlantic part of the left and right VAs in human fetuses [114]. *Case 1*: Left VA is located on the posterior arch of the atlas (*CI*); distribution of its spinal branch (*black arrows*) at the level of the first cervical intervertebral foramen. *Case 2*: A nutrient artery (*na*) of the left VA for the posterior arch; distribution of VA spinal branch (*black arrows*) at the level of the first cervical intervertebral foramen. *Case 3*: Relation of the left VA muscular branch (*mb*) with the occipital artery (*OA*) in the suboccipital region

from the large profound vein within the posterior cervical muscles, from adjacent vertebrae, and from the internal vertebral plexus via the intervertebral foramina [98].

A special proximity of the VA to the venous plexus predisposes to the development of the arteriovenous fistulas [13]. Left vertebral arteriogram in a 20-month-old boy revealed a high-flow fistula at the level of CI–CII, communicating with the posterior venous plexus, with faint opacification of the VA distal to the fistula [99]. There was a large vertebral arteriovenous malformation just below the foramen magnum with a major supply from the right VA in a 5-year-old boy [35]. Also, there was an efferent vein from the vertebral fistula in the gap between the superior and inferior oblique muscles in a 20-year-old male with diagnosed suboccipital arteriovenous aneurysm [40].

Histology

Mann and Refsauge [60] noted that the composition of the VA varies both among its layers and along its length, probably in response to the different demands along its course.

The tunica intima is the most elastic, being composed of a single layer of endothelial cells and a network of elastic fibers [86]. Results of Charpie et al. [16] showed that human infant VAs (0–2 years) with an intact endothelium did not sustain

Table 1 Values of the vertebral artery (VA) caliber from prenatal to postnatal period

References	Human subjects (age)	Left VA (mm)	Right VA (mm)	Left/right VAs (mm)
Vasović [114]	Human fetuses (17–26 weeks)	0.61	0.53	
Wang et al. [125]	Healthy children (2.5–14 years)			3.45
	Affected children			3.48
Aranđelović-Minić et al. [3]	Healthy male subjects (≥17 years)			4.18
Dodevski et al. [21]	Patients (≥19 years)	3.35	3.19	
Argenson et al. [4]	Black African subjects (≥20 years)	5.30	4.40	
	European subjects (≥21 years)	4.70	4.30	

contractile responses to endothelin-1 and serotonin, i.e., that endothelium-dependent contractions in VAs are attenuated because of an increased prostaglandin activity.

The tunica media contains a few collagen fibers and a smooth muscle that is sparsely interposed with some elastic fibers; the tunica adventitia is comprised mainly of collagen fibers arranged longitudinally in the inner aspect and circumferentially in the external layer [86]. Histological examination of the VA 1 cm proximal and distal to the site of penetration of the dura mater found that the adventitia and media thinned to approximately half the thickness after penetration, but that the thickness of the intima and internal elastic lamina remained unchanged [93].

The adventitia of the VA is fixed at the point of dural penetration, and consequently this anatomical feature prevents injury to the VA from various neck movements [77]. However, a focal VA dissection involving the left atlantic part in a 5-year-old [26] and 12-year-old boys [95] was described.

Caliber

The one measure of constancy is that the size of any given VA changes only gradually along its course [91]. Unilateral segmental narrowing of the VA was found in 12 % of the cadavers aged 16 years and older [45].

David et al. [19] described that diameters of VAs were "asymmetric" in four human embryos (45, 50, 53, and 58 days) and in a 77-day-old fetus. In selected 95 cases of a single vertebral trunk in fetuses, both VAs were equaled in 57.9 %, the left and right VAs were larger in 29.4 and 11.7 % of the cases, respectively [114].

Table 1 shows values of average calibers of the VA in prenatal and postnatal period noted by some authors. It could be calculated that the caliber of the VA in adult status up to 19 years is almost seven times larger than in fetal status and eight times after the 19th year.

The concept of a dominating or single VA now appears to be an accepted fact in the anatomic and radiologic literature. In general population, the left VA is dominant in approximately 50 %, the right in 25 %, and two VAs of similar caliber in 25 % of cases [17]. However, the left VA was dominant in 31.2 %, whereas both VAs were of same caliber in 47.9 % of healthy 48 men (conscripts) aged 17–26 years [3]. Opposite to previous finding, the left VA was larger in 46.6 % of the patients aged 19 years and older, whereas the right VA was larger in 30 % of cases [21].

Hypoplasia

Khodadad [47], in his study of PPHA based on 50 dissected fetal brains, described that in 90 % of the specimens, one of the VAs was hypoplastic while the opposite VA was absent or both VAs were hypoplastic. An extreme and relative hypoplasia of the fetal VA was found in 7.1 and 11.5 %, respectively [114].

Postnatal, an extremely small left VA in a 7-week-old infant was associated with a hypoplastic left ICA, mild aortic coarctation, cardiac maldevelopment, and a ductal aneurysm [106]. Six infants from 2 months to 4 years with PHACES syndrome had hypoplastic vertebrobasilar system in three cases, hypoplastic right VA in two cases, and left VA in one case [37].

In up to 15 % of the healthy population, the caliber of one VA is less than 2 mm [17]. However, hypoplasia of the VA was found in 6.67 % of Macedonian subjects (patients) aged 19 years and older [21], as well as a bilateral hypoplasia was found in two cases among 54 African subjects aged 20 years and older [4].

Physiology

Because of the peculiar mode of embryonic formation, the VA has been described as a "hemodynamic solution" rather than a true vessel [10].

Differences in anatomy of the VA and ICA may well reflect in dissimilar flow dynamics between the origins of the carotid and vertebrobasilar circulations [17]. The VA is a high-resistance artery compared to the ICA [11]. Circular collagen fibers of the dura mater and arachnoidea are incorporated in the tunica adventitia of the intracranial VA, giving resistance to the vascular wall [86]. Values for the 50th percentile for the resistance index in the VA were higher at 22–26 weeks' gestational age (0.87) than they were at the beginning of the second trimester (0.85) and at the end (0.75) of gestation [69].

The extracranial VA resists tensile forces, whereas the intracranial section maintains transmitted blood pressure [60]. Tensile strength of the left VA is larger than of the right VA in fetuses and newborns [43]. Pronounced hypoplasia is impressive because the signal amplitude is significantly lower, the flow velocity is reduced, and the flow resistance can be greater than normal [73].

Elmaci et al. [25] presented a case of a 5-years-old girl with a hypoplastic aortic arch and an unusually located coarctation of the aorta, which were associated with reversal blood flow in the left vertebral artery.

Blood flow through the whole brain of the child is 105 ml/100 g/min [15]. Cerebral perfusion rises markedly during the first 2 weeks of life in preterm neonates [46]. An average VA volume of 112.89±47.97 ml/min was measured in healthy infants from 2.5 to 14 years [125]. Although the absolute reduction in the bilateral ICA and VA flow volumes from childhood to adulthood was equal, the proportion of VA flow volume in total cerebral blood flow volume decreased from 31 % at the age of 4 years to 24 % at the age of 18 years [94]. Localized segmental narrowing of the cervical arteries as well as general narrowing and tortuosity of the vessels have an effect on the amount of blood running through them [45]. When blood flow on one side of the VA is temporarily reduced, the opposite side can fill the BA to compensate; thus, consequential symptoms do not occur [125]. The absence of neurological deficit after thrombosis of the VA in 2 of 43 children may be attributed to the younger age group and the possible establishment of an adequate collateral circulation [34].

Conclusion

Some key points of morphofunctional features of the extracranial VA are as follows:

1. Subclavian origin of the VA is more frequent in fetal, as well as in young people, independent from the gender.
2. The caliber of the VA after 19 years of age is almost eight times larger than in fetal status.
3. The incidences of variable VA origins and domination of left or right VA are different from one series of human specimens to another one.
4. Developmental anomalies of the VA, presenting at fetal status or at birth, will not change with age.
5. Anomalous origin and/or variable course of the extracranial VA had little or did not result in clinical symptoms.
6. The true value of discovery of anomalous VA origin is in the diagnostic gain before vascular surgery of supra-aortic arteries.

Proposals for the Future

The aim of this chapter is following (ab)normal developmental changes of the VA only to the age 21 when each human in most European countries becomes full of age.

A relative low number of available papers based on investigation of the VA in young humans will inspire us for future review, which will base on anomalous origins of the VA from literature case reports independent from age. On this manner, singular cases in a "new" group of variable VA origins in prenatal and postnatal status could be compared and classified according to the persistence of corresponding primitive vessels, as well as in relation to the age, the gender, and associated vascular variants and/or pathology.

Acknowledgment This work is supported by Ministry of Science and Technological Development of the Republic of Serbia (contract grant number: 175092).

References

1. Abe K, Suzuki T (1964) Persistence of embryonic carotid–vertebrobasilar anastomoses. Folia Psychiatr Neurol Japonica 18:257–276
2. Achiron R, Zimand S, Hegesh J, Lipitz S, Zalel Y, Rotstein Z (2002) Fetal aortic arch measurements between 14 and 38 weeks' gestation: in-utero ultrasonographic study. Ultrasound Obstet Gynecol 15:226–230
3. Aranđelović-Minić G, Vasović L, Marković N, Rakočević R (1996) Mikroanatomska i Doppler studija u istraživanju vertebralnih arterija. In: Abstract book of the IVth Congress of neurologists of Yugoslavia. Prosveta, Niš, p 48 (In Serbian)
4. Argenson C, Francke JP, Sylla S, Dintimille H, Papasian S, di Marino V (1980) The vertebral arteries (segments V1 and V2). Anat Clin 2:29–41
5. Atay Y, Engin C, Posacioglu H, Ozyurek R, Ozcan C, Yagdi T, Ayik F, Alayunt EA (2006) Surgical approaches to the aberrant right subclavian artery. Tex Heart Inst J 33:477–481
6. Babin E, Haller M (1974) Correlation between bony radiological signs and dolichoarterial loops of the cervical vertebral artery. Neuroradiology 7:15–17
7. Barry A (1951) The aortic arch derivatives in the human adult. Anat Rec 111:221–238
8. Bernini FP, Elefante R, Smaltino F, Tedeschi G (1969) Angiographic study on the vertebral artery in cases of deformities of the occipitocervical joint. AJR Am J Roentgenol 107: 526–529
9. Borenstein M, Minekawa R, Zidere V, Nikolaides KH, Allan LD (2010) Aberrant right subclavian artery at 16 to 23+6 weeks of gestation: a marker for chromosomal abnormality. Ultrasound Obstet Gynecol 36:548–552
10. Burger IM, Siclari F, Greggb L, Gailloud P (2007) Bilateral segmental agenesis of the vertebrobasilar junction: developmental and angiographic anatomy. AJNR Am J Neuroradiol 28:2017–2022
11. Cairney J (1925) The anomalous right subclavian artery considered in the light of recent findings in arterial development; with a note on two cases of an unusual relation of the innominate artery to the trachea. J Anat 59:265–296
12. Camacho A, Villarejo A, de Aragón AM, Simón R, Mateos F (2001) Spontaneous carotid and vertebral artery dissection in children. Pediatr Neurol 25:250–253
13. Carney AL (1981) Vertebral artery surgery: historical development, basic concepts of brain hemodynamics, and clinical experience of 102 cases. Adv Neurol 30:249–282
14. Castelana C, Kósa F (1999) Morphology of the cervical vertebrae in the fetal-neonatal human skeleton. J Anat 194:147–152
15. Cerebral blood flow and metabolism (2012) http://www.neurosurg.cam.ac.uk/pages/brainphys/02-Cerebral_blood_flow.pdf
16. Charpie JR, Schreur KD, Papadopoulos SM, Webb RC (1994) Endothelium dependency of contractile activity differs in infant and adult vertebral arteries. J Clin Invest 93:1339–1343
17. Cloud GC, Markus HS (2003) Diagnosis and management of vertebral artery stenosis. QJM 96:27–54
18. Cross KW, Dear PRF, Hathorn MKS, Hyams A, Kerslake DMK, Milligan DWA, Rahilly PM, Stothers JK (1979) An estimation of intracranial blood flow in the new-born infant. J Physiol 289:329–345
19. David KM, McLachlan JC, Aron JF, Whiten SC, Smart SD, Thorogood PV, Crockard HA (1998) Cartilaginous development of the human craniovertebral junction as visualized by a new three-dimensional computer technique. J Anat 192:269–277
20. Development of the circulatory system (2012) http://www.slideserve.com/galya/development-of-the-circulatory-system
21. Dodevski A, Lazareska M, Tosovska-Lazarova D, Zhivadinovik J, Aliji V (2011) Morphological characteristics of the first part of the vertebral artery. Prilozi 32:173–188 (In FYROM)

22. Drozdova MM (1968) K voprosu o stroenii kanala poperečnih otrostkov šeĭnih pozvonkov. Arh Anat Gist Embriol 55:16–21 (In Russian)
23. Duan SY, Lu SM, Feng YE, Ling QC, Chen LB (2009) Three-dimensional CT angiography study on the relations between the vertebral artery and atlantoaxial joint. Chin Med J 122:917–920
24. Dubousset J (1986) Torticollis in children caused by congenital anomalies of the atlas. J Bone Joint Surg Am 68:178–188
25. Elmaci TT, Onursal E, Aydoan U, Dindar A (2000) Congenital subclavian aortic steal syndrome: hypoplastic aortic arch with severe coarctation of the aorta of unusual location. Ann Thorac Surg 70:291–292
26. Fan TW, Tang KW, Chan KF, Wu SP (2003) Vertebral artery dissection in a 5-year-old child: serial magnetic resonance angiography appearance. J Hong Kong Coll Radiol 6:158–161
27. Felsont B, Strife JL (1989) Cervical aortic arch: a commentary. Semin Roentgenol 24: 114–120
28. Fraser RAR, Zimbler SM (1975) Hindbrain stroke in children caused by extracranial vertebral artery trauma. Stroke 6:153–159
29. Fujimoto K (1996) 'Medial defects' in the prenatal human cerebral arteries. An electron microscopic study. Stroke 27:706–708
30. Ganesan V, Chong WK, Cox TC, Chawda SJ, Prengler M, Kirkham FJ (2002) Posterior circulation stroke in childhood. Risk factors and recurrence. Neurology 59:1552–1556
31. Gielecki JS, Wilk R, Syc B, Musiał-Kopiejka M, Piwowarczyk-Nowak A (2004) Digital-image analysis of the aortic arch's development and its variations. Folia Morphol 63: 449–454
32. Giuffrè R, Sherkat S (2000) Maldevelopmental pathology of the vertebral artery in infancy and childhood. Childs Nerv Syst 16:627–632
33. Goray VB, Joshia AR, Garga A, Merchanta S, Yadava B, Maheshwaria P (2005) Aortic arch variation: a unique case with anomalous origin of both vertebral arteries as additional branches of the aortic arch distal to left subclavian artery AJNR Am J Neuroradiol 26:93–95
34. Govender S, Kumar KPS (2002) Staged reduction and stabilisation in chronic atlantoaxial rotatory fixation. J Bone Joint Surg Br 84-B:727–731
35. Greenberg J (1970) Spontaneous arteriovenous malformations in the cervical area. J Neurol Neurosurg Psychiatry 33:303–309
36. Gupta M, Gupta R, Seith A (2010) Persistent primitive hypoglossal artery associated with Chiari II malformation: diagnosis and clinical implications. Indian J Radiol Imaging [serial online] 20:258–260
37. Heyer GL, Dowling MM, Licht DJ, Tay SK-H, Morel K, Garzon MC, Meyers P (2008) The cerebral vasculopathy of PHACES syndrome. Stroke 39:308–316
38. Hoh BL, Rabinov JD, Pryor JC, Hirsch JA, Dooling EC, Ogilyv CS (2004) Persistent nonfused segments of the basilar artery: longitudinal versus axial nonfusion. AJNR Am J Neuroradiol 25:1194–1196
39. James CA, Glasier CM, Angtuaco EE (1995) Altered vertebrobasilar flow in children: angiographic, MR, and MR angiographic findings. AJNR Am J Neuroradiol 16:1689–1695
40. Jefferson G, Bailey RA, Kerr AS (1956) Suboccipital arteriovenous aneurysms of the vertebral artery. J Bone Joint Surg Br 38B:114–127
41. Johnson CP, Baugh R, Wilson CA, Burns J (2001) Age related changes in the tunica media of the vertebral artery: implications for the assessment of vessels injured by trauma. J Clin Pathol 54:139–145
42. Jung A, Kehr P (1968) Syndrome de l'artère vertébrale et syndrome des scalènes. J Chir (Paris) 95:437–456
43. Kalmin OV (1995) Deformativno-pročnostie svoĭstva pozvonočnoĭ i obščeĭ sonnoĭ arteriĭ plodov i novoroždennih deteĭ. Morfologia 108:25–29 (In Russian)
44. Kandelĭ EI, Saribekian AS (1978) Sočetanie persistiruiuščeĭ primitivnoĭ trigeminalĭnoĭ arterii s anevrizmoĭ sredneĭ mozgovoĭ arterii. Vopr Neĭrohir 2:50–52 (In Russian)

45. Kauppila LI, Penttila A (1994) Postmortem angiographic study of degenerative vascular changes in arteries supplying the cervicobrachial region. Ann Rheum Dis 53:94–99
46. Kehrer M, Blumenstock G, Ehehalt S, Goelz R, Poets C, Schönin M (2005) Development of cerebral blood flow volume in preterm neonates during the first two weeks of life. Pediatr Res 58:927–930
47. Khodadad G (1977) Persistent hypoglossal artery in the fetus. Acta Anat 99:477–481
48. Korneev GI (1969) Vozrastnie izmenenĭa magistralnih arteriĭ šei. Arh Anat Gist Embriol 9:89–92 (In Russian)
49. Kowada M, Yamaguchi K, Takahashi H (1972) Fenestration of the vertebral artery with a review of 23 cases in Japan. Radiology 103:343–346
50. Kunc Z, Bret J (1976) Persisting embryonal arterial communication between vertebral artery and subclavian vein. J Neurosurg 44:632–637
51. Lamberty BGH, Živanović S (1973) The retro-articular vertebral artery ring of the atlas and its significance. Acta Anat 85:113–122
52. Lang J (2001) Skull base and related structures: atlas of clinical anatomy, 2nd edn. Schattauer, Sttutgart, pp 24–25
53. Lansing AM, Murphy J (1968) Origin of the left subclavian artery from the pulmonary artery with congenital subclavian steal. Surgical implications in cyanotic patients. Ann Thorac Surg 5:146–152
54. Lasjaunias P, Theron J, Moret J (1978) The occipital artery. Anatomy – normal arteriographic aspects – embryological significance. Neuroradiology 15:31–37
55. Lasjaunias P, Moret J, Theron J (1978) The so-called anterior meningeal artery of the cervical vertebral artery. Neuroradiology 17:51–55
56. Lie TA (1972) Congenital malformations of the carotid and vertebral arterial systems, including persistent anastomoses. In: Vinken PJ, Bruyn GW (eds) Handbook of clinical neurology, vol 12. North Holland, Amsterdam
57. Loukas M, Louis RG Jr, Gaspard J, Fudalej M, Tubbs RS, Merbs W (2006) A retrotracheal right subclavian artery in association with a vertebral artery and thyroidea ima. Folia Morphol 65:236–241
58. Macalister A (1893) Notes on the development and variations of the atlas. J Anat 27: 519–542
59. Machii M, Becker AE (1997) Morphologic features of the normal aortic arch in neonates, infants, and children pertinent to growth. Ann Thorac Surg 64:511–515
60. Mann T, Refsauge KM (2001) Causes of complications from cervical spine manipulation. Aust J Physiother 47:255–266
61. Mansone AJ (1988) Hirurgičeskaĭa anatomiĭa anastomičeskoĭ vetvi meždu zatiločnoĭ i pozvonočnoĭ arteriĭami. Arh Anat Gist Embriol 7:38–41 (In Russian)
62. Mart CR, Kaza AK (2011) Left subclavian artery stenosis in neonatal coarctation: diagnosis and treatment. J Clin Exp Cardiol 2:3. http://www.omicsonline.org/2155-9880/2155-9880-2-126.pdf
63. Menck J, Lierse W (1990) The arterial supply of the cervical vertebral body in newborns. In: Abstract. Acta Anat (Basel) 137:165–169 (In German)
64. Mendonça RA (2009) Spinal infection and inflammatory disorders. In: Atlas SW (ed) Magnetic resonance imaging of the brain and spine, 4th edn. Lippincott Williams & Wilkins, Philadelphia
65. Menezes AH (2008) Craniocervical developmental anatomy and its implications. Childs Nerv Syst 24:1109–1122
66. Mitchell JA (2003) Changes in vertebral artery blood flow following normal rotation of the cervical spine. J Manipulative Physiol Ther 26:347–351
67. Mitchell JA (2004) An investigation of an autonomic innervation of the vertebral artery using monoamine histofluorescence. Eur J Histochem 48:115–120
68. Miyake N, Hayashi S, Kawase T, Cho BH, Murakami G, Fujimiya M, Kitano H (2010) Fetal anatomy of the human carotid sheath and structures in and around it. Anat Rec 293: 438–445

69. Morales-Roselló J (2002) Doppler sonography of normal fetal vertebral and internal carotid arteries during pregnancy. J Clin Ultrasound 30:257–263
70. Müller M, Schmitz BL, Pauls S, Schick M, Röhrer S, Kapapa T, Schlötzer W (2011) Variations of the aortic arch – a study on the most common branching patterns. Acta Radiol 52:738–742
71. Napoli C, Witztum JL, de Nigris F, Palumbo G, D'Armiento FP, Palinski W (1999) Intracranial arteries of human fetuses are more resistant to hypercholesterolemia-induced fatty streak formation than extracranial arteries. Circulation 99:2003–2010
72. Natsis IK, Tsitouridis AI, Didagelos VM, Fillipidis AA, Vlasis GK, Tsikaras DP (2009) Anatomical variations in the branches of the human aortic arch in 633 angiographies: clinical significance and literature review. Surg Radiol Anat 31:319–323
73. Nicolau C, Gilabert R, Chamorro A, Vázquez F, Bargalló N, Brú C (2000) Doppler sonography of the intertransverse segment of the vertebral artery. J Ultrasound Med 19:47–53
74. Núñez F, Martínez-Costa C, Soler F, Guijarro-Martínez R, Castelló ML, Brines J (2010) Arteriovenous fistula of the vertebral artery in a female infant with hypotonia and cephalocorporal disproportion. Acta Paediatr 99:1434–1436
75. O'Rahilly R, Muller F, Meyer DB (1983) The human vertebral column at the end of the embryonic period proper 2. The occipitocervical region. J Anat 136:181–195
76. Oguz B, Yigit AE, Oguz KK, Haliloglu M (2010) MDCT angiography of right-sided aortic arch with aberrant left subclavian artery and duplicated left vertebral artery. Int J Anat Variat 3:15–18
77. Ohata K, Goto T (2011) Vertebral artery management in craniovertebral junction surgery. In: Goel A, Cacciola F (eds) The craniovertebral junction: diagnosis, pathology, surgical techniques. Georg Thieme Verlag, Stuttgart
78. Okumura A, Lee T, Shimojima K, Hisata K, Shoji H, Takanashi J, Yamamoto T, Shimizu T, Barkovich AJ (2009) Brainstem disconnection associated with nodular heterotopia and proatlantal arteries. In: Abstract. AJMG Am J Med Genet 149A:2479–2483
79. Onizuka M, Kazekawa K, Tsutsumi M, Kodama T, Aikawa H, Ikou M, Tomokiyo M, Matsubara S, Nii K, Tanaka A (2006) Hyperform remodeling balloon for the balloon occlusion test of persistent primitive trigeminal artery aneurysm—case report. Neurol Med Chir (Tokyo) 46:541–543
80. Oppido G, Napoleone CP, Gabbieri D, Giardini A, Formigari R, Martin-Suarez S, Picchio FM, Gargiulo G (2005) Left common carotid artery isolation in a newborn with tetralogy of Fallot and DiGeorge syndrome. Circulation 111:e4–e5
81. Oviedo JDR (2009) Variations in number of branches of aortic arch in Colombian fetus. Repletion with polyester resin. http://www.anato.cl/global/5-angiologia/5c-cor/5cHgt00002/5cHgt00002.pdf
82. Özgen S, Pait TG, Çağlar YS (2004) The V2 segment of the vertebral artery and its branches. J Neurosurg Spine 1(3):299–305
83. Padget DH (1954) Designation of the embryonic intersegmental arteries in reference to the vertebral artery and subclavian stem. Anat Rec 119:349–356
84. Pamphlett R, Murray N (1996) Vulnerability of the infant brain stem to ischemia: a possible cause of sudden infant death syndrome. J Child Neurol 11:181–184
85. Paraskevas G, Papaziogas B, Tsonidis C, Kapetanos G (2005) Gross morphology of the bridges over the vertebral artery groove on the atlas. Surg Radiol Anat 27:129–136
86. Piffer CR, Zorzetto NL (1980) Microscopy anatomy of the vertebral artery in the suboccipital and intracranial segments. Anat Anz 147:382–388
87. Plaugher G, Alcanatara J (1997) Adjusting the pediatric spine. Top Clin Chiropr 4:59–69
88. Prescher A (1998) Anatomy and pathology of the aging spine. Eur J Radiol 27:181–195
89. Purkayastha S, Gupta AK, Varma R, Kapilamoorthy TR (2005) Proatlantal intersegmental arteries of external carotid artery origin associated with Galen's vein malformation. AJNR Am J Neuroradiol 26:2378–2383
90. Ravichandran D, Shanthi KC, Srinivasan V (2011) Vertebral artery groove in the atlas and its clinical significance. J Clin Diagnostic Res 5:542–545

91. Saneli PC, Tong S, Gilberto Gonzalez R, Eskey CJ (2002) Normal variation of vertebral artery on CT angiography and its implications for diagnosis of acquired pathology. J Comput Assist Tomogr 26:462–470
92. Sartor K, Freckman N, Böker D-K (1980) Related anomalies of origin of left vertebral and left thyroid arteries. Neuroradiology 19:27–30
93. Sato T, Sasaki T, Suzuki K, Matsumoto M, Kodama N, Hiraiwa K (2004) Histological study of the normal vertebral artery. Etiology of dissecting aneurysms. Neurol Med Chir (Tokyo) 44:629–636
94. Schöning M, Hartig B (1996) Age dependence of total cerebral blood flow volume from childhood to adulthood. J Cereb Blood Flow Metab 16:827–833
95. Sedney CL, Rosen CL (2011) Cervical abnormalities causing vertebral artery dissection in children. Report of 2 cases. J Neurosurg Pediatr 7:272–275
96. Seeger JF, Gabrielsen TO, Latchaw RE (1974) Some technique-dependent patterns of collateral flow during cerebral angiography. Neuroradiology 8:149–155
97. Sharatt GP, Leanage R, Monro JL, Shinebourne EA (1979) Aortic arch interruption presenting with absence of all limb pulses. Arch Dis Child 54:49–53
98. Sher MH, Meyer NI, Lenhardt HR, Trummer MJ (1966) Arteriovenous fistula involving the vertebral artery: report of three cases. Ann Surg 163:408–413
99. Shownkeen H, Bova D, Chenelle AG, Origitano TC (2003) Pediatric congenital vertebral artery arteriovenous malformation. Pediatr Radiol 33:354–356
100. Siclari F, Burger IM, Fasel JHD, Gailoud P (2007) Developmental anatomy of the distal vertebral artery in relationship to variants of the posterior and lateral spinal arterial systems. AJNR Am J Neuroradiol 28:1185–1190
101. Singh AP (2011) Development and blood supply of odontoid. http://boneandspine.com/category/spine/cervical-spine/
102. Son JS, Hong KB, Chung DCW (2008) Pseudocoarctation of the aorta associated with the anomalous origin of the left vertebral artery: a case report. Korean J Radiol 9:283–285
103. Szpinda M, Flisiński P, Elminowska-Wenda G, Flisiński M, Krakowiak-Sarnowska E (2005) The variability and morphometry of the brachiocephalic trunk in human fetuses. Folia Morphol 64:309–314
104. Szpinda M, Flisiński P, Szwesta A, Wiśniewski M, Dombek M, Krakowiak-Sarnowska E (2008) Quantitative morphology of the left subclavian artery in human fetuses. Adv Med Sci 53:69–75
105. Tahta K, Akkurt C, Bertan V (1990) A pro-atlantal intersegmental artery between the vertebral and occipital arteries. Turk Neurosurg 1:171–173
106. Taintor AR, Juern AM, Drolet BA (2010) A 7-week-old infant with a large facial haemangioma. http://www.medscape.com/viewarticle/715477
107. Takemura A, Okuda H, Oda K, Fang YR, Hsieh HM, Ohta Y (1990) A case of the right subclavian artery as the last branch of the aortic arch in the human fetus and a new classification on these variations. In: Abstract. Kaibogaku Zasshi 65:374–380 (In Japanese)
108. Tanaka T, Uhthoff HK (1981) The pathogenesis of congenital vertebral malformations. A study based on observations made in 11 human embryos and fetuses. Acta Orthop Scand 52:413–425
109. Tsai I-C, Lee T, Chen M-C, Lin P-C, Chen CC-C (2007) Vertebral and carotid artery anomalies in patients with aberrant right subclavian arteries. Pediatr Radiol 37:1007–1012
110. Tubbs RS, Shoja MM, Shokouhi G, Farahani RM, Loukas M, Oakes WJ (2007) Simultaneous lateral and posterior ponticles resulting in the formation of a vertebral artery tunnel of the atlas: case report and review of the literature. Folia Neuropathol 45:43–46
111. Ultrasonic analysis of the anatomical relationships between vertebral arteries and internal jugular veins in children (2012). http://scienceindex.com/stories/2111093/Ultrasonic_analysis_of_the_anatomical_relationships_between_vertebral_arteries_and_internal_jugular_veins_in_children.html
112. Vanhatalo S, Nikolajev K, Kiekara O, Seuri R, Riikonen R (2003) Vertebral artery insufficiency as a possible mechanism for sudden infant death – in vivo evidence does not support findings from postmortem studies. Brain Dev 25:322–325

113. Vasiljević B, Gojnić M, Maglajlić-Đukić S, Antonović S (2010) Normalne vrednosti brzine cerebralnog vaskularnog protoka kod novorođenčadi [In Serbian]. Srp Arh Celok Lek 138:186–191
114. Vasović L (1986) Varijacije vanlobanjskog dela kičmene arterije – put, odnosi i grane. Master thesis, Faculty of Medicine, Niš (In Serbian)
115. Vasović L (1990) Morfološke karakteristike moždanog arterijskog prstena kod različitog porekla kičmenih arterija. Doctoral thesis, Faculty of Medicine, Niš (In Serbian)
116. Vasović LP (2004) Reevaluation of the morphological parameters according to 11 different duplications of the fetal vertebral artery at prevertebral (V1) and intracranial (V4) parts. Cells Tissues Organs 176:195–204
117. Vasović L, Arsić S, Vlajković S, Zdravković D (2004) Morphological aspect of the thyroid ima artery in human fetuses. Int J Anat Embryol 109:189–197
118. Vasović L, Milenković Z, Jovanović I, Čukuranović R, Jovanović P, Stefanović I (2008) Hypoglossal artery: a review of normal and pathological features. Neurosurg Rev 31: 385–395
119. Vasović L, Mojsilović M, Anđelković Z, Jovanović I, Arsić S, Vlajković S, Milenković Z (2009) Proatlantal intersegmental artery: a review of normal and pathological features. Childs Nerv Syst 25:411–421
120. Vasović L, Arsić S, Vlajković S, Jovanović I, Jovanović P, Ugrenović S, Anđelković Z (2010) Otic artery: a review of normal and pathological features. Med Sci Monit 16:RA101–RA109
121. Vasović L, Jovanović I, Ugrenović S, Vlajković S, Jovanović P, Stojanović V (2012) Trigeminal artery: a review of normal and pathological features. Childs Nerv Syst 28:33–46
122. Veleanu C (1974) Der Sperrmechanismus der Halswirbelsäule beim Foetus und Neugeborenen in Vergleich zum erwachsenen Menschen. Anat Anz Bd 136:401–405
123. Veleanu C, Barzu S, Milos A, Badulescu F (1974) Aspects of ontogenetic evolution of the osteo-vasculo-nervous space relationships at the height of the cervical intervertebral canal in man. Anat Anz Bd 136:412–416
124. Vogelberg C, Taut-Sack H, Friebel D, Maier U, Rupprecht E (2004) Bradycardia and hypoxaemia due to position-dependent hypoperfusion of the brain stem in a preterm infant. Acta Paediatr 93:275–282
125. Wang Y, Cai A, Liu L, Wang Y (2009) Sonographic diagnosis of congenital variations of the extracranial vertebral artery and assessment of its circulation. J Ultrasound Med 28: 1481–1486
126. Weon Y-C, Chung J-I, Kim H-J, Byun H (2005) Agenesis of bilateral internal carotid arteries and posterior fossa abnormality in a patient with facial capillary hemangioma: presumed incomplete phenotypic expression of PHACE syndrome. AJNR Am J Neuroradiol 26: 2635–2639
127. Westaby S, Kendall SWH, Osman-Smith I (1993) Congenital septation of the aortic arch with carotid stenosis. Ann Thorac Surg 56:550–552
128. Wiedner F, Schreyer H (1976) Seltene Anomalien zerebraler Gefäβe (einseitige Aplasie der A. carotis interna, Persistenz der A. Hypoglossica). Fortschr Röntgenstr 124:245–249
129. Yamazaki M, Okawa A, Aramomi M, Hashimoto M, Masaki Y, Koda M (2004) Fenestration of vertebral artery at the craniovertebral junction in Down syndrome: a case report. In: Abstract. Spine 29:E551–E555
130. Zaĭceva RL, Čudnovskiĭ NA (1983) Osobenosti topografo-anatomičeskih vzaimootnošenii pozvonočnoĭ arterii, mišc, soedinitelĭno-tkanih i nervnih obrazovanii v oblasti atlantozatiločnogo sustava [In Russian]. Arh Anat Gist Embriol 84:23–29
131. Zaidi Z (2012) The aortic arches. http://www.google.rs/search?q=%28ppt%29%20aortic%20arches&ie=utf-8&oe=utf-8&aq=t&rls=org.mozilla:en-US:official&client=firefox-a&source=hp&channel=np
132. Zlotnik EI, Gitkina LS (1963) Sindrom prehodĭaščeĭ vertebro-bazilĭarnoĭ nedostatočnosti pri lateralĭnom smeščenii ustĭa pozvonočnoĭ arterii. Vopr Neĭrohir 1:44–46 (In Russian)

Imaging of the Craniovertebral Junction Anomalies in Children

Matylda Machnowska and Charles Raybaud

Contents

M. Machnowska, MD, FRCPC
Division of Neuroradiology, Sunnybrook Health Sciences Centre,
University of Toronto, 2075 Bayview Avenue,
Toronto, ON M4N3M5, Canada
e-mail: mmachnowska@gmail.com

C. Raybaud, MD, FRCPC (✉)
Division of Neuroradiology, Hospital for Sick Children,
University of Toronto, 555 University Avenue,
Toronto, ON M5G1X8, Canada
e-mail: charles.raybaud@sickkids.ca

C. Di Rocco, N. Akalan (eds.), *Pediatric Craniovertebral Junction Diseases*,
Advances and Technical Standards in Neurosurgery 40,
DOI 10.1007/978-3-319-01065-6_4,

Abstract The craniovertebral junction (CVJ) is interposed between the unsegmented skull and the segmented spine; it is functionally unique as it allows the complex motion of the head. Because of its unique anatomy, numerous craniometric indices have been devised. Because of its complex embryology, different from that of the adjacent skull and spine, it is commonly the seat of malformations. Because of the mobility of the head, and its relative weight, the craniovertebral junction is vulnerable to trauma. Like the rest of the axial skeleton, it may be affected by many varieties of dysplasia. In addition, the bony craniovertebral junction contains the neural craniovertebral junction and its surrounding CSF: any bony instability or loss of the normal anatomic relationships may therefore compromise the neural axis. In addition, the obstruction of the meningeal spaces at this level can compromise the normal dynamics of the CSF and result in hydrocephalus and/or syringohydromyelia. To image the CVJ, plain X-rays are essentially useless. MR is optimal in depicting the soft tissues (including the neural axis) and the joints, as well as the bone itself. CT still may be important to better demonstrate the bony abnormalities.

Keywords Imaging • Craniovertebral junction • Malformations • Inflammation • Trauma

Imaging of the craniovertebral junction in children requires alternate considerations from imaging of this region in adults due to the normal anatomic features, unique to infants and children, of ligamentous laxity and hypermobility and the specific subset of congenital and genetic abnormalities that present in the pediatric age group [6, 7]. This chapter will attempt to elucidate current methods in the radiological assessment of the craniovertebral junction including a review of both normal anatomy and radiographic findings in trauma, congenital, developmental, and neoplastic entities.

Embryology

A basic understanding of the embryologic development of the cranial base and craniovertebral junction is helpful when considering pathologies that may subsequently affect this region. The craniovertebral junction, which allows the mobility of the head in relation to the spine, is interposed between the unsegmented sclerotomes of the occipital bone and the sequentially re-segmented sclerotomes of the spine; it presents its own specific pattern of segmentation [94]. Central to this discussion is the fate of the fourth occipital sclerotome, or proatlas, and first two spinal sclerotomes [71]. The proatlas is divided into three parts: the hypocentrum, the centrum, and the neural arch. The hypocentrum forms the anterior tubercle of C1 (while the anterior arch of C1 is formed by the hypocentrum of the first spinal sclerotome). The centrum forms the apical cap of the dens and the apical ligament. The neural arch divides into rostroventral and caudodorsal segments. The anterior margin of the foramen magnum and occipital condyles forms from the rostroventral segment, while the caudodorsal segment gives rise to the lateral atlantal masses and the superior portion of the posterior arch of the atlas. The inferior segment of the posterior arch of the atlas is formed from the neural arch of the first spinal sclerotome. The caudodorsal segment of the neural arch of the proatlas gives rise to the cruciate, transverse, and alar ligaments [23, 71]. The inferior segment of the C1 arch is formed from the neural arch of the first spinal sclerotome, while its centrum gives rise to the dens. The body and posterior arch of the axis are formed from the centrum and neural arch of the second spinal sclerotome, respectively [71].

Anatomy and Craniometry

Normally, the tip of the dens projects to the level of the spinomedullary junction and the spheno-occipital synchondrosis projects to the midportion of the pons. Neural tissue is separated from the osseous walls of the cervicovertebral junction by wide subarachnoid spaces that are maintained by multiple arachnoid trabeculations that attach to the pia and the inner dural layer separating the posterior fossa into cisterns [96]. The spinal cord is attached by the posterior subarachnoid septum (septum posticum), the anterior linea splendens, and the lateral dentate ligaments [94].

The craniovertebral junction is a unique region of the neuromuscular spine in that it lacks intervertebral discs and has horizontally aligned articular facets, facilitating its primary function of providing mobility to the head at the expense of the stability conferred by these structures. The role of stabilizing the craniocervical junction is therefore delegated to ligaments and membranes [23]. The supporting ligaments of the craniovertebral junction can be separated into extrinsic and intrinsic. The *extrinsic ligaments* include the fibroelastic membranes that represent the cranial continuation of the anterior longitudinal ligament, the segment of the ligamentum flavum between the axis and atlas, and the nuchal ligament. The *intrinsic ligaments* from ventral to dorsal include the anterior atlanto-occipital membrane, the alar and apical odontoid ligaments, the cruciate, the accessory atlantoaxial, and the tectorial membrane. The capsular joint ligaments are located in the lateral region of the spinal canal and the posterior atlanto-occipital membrane is located at the posterior aspect of the spinal canal [23].

Numerous radiographic criteria have been established for assessing the relationships of the osseous structures comprising the craniovertebral junction [105]. A detailed review of all of the craniometric indicators of normal anatomy is beyond the scope of this chapter. However, several easily measured lines, angles, and distances, which in our experience are most pertinent to daily clinical practice, will be discussed further.

While many distances and angles can be assessed on a lateral cervical spine radiograph, they are far more easily and accurately demonstrated with cross-sectional imaging methods. Although interpretation of images from any examination of the cervical spine should be performed with three plane reconstruction using CT, and in at least two planes using MRI, most of these measurements can be seen on a single midline sagittal image, with a few requiring assessment in the coronal plane (Figs. 1 and 2).

Measurements seen on the midline sagittal image include Wackenheim's line, Chamberlain's line, McGregor's line, the basal angle, the basion-dens distance, the basion-posterior-axial line interval, and the Powers' ratio. Measurements assessed in the coronal plane include the atlanto-occipital joint axis angle and the widths of the occipital-C1 joints [56, 105]. Wackenheim's clivus baseline is a line drawn along the posterior aspect of the clivus which should fall tangent to the posterior portion of the apex of the dens, irrespective of a flexed, extended, or neutral position. It is useful in assessing congenital or developmental conditions leading to basilar impression or basilar invagination, as any intersection of the line with the dens is abnormal, and in the traumatic setting, particularly if dynamic flexion-extension radiography is required [56, 105, 114] (Fig. 2a).

Chamberlain's line [11] and McGregor's line [66] are drawn from the tip of the hard palate to the opisthion and the lowest point of the occipital squamosal surface respectively (Fig. 2b); projection of the dens 5 mm above Chamberlain's line and 7 mm above McGregor's line is considered abnormal. These lines are useful in determining the degree of basilar impression or invagination. The basal angle can be measured as the intersection of the nasion-tuberculum sellae and tuberculum sellae-basion tangents [105]. The minimum angle is 121° and the maximum 149° (Fig. 2c).

Harris and colleagues defined the normal basion-dens interval (or measurement from the basion to the tip of the dens) on a lateral radiograph of the cervical spine, as less than 12 mm [40, 41] (Fig. 2d). Although this measurement was performed in adults and children over 13 years of age, it is generally used in our clinical practice for evaluation of lateral radiographs as well as midline sagittal cross-sectional images of the cervical spine in younger children. Harris et al. also defined the basion-posterior-axial interval or distance between the basion and a line drawn tangential to the posterior border of the dens as abnormal if more than 12 mm anterior and 0 mm posterior to the posterior axial line in children (12 mm anterior and 4 mm posterior in adults) [41] (Fig. 2d).

The Powers' ratio is defined as the ratio of the distance from the basion to the posterior arch of the atlas and the distance from the opisthion to the anterior arch of the atlas [92] (Fig. 2e). A ratio of greater than 1.0 is considered abnormal. While the Powers' ratio may be used for assessing the presence of anterior atlanto-occipital dissociation in the traumatic setting, it is unable to diagnose the rare posterior variant [56].

In the coronal plane, the tangents drawn parallel to the atlanto-occipital joints should intersect at the center of the odontoid process if the condyles are symmetric (Fig. 2f). The average angle measures between 124° and 127° [113], and a more obtuse angle suggests occipito-condylar hypoplasia.

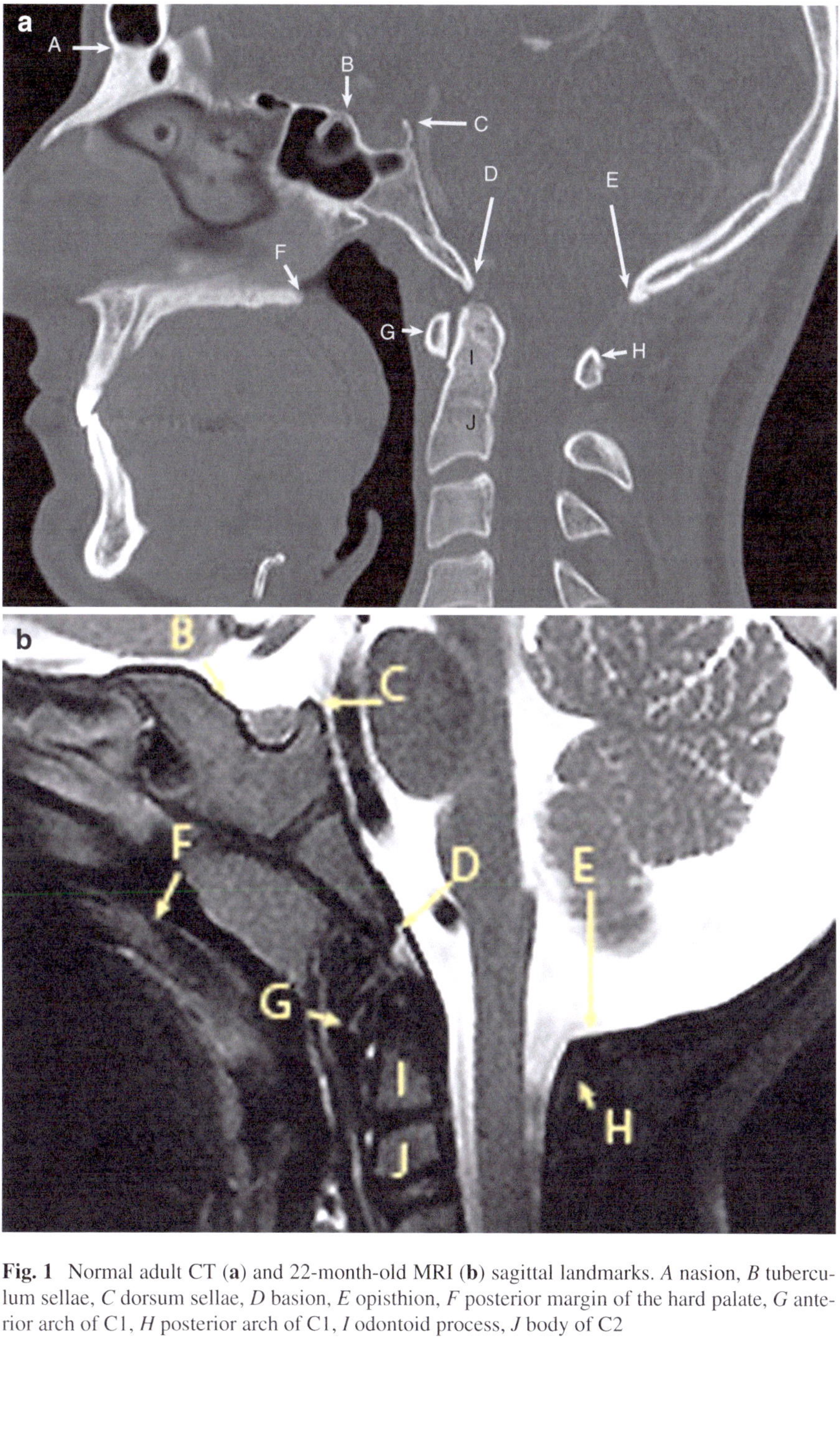

Fig. 1 Normal adult CT (**a**) and 22-month-old MRI (**b**) sagittal landmarks. *A* nasion, *B* tuberculum sellae, *C* dorsum sellae, *D* basion, *E* opisthion, *F* posterior margin of the hard palate, *G* anterior arch of C1, *H* posterior arch of C1, *I* odontoid process, *J* body of C2

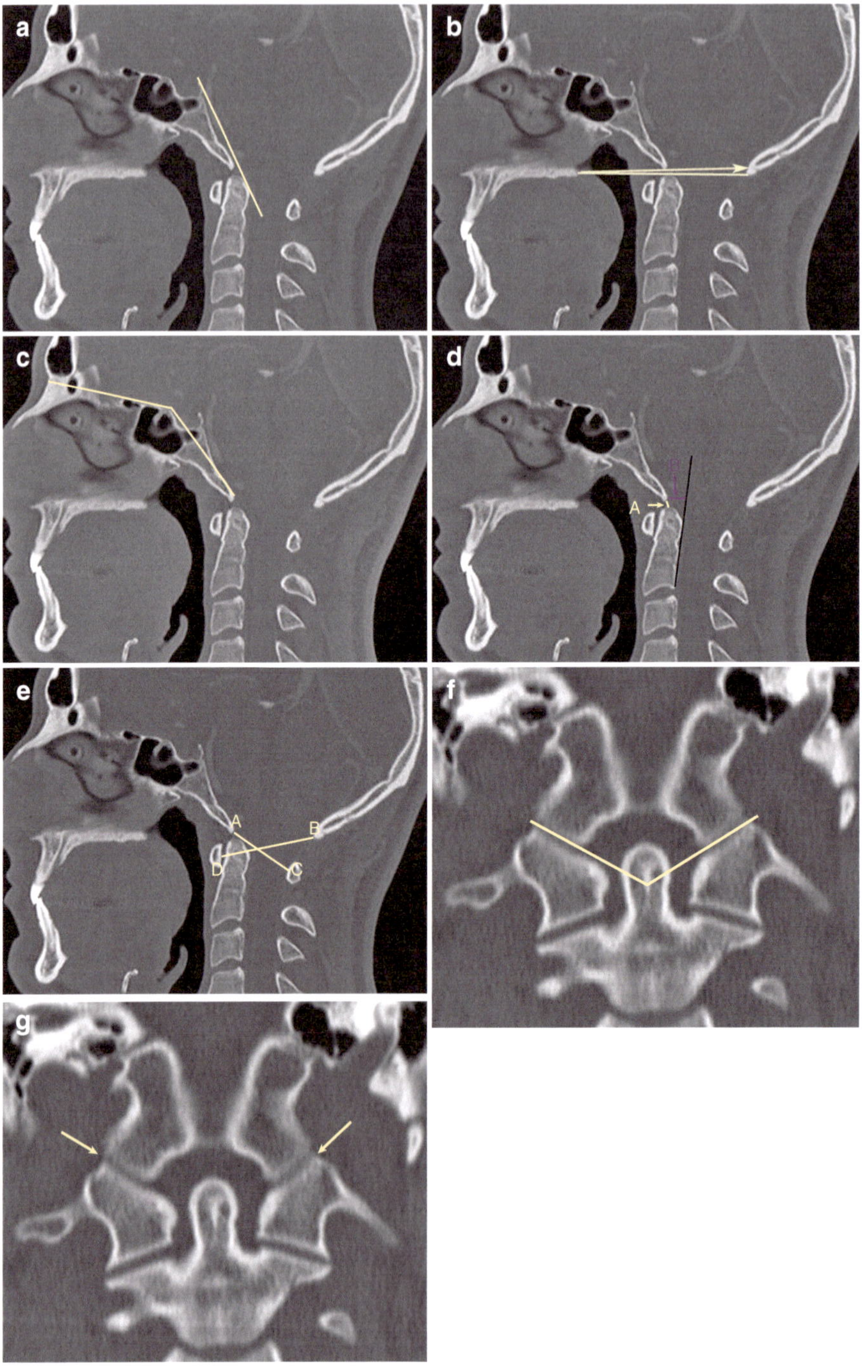

Fig. 2 Normal lines, angles, and interspaces. (**a**) Wackenheim's clivus baseline; (**b**) Chamberlain's line (drawn from the tip of the hard palate to the opisthion); McGregor's line (drawn from the tip of the hard palate to the lowest occipital squamosal surface); (**c**) basal angle (minimum = 121°, maximum = 149°); (**d**) *A*: basion-dens interval (normal is <12 mm); *B*: basion-posterior axial interval (normal is <12 mm); (**e**) Powers' ratio (normal *AC*/*BD* ratio is <1.0); (**f**) atlanto-occipital joint axis angle (normal 124–127°); (**g**) normal occipital-C1 joints (normal joint space is <2 mm)

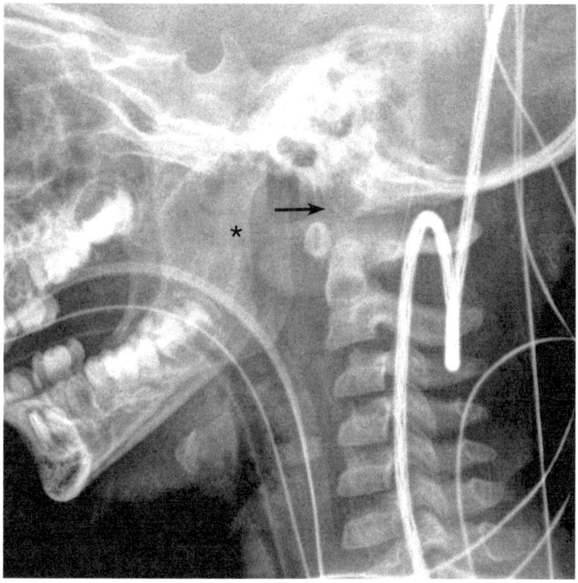

Fig. 3 Atlanto-occipital dislocation. Note the increased basion-dens interval and marked nasopharyngeal soft tissue prominence

Pang and colleagues determined that the widths of the normal occipital-C1 joints should be less than 2 mm and that there is strong left-right symmetry [90, 91] (Fig. 2f). Occipital-C1 joint distances greater than 4 mm were considered strongly suggestive of atlanto-occipital dislocation [91].

Trauma

The four major injury patterns of the pediatric craniocervical junction include longitudinal subluxation with failure of the major unit stabilizers across the occiput-C2 unit more commonly referred to as atlanto-occipital subluxation, translational atlantoaxial subluxation, atlantoaxial rotatory fixation, and fractures [56].

Evaluation of cervical spine trauma typically begins with plain radiographs (Fig. 3). It is important to note, however, that radiographic evaluation has significant limitations and low sensitivity. Woodring and Lee found that "trauma series" cervical spine radiographs including lateral, anteroposterior, and odontoid views failed to detect 61 % of fractures and 36 % of subluxations in a series of adult patients [119]. Therefore, further evaluation with high-resolution CT and MRI in many cases is necessary (Fig. 4).

The drawbacks of CT include poorer evaluation of ligamentous structures. And while the clinical relevance of subtle MRI findings of slightly increased high signal in the transverse or alar ligaments with a normal CT scan is not yet well understood, a study in a pediatric imaging center showed that the use of MR imaging in obtunded patients resulted in decreased time to C-spine clearance with resultant decreased ICU and hospital stays, without a significant increase in diagnosis of injuries [32]. Therefore both CT and MRI are useful adjuncts in the setting of pediatric cervical trauma.

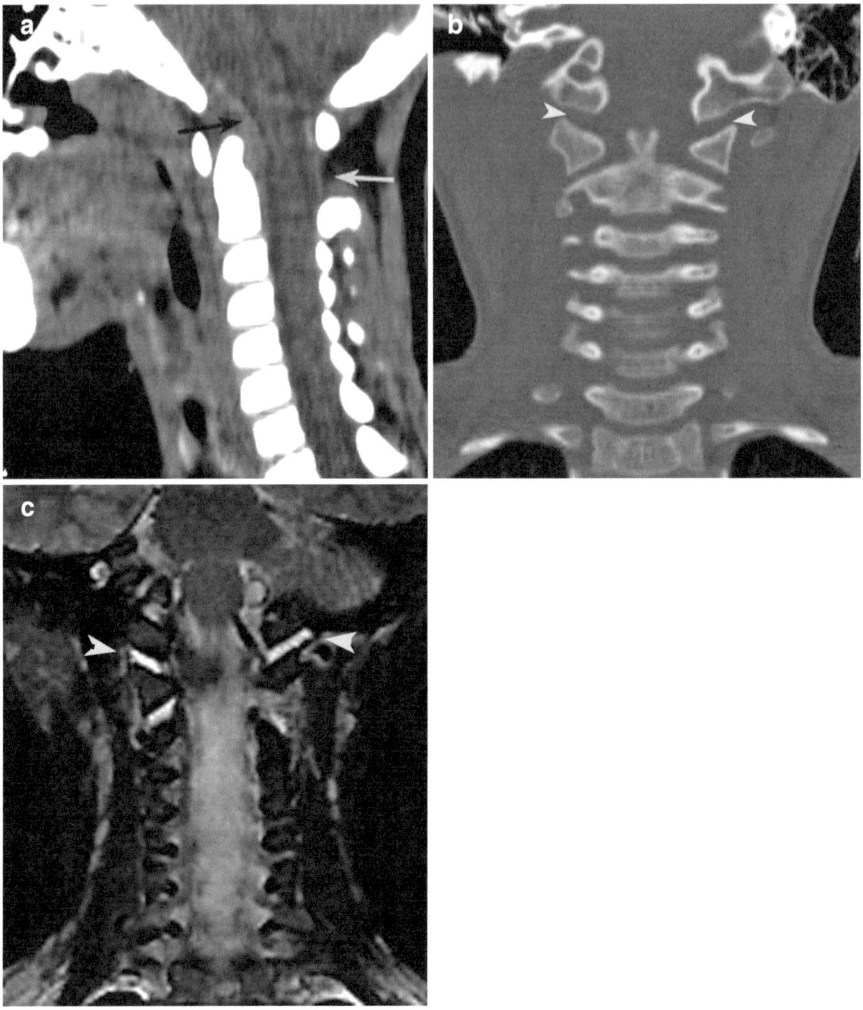

Fig. 4 Atlanto-occipital dislocation. The basion-dens interval in this child was 9 mm (normal <12 mm). However, the midline sagittal CT (**a**) shows a retrodental epidural hematoma (*black arrow*) and an increased posterior interspace between C1 and C2 (*grey arrow*). Coronal CT (**b**) shows bilaterally widened atlanto-occipital joints (*grey arrowheads*) to 4.2 mm (normal <2 mm). Coronal MRI (**c**) confirms injury to the atlanto-occipital joints evidenced by high T2 fluid signal (*grey arrowheads*). Note also the abnormal T2 signal in the visualized right atlantoaxial joint

Atlanto-occipital subluxation results from disruption of the ligaments connecting the occiput to the atlas and axis. It is often a result of high-speed motor vehicle accidents or pedestrian accidents. Children, particularly those younger than ten, are predisposed to this injury due to a greater head weight to body weight ratio and smaller, more horizontally oriented atlanto-occipital joints [56] (Figs. 3 and 4).

In a review of 16 patients aged 3–17 years of age who satisfied one or more known radiographic criteria or presented with well-known clinical and MRI features of atlanto-occipital dissociation, Pang and colleagues compared measurements of the occipital condyle-C1 interval (taking an abnormal value to be greater than 4 mm) with five radiographic criteria including a dens-basion interval of more than 12 mm, a Powers' ratio of greater than 1, Harris' basion-posterior-axial interval of greater than 12 mm or less than 0 mm, and an abnormal Sun's interspinous ratio where the ratio of the interspinous distances between C1–C2 and C2–C3 is greater than 2.5 using high-resolution CT. They found that only the occipital condyle-C1 interval joint distance had a sensitivity and specificity of 100 % for detecting atlanto-occipital dislocations with the sensitivities of the other tests ranging from 25 % for the Sun's interspinous ratio (C1–C2/C2–C3 distance, should be less than 2.5) to 50 % for an abnormal dens-basion interval and false-positive rates ranging from 10 % for the Powers' ratio to 60 % for Sun's interspinous ratio [90, 91] (Fig. 4).

Additional CT and MRI findings of atlanto-occipital dislocation include extra-axial and perimedullary blood, tectorial membrane rupture, alar ligament rupture, blood and edema in between the dens and clivus, blood in the predental soft tissues, edema in the C1–C2 prevertebral fascia, and edema in the posterior soft tissue between the occiput and C2 [90, 91]. Severe cases may result in transection of the brainstem and cervicomedullary junction or acute and delayed hydrocephalus with syringomyelia [74, 95].

Translational atlantoaxial subluxation without fracture occurs due to loss of the transverse ligament resulting in compression of the spinal cord between the odontoid and the posterior arch of the atlas. When traumatic in nature, this usually results from a flexion injury incurred during violent trauma [62]. (Nontraumatic causes due to ligamentous laxity of the transverse ligament or dens hypoplasia include Down syndrome, Klippel-Feil syndrome, and skeletal dysplasias which will be discussed further in the chapter [56].)

Dickman and colleagues differentiated injuries of the transverse ligament into two types with differing clinical consequences. *Type I injuries* disrupt the ligament substance in its midportion (IA) or at its periosteal insertion (IB); these injuries were found to necessitate internal fixation. *Type II injuries* disconnect an intact transverse ligament from the C1 lateral mass involving comminution of the C1 lateral mass (*IIA*) or avulsion of the tubercle from an intact lateral mass (IIB) and had a 74 % recovery rate with nonoperative treatment [24].

An atlantodental distance of greater than 4 mm in children is considered abnormal on plain lateral radiographs [24, 56]. CT allows for detailed evaluation of fractures of the atlas and avulsions of the C1 tubercles. MRI findings of transverse ligament disruption include loss of continuity of the ligament, high-signal intensity in the ligament, or blood separating the ligament from its insertion [24]. Additional imaging features on CT and MRI include widening and edema in the retropharyngeal soft tissues.

Atlantoaxial rotatory subluxation refers to a range of abnormalities involving the atlas and axis from mild abnormalities of rotation to complete fixation. Trauma is responsible for about 30 % of cases and is usually minor [55, 56]. Other causes include head and neck infections, surgery, and neoplasms. Pang and Li have described the normal rotational motion of C1 with respect to C2 [86, 87]. They suggest that atlantoaxial rotatory subluxation is a "stickiness," or resistance to turning of C1 with respect to C2, and therefore cannot be evaluated with a static image alone. They describe the normal physiologic movements of C1 and C2 as follows: crossover of C1 with respect to C2 occurs at O° or with the nose pointing forward, for the first 23° of rotation C1 moves in isolation with respect to C2 mainly due to the horizontal orientation of the C1–C2 facets, and at about 23° of rotation tightening of the alar ligaments results in pull and rotation of the dens, which for the next 42° rotates nonlinearly with respect to C1 approaching its speed. At about 65° away from the neutral position, the two vertebrae rotate in unison [86, 87]. The movements on the right and left side of the head are mirror images of each other. Having described the normal physiology of the atlantoaxial joints, the group went on to develop a four-point system which requires CT imaging in three planes: the plane of rotation most comfortable to the patient, the neutral position in which the head is perpendicular to the CT table, and head rotation as far as possible to the contralateral side. *Grade I injuries* are those which show a locked C1–C2 articulation. *Grade 2 injuries* have reduction of the C1–C2 angle with forced correction, but no crossing of C1 with respect to C2. *Grade 3 injuries* have C1–C2 crossover only when the head is turned far to the opposite side, and not in the expected neutral position. A fourth type of injury shows dynamics in between the range of normal and grade 3 injuries and has been termed the "diagnostic grey zone" [86–88].

A fracture at the craniocervical junction specific to children involves the dens synchondrosis (Fig. 5). This synchondrosis normally fuses by 5–7 years of age but may remain open into adolescence [2]. True fractures will result in an anteriorly displaced and angulated odontoid process with a preserved atlantodental interval [16, 29]. However, nondisplaced fractures of the synchondrosis (odontoid epiphysiolysis) may be difficult to detect. According to one series, nondisplaced fractures occur less than 10 % of the time. The same series showed that 53 % of displaced or nondisplaced odontoid synchondrosis fractures have been shown to be associated with spinal cord injury, usually at the cervicothoracic junction. It is therefore important to reevaluate the synchondrosis for subtle widening on CT in cases of seemingly isolated spinal cord injury [29]. Contributory MRI findings include increased signal in the synchondrosis and prevertebral soft tissue changes at the C1–C2 level (Fig. 5d).

True odontoid adult type fractures may occur in older children [56].

The neurocentral synchondrosis, which closes between 3 and 6 years of age, is another radiologic pitfall, and its presence on oblique radiographs may be misinterpreted as a pars interarticularis or hangman's fracture [65, 78, 107]. Note should be made that true fractures through this synchondrosis have been reported and are analogous to odontoid epiphysiolysis. In one of the cases reported, initial radiographs, CT, and bone scan were attributed to congenital defects with subsequent subluxation at the pedicular level uncovering the underlying fracture [38].

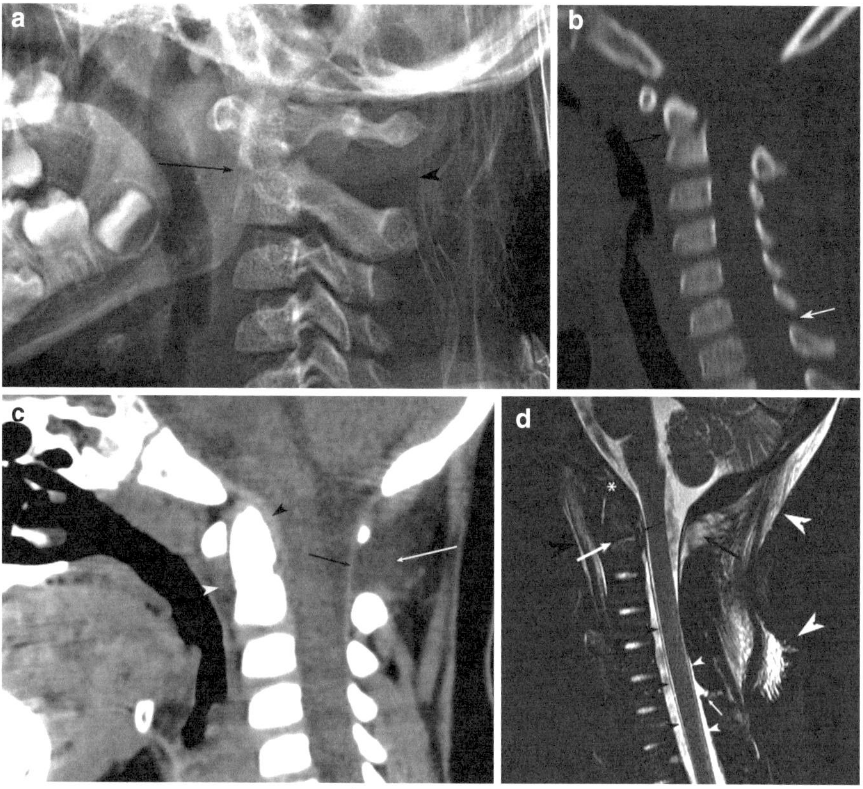

Fig. 5 A 6-year-old male with odontoid synchondrosis fracture. (**a**) Lateral radiograph demonstrates mild widening of the odontoid synchondrosis and of the C1–C2 spinous interspace. (**b**) Sagittal CT image with bone windows just off midline demonstrates angulation at the occipital synchondrosis (*black arrow*); subtle widening of the C5–C6 spinous processes (*grey arrow*). (**c**) Midsagittal CT image with soft tissue windows demonstrates small retrodental epidural hematoma (*black arrowhead*), widening of the spinous processes interspace (*black arrow*), retropharyngeal tissue edema (*grey arrowhead*), posterior soft tissue edema/hematoma (*grey arrow*). (**d**) MRI in the same patient shows the extent of injuries including a synchondrosis fracture and edema (*grey arrow*), C1–C2 interspinous ligament tear (*black arrow*), anterior and posterior soft tissue edema (*large black* and *grey arrowheads* respectively), small retrodental epidural hematoma (*small black arrow*), C5–C6 interspinous ligament tear and suspected dural tear (*small grey arrow*), lifting off of the anterior (*small black arrowheads*) and posterior dura (*small grey arrowheads*), and extensive CSF isointense epidural collection

True fractures of the pars interarticularis are generally classified according to the Effendi classification based on the degree of displacement of the anterior and posterior C2 fragments [26]. Type I fractures are either hairline fractures or have minimal anterior displacement or angulation of the axis. Fractures with greater than 3 mm of anterior translation of C2 with respect to C3 are considered type II. Type III fractures are the rarest and involve a displaced anterior fracture fragment with dislocated or subluxed unilateral or bilateral facet joints [26].

Craniovertebral Junction Bone Anomalies

The subsequently described anomalies of the craniovertebral junction may occur in isolation or as part of congenital syndromes; the latter will be described in greater detail further in the chapter.

Some authors have separated anomalies of the craniovertebral junction into those present at birth and those which, although resulting from an underlying faulty embryology, become symptomatic in childhood or early adulthood. The former group includes entities such as proatlas segmentation failures, congenital basilar impression, basilar invagination, atlas assimilation, condylar hypoplasia, absent components of the atlas, spondylolysis, and segmentation failures resulting in hemivertebrae. The second group includes entities such as acquired basilar impression, rotatory dislocation in the nontraumatic setting, os odontoideum, syndromic abnormalities, and osteogenesis imperfecta [71]. Note should be made of the fact that implied meaning of the terms "basilar invagination" and "basilar impression" has varied in literature, with certain authors reserving the term "basilar impression' for congenital entities and basilar invagination for acquired entities [105] and others differentiating primary or congenital basilar impression from secondary or acquired basilar impression [66, 89].

For the purposes of the following discussion, we will use the term "congenital basilar impression" to define occipital dysplasia which results in a shallow occipital "box" resulting in a drop of posterior fossa contents and an abnormally high position of the vertebral column with respect to the foramen magnum [89]. "Acquired basilar impression" involves similar morphologic abnormalities but is due to softening conditions of the skull base such as osteogenesis imperfecta, hyperparathyroidism, rickets, and Paget's disease [105]. The term "basilar invagination" on the other hand is reserved for the invagination of the opisthion into the cranial aperture, which may occur as a result of the posterior form of congenital basilar impression in which the exoccipital bones are elevated into the foramen magnum, without lordosis or retroflexion of the dens [89].

Congenital abnormalities may be further subdivided into those that involve the central pivot of the craniocervical junction and those that involve the two-ringed structures that surround this pivot, reflecting the previously discussed embryologic fates of the axial and lateral components of the proatlas and first two cervical sclerotome segments. The structures which form the central pillar are the dens, C2 vertebral body, and the clivus which is embryologically and functionally in vertical linearity with the central pillar. As already discussed, these structures arise from the centra of the proatlas and first two cervical sclerotomes. Structures arising from the neural arches of the same sclerotomes, and hypocentra of the proatlas and first cervical sclerotome, develop into the ringed structures surrounding the pivot and include the lateral portion of the clivus, the exoccipital bones and the opisthion, the anterior arches, posterior arches, and lateral masses of the atlantal ring [89]. Malformations of the central pillar include basiocciput hypoplasia, congenital basilar impression, basilar invagination, platybasia, basilar kyphosis, os avis, aplasia or hypoplasia of the dens, retroflexed dens, disturbance of the odontoid synchondroses, and bifid dens. Malformations of the surrounding rings include third

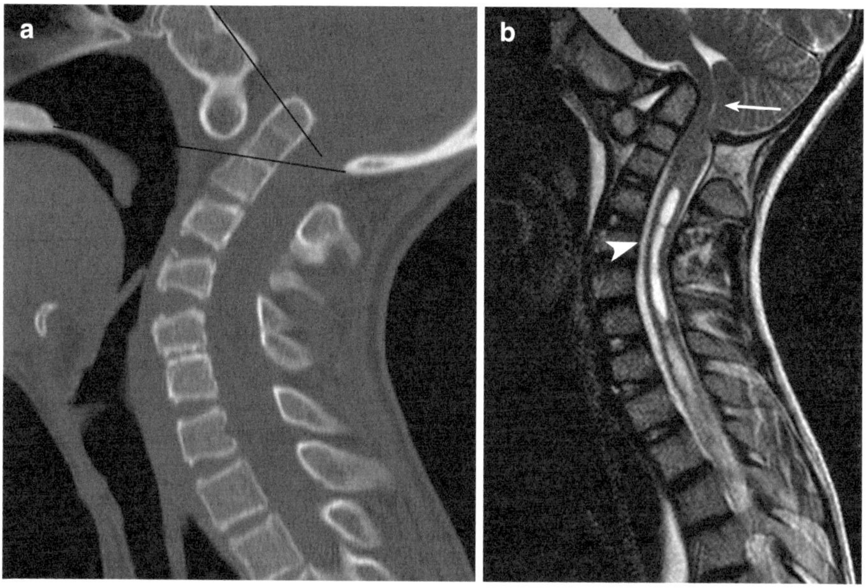

Fig. 6 Midline sagittal CT (**a**) and MRI (**b**) in a 14-year-old male with VACTERL syndrome and congenital basilar impression. The dens projects 18 mm above Chamberlain's line and abnormally intersects Wackenheim's clivus baseline. This results in severe compression of the cervicomedullary junction (*grey arrow*) and cervical syringohydromyelia (*white arrowhead*). There is fusion of the occipital ring to C1. A rudimentary disc space is seen at C5–C6

occipital condyle, preoccipital arch, hyperplasia or hypoplasia of the occipital condyles, atlas assimilation, and aplasia and hypoplasia of the anterior or posterior C1 arches [89]. Appreciating these two ontogenetic categories is helpful in understanding the frequent associations seen between clival and odontoid craniocervical junction abnormalities such as platybasia, basilar kyphosis, retroflexed dens, and cerebellar ectopia, which affect both the clival and odontoid primordia. Note is made of the fact, however, that, as in basioccipital dysplasia which is often associated with occipital condyle hypoplasia, defects of the axial and ring components of the craniocervical junction are not mutually exclusive and not infrequently occur together [89, 105].

The following is a discussion of possible congenital anomalies of the craniocervical junction with reference to this ontogenetic classification.

Basioccipital Dysgenesis

Congenital basilar impression results from hypoplasia of the basiocciput and exocciput with obligatory constriction of the supraoccipital bone, the enchondral growth of which depends on the chondrocranial molds of the other two parts [89]. On imaging studies basilar impression is defined as elevation of the tip of the odontoid 5 mm above Chamberlain's line and 7 mm above McGregor's line (Fig. 6). Because this occipital hypoplasia results in a small posterior fossa, it is often associated with a Chiari I deformity of the cerebellum.

Studies have shown that patients with basilar impression have significantly shorter clivus lengths than control groups [84]. Normally, the basioccipital clivus measures more than 3.2 cm from the spheno-occipital synchondrosis in adults and should terminate at the cervicomedullary junction [84, 89, 94]. *Anterior congenital basilar impression* results from changes in the axial occipital sclerotomes and can lead to platybasia, often accompanied by basiocciput hypoplasia. (As previously described platybasia is defined as flattening of the basal angle to greater than 150°.) This results in elevation of the basion and an upward tilting of the foramen magnum and condyle-atlas articulations. The lordotic deformity of the skull base often results in a compensatory lordotic curve of the dens, which may cause significant impression on the adjacent brainstem (Fig. 6).

Posterior basilar impression involves the elevation of the exoccipital bones with secondary elevation of the dens towards the cranial cavity without retroflexion. It is this type of basilar impression that often results in basilar invagination or the projection of the opisthion into the cranial aperture [89].

Abnormalities of the Dens

The dens forms from the centra of the proatlas and first spinal sclerotome which fuse to the centrum of the second spinal sclerotome [71]. Therefore there are two embryologic dental segments, the apical and basal, both of which may fail to form. The most common variety of dens agenesis is absence of only the apical segment resulting in a short dens, but with adequate support for the cruciate ligament, which prevents instability. On the other hand, agenesis of both dental segments or only the basal segment will result in instability [89]; furthermore, lesions resulting in instability of this region have been associated with irregularities of the vertebral arteries leading to posterior fossa infarcts [4, 76]. Because sporadic congenital defects in the primordia of two centra are unusual, complete agenesis of both dental components results rather from collagenopathy syndromes such as spondyloepiphyseal and spondylometaphyseal dysplasias or mucopolysaccharidoses where there is a failure of ossification rather than of chondrification [89].

The os odontoideum is defined as an independent bone in the place of the dens, cranial to the axis vertebra (Fig. 7). Controversy exists in the literature as to whether the etiology of this condition is traumatic, the result of a non-united odontoid fracture, or developmental [18, 43, 45, 47, 89]. In support of a post-traumatic etiology, in one series of children aged 1–4 years, several cases of os odontoideum were identified in patients who had previously had radiographically documented normal odontoid processes [70]. Proponents of the traumatic theory also suggest that often there is a small bony cupola attached to the base of the dens that is thought to represent the fractured base of the dens [70, 71, 105]. On the other hand, os odontoideum has been identified in families, identical twins, and children with epiphyseal

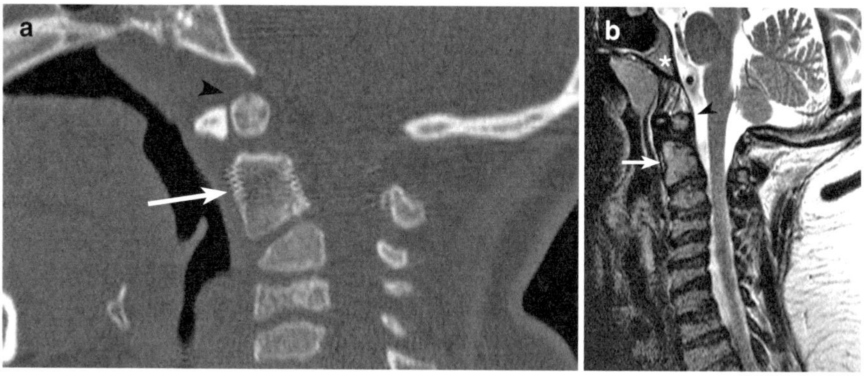

Fig. 7 Os odontoideum in a child with Kniest dysplasia. Midline sagittal CT (**a**) and T2-weighted MRI (**b**) show hypoplasia of the dens (*grey arrows*) and an os odontoideum (*black arrowheads*). There is hypoplasia of the clivus (*white asterisk*). Note also the mild cervical kyphosis centered at C3–C4, platyspondyly, and undulating vertebral body endplates

dysplasias suggesting a developmental nature [53, 77, 80]. Some authors point out that the current literature likely includes a heterogenous group of disorders, arising from both post-traumatic and developmental etiologies, discussed under the umbrella term of os odontoideum [89].

Irrespective of etiology, however, the clinical implications of os odontoidea are similar. Because of the gap between the os and the body of C2, there may be incompetence of the cruciate ligament resulting in atlantoaxial instability. While patients may be asymptomatic, symptoms can occur and range from neck pain, paretic episodes, and brainstem strokes resulting from vertebral artery stretching to compression of the cervicomedullary junction [4, 76, 105, 109].

An abnormality separate from the os odontoideum is the ossiculum terminale, which is felt to represent nonunion of the apical-dental segment derived from the centrum of the proatlas [21, 22]. The abnormality may be misinterpreted as a fracture, although its well corticated border should point to its congenital nature. As there is enough room on the base of the dens for the insertion of the cruciate ligament, instability has only been seen in cases where there is hypoplasia of the basal dental segment [89, 105].

Disturbance of the Craniovertebral Ring Structures

In morphometric studies on 404 occipital condyles, Naderi and colleagues have determined that normal condylar length is 23.4 mm, the normal condylar width is 10.6 mm, and the normal condylar height is 9.2 mm [81].

Hyperplasia of the proatlas hypocentrum is a rare anatomic abnormality which can result in a bony spur that projects obliquely backwards from the occipital bone. This bony spur has the potential of forming synovial joints with the anterior arch of

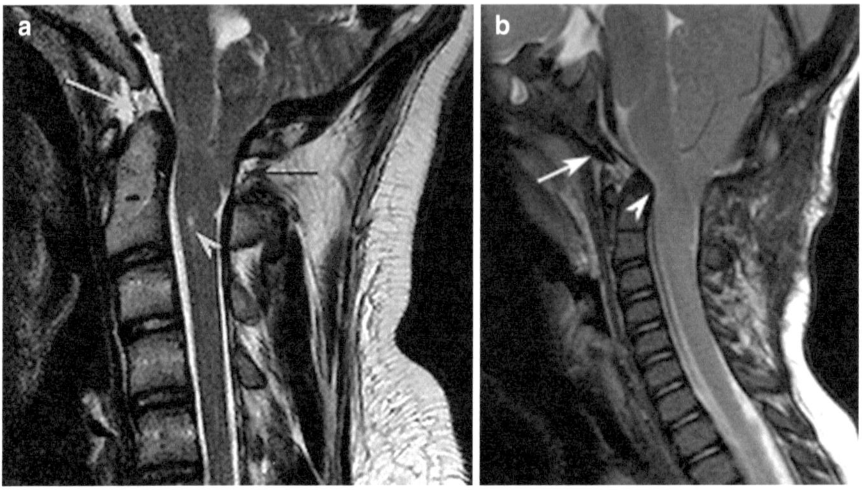

Fig. 8 Chiari I malformation in two different patients. (**a**) Midline sagittal T2-weighted MRI shows cerebellar tonsillar descent to below the level of the posterior C1 arch (*black arrow*) resulting in crowding of structures at the cervicomedullary junction. There is only very minimal retroversion of the dens (*grey arrow*). There is a tiny syrinx of the upper cervical cord (*white arrowhead*). (**b**) Midline sagittal T2-weighted MRI shows cerebellar tonsillar descent to the level of the posterior C1 arch. There is hypoplasia of the clivus (*white arrow*) which terminates at the mid-medullary level and mild retroversion of the odontoid which results in medullary compression and crowding at the foramen magnum

C1 and has therefore been termed the third occipital condyle. There are reports of this abnormality causing significant symptoms resulting from compression and myelopathy at the craniocervical junction [58, 73]. Similarly, hyperplasia of the lateral sclerotome of the proatlas leads to hyperplastic and overgrown occipital condyles. Bilateral hyperplasia of the occipital condyles leads to early symptoms, generally presenting in the first two decades of life [73].

Hypoplasia of the occipital condyles often results in basilar impression and has been discussed in the section describing anomalies of the basiocciput.

Studies have shown that that there is about a 33–39 % association between abnormalities of proatlas segmentation and Chiari I deformity [71, 73] (Fig. 8).

Atlas Anomalies

One of the most common anomalies of the craniocervical junction is assimilation of the atlas, which has been reported to have a prevalence rate of 0.08–2.8 % in the general population [12, 61] (Fig. 6). Assimilation can occur at the site of the anterior or posterior arches or lateral masses, or any combination of the above. While symptoms usually present in adulthood, a recent study of pediatric patients revealed that symptoms can occur in children and range from neck pain, torticollis, and motor and sensory symptoms to incontinence [34]. Assimilation of the atlas has been associated with increase in the atlantodental interval in as many as 57 % of patients [34], fusions of other cervical vertebrae, basilar invagination, os odontoideum, Chiari I deformity, and spinal canal encroachment [3, 28, 34, 68, 69].

Assimilation of the atlas was also associated with failures of the posterior arch of the atlas to form, arising from malformations from the lateral C1 sclerotome. Complete or partial agenesis of the posterior arch of the atlas can also occur in isolation and is ten times more common than abnormalities of the anterior arch, likely due to a developmental failure of chondrogenesis. In general, isolated agenesis or aplasia of the posterior arch does not affect the dental pivot and cruciate ligament and is more stable than its anterior counterpart [89]. However there are several reports of posterior arch anomalies causing a Lhermitte's sign with neck extension, transient quadriparesis, and chronic neck pain [19, 54, 98, 100, 102].

Anomalies of the anterior arch of the atlas are said to be exceedingly rare, with only a few case reports existing in the literature [33, 113]. Much more common than aplasia or hypoplasia of the atlas arches are clefts, with posterior arch clefts occurring 4 % of the time.

Syndromes Affecting the Craniocervical Junction

Numerous syndromes have been associated with abnormalities of the cervical junction. The most common ones include Down syndrome, Chiari type I, Klippel-Feil, osteogenesis imperfecta, Conradi, Goldenhar, the mucopolysaccharidoses, Weaver, achondroplasia, and spondyloepiphyseal dysplasia.

Down Syndrome

Trisomy 21 is the most frequent of chromosomal disorders, occurring in 1:660 live births [51]. The primary abnormalities observed at the craniocervical junction in children with Down syndrome include atlantoaxial and atlanto-occipital instability. Atlantoaxial instability is attributed primarily to the laxity of the transverse ligament, resulting in a widened atlantodental interval of greater than 5 mm, found in about 10–30 % of patients [10, 25, 30, 93]. In addition to the craniometric measurements used to assess atlanto-occipital instability described earlier in the chapter, including the Powers' ratio and the apical-dental interval, one may assess the Wiesel-Rothman ratio. This is a dynamic measurement requiring radiography in both flexion and extension. The distance is measured between two perpendicular lines to the atlantal line, one tangential to the posterior cortex of the anterior arch of the atlas, and the other tangential to the posterior point of the basion. A difference of greater than 1 mm in flexion and extension is considered significant [118]. A recent study found the apical-dental interval and Wiesel-Rothman method to be the most reproducible when assessing atlanto-occipital instability [116]. Using the Wiesel-Rothman method, children with Down syndrome were shown to have a 79 % rate of hypermobility at the occiput-C1 level compared with a 21 % rate among control subjects [63]. A recent study with high-resolution CT of children with greater than 8 mm subluxation on flexion-extension radiographs using the Wiesel-Rothman method proposed a morphometric analysis of the occipitocervical joints that involved measuring the ratio of the depth of the curvature of the superior articular surface of C1 and the length of the joint. It was found that the mean ratio in children with Down syndrome was 0.08 and in aged matched controls was 0.2, suggesting a much shallower joint in patients with Down syndrome [9]. This may suggest that abnormal biomechanics at the joint may lead to capsular ligament instability and further contribute to atlanto-occipital instability in the region, which has been shown to be progressive in children with Down syndrome, necessitating serial radiographic evaluation [9]. Additional abnormalities seen in children with Down syndrome include os odontoideum and odontoid hypoplasia [10, 63, 64, 101].

Chiari I Deformity

Chiari I deformity (or malformation) has classically been described as tonsillar descent below the foramen magnum. Mikulis proposed for criteria for tonsillar ectopia when tonsillar descent extends below the foramen magnum by 6 mm in the first decade and 5 mm in the subsequent two decades [75]. In reality Chiari I deformity may develop or disappear in a given patient, and its development probably depends on a predisposing anatomy (shallow posterior fossa, basilar impression, progressive bony thickening of the skull) associated with the effects of the CSF dynamics across a foramen magnum partly obstructed by the cerebellar tissue. In this way, a Chiari I deformity is pathogenetically different from a Chiari II malformation which, by definition, results from a neural tube defect (commonly a lumbosacral myelomeningocele) and from a Chiari III malformation which is an occipitocervical meningoencephalocele. In the authors' opinion, terms like "Chiari 0" malformation [111] or "Chiari 1.5" malformation [112] are misleading as they suggest that instead of different pathogeneses, the Chiari I, II, III classifications would reflect a degree of tonsillar/brainstem descent. A cervical syringomyelia without a tonsillar malposition ("Chiari 0") [111] should not be called a Chiari malformation at all; a low position of the medulla (obex) associated with the tonsillar malposition ("Chiari 1.5") [112] only reflects the shallowness of the posterior fossa (or the obliquity of the foramen in case of hypoplastic clivus) and therefore should be considered one particular presentation of Chiari I.

Chiari I deformities may be associated with a variety of symptoms including pain, motor and sensory disturbances, and scoliosis [39]. In this chapter, we would specifically like to touch on complex Chiari I deformities associated with osseous abnormalities including a retroflexed odontoid process, basilar impression, and

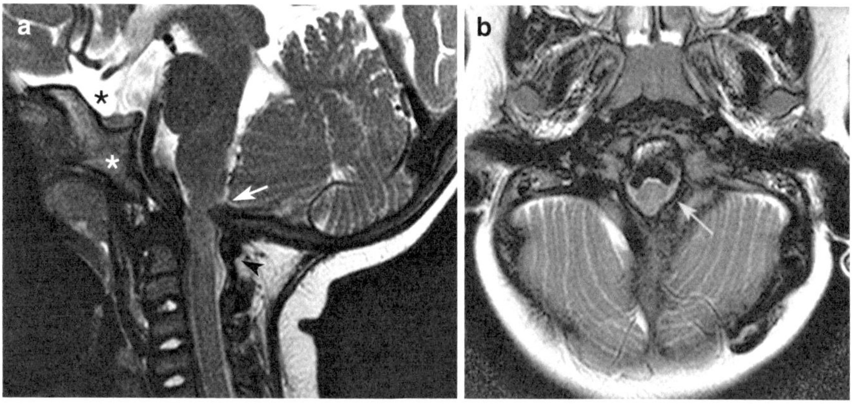

Fig. 9 Achondroplasia. Midline sagittal T2-weighted MRI (**a**) shows the overgrowth of the opisthion (*grey arrow*) and anterior position of the posterior C1 arch (*black arrowhead*), resulting in significant medullary-cord junction compression. There is hypoplasia of the clivus (*white asterisk*) and hydrocephalic prominence of the basilar cisterns (*black asterisk*). (**b**) Axial T2-weighted MRI shows the "teardrop" shape configuration of the foramen magnum

platybasia, seen usually in patients younger than age 2 and associated with ventral brainstem compression [5] (Fig. 8).

Craniometric measurements developed to assess the degree of odontoid retroversion and brainstem compression include the clivoaxial angle [104] and pB-C2 line [37]. The clivoaxial angle is defined as the angle formed by the intersection of Wackenheim's clivus baseline and a line drawn along the posterior aspect of the body of the axis and the odontoid process and should normally range from 150° to 180° [104]. The pB-C2 line is defined as a line drawn perpendicularly (p) to a line drawn from the basion (B) to the inferoposterior aspect of C2, through the odontoid tip to the ventral dura [37]. A pB-C2 line greater than or equal to 9 mm was found to be compatible with brainstem compression.

Tonsillar descent associated with basilar impression, or a clivoaxial angle of <125°, increases the risk of requiring occipitocervical fusion in adjunct to surgical decompression.

Achondroplasia

Achondroplasia results from a point mutation in the fibroblast growth factor receptor 3 gene (*FGFR3*). About 80 % of cases are sporadic, while the mutation has an autosomal dominant inheritance [49]. The classic appearance of the cervical junction is a teardrop configuration of the foramen magnum in the axial plane, resulting from underdevelopment of bones undergoing enchondral ossification and causing compression of the cervicomedullary junction [52, 99, 115] (Fig. 9). Other findings include a horizontalized occiput, prominent basal cisterns, anterior extension of the opisthion, hypoplasia of the basiocciput, and odontoid dysplasia [99] (Fig. 9a).

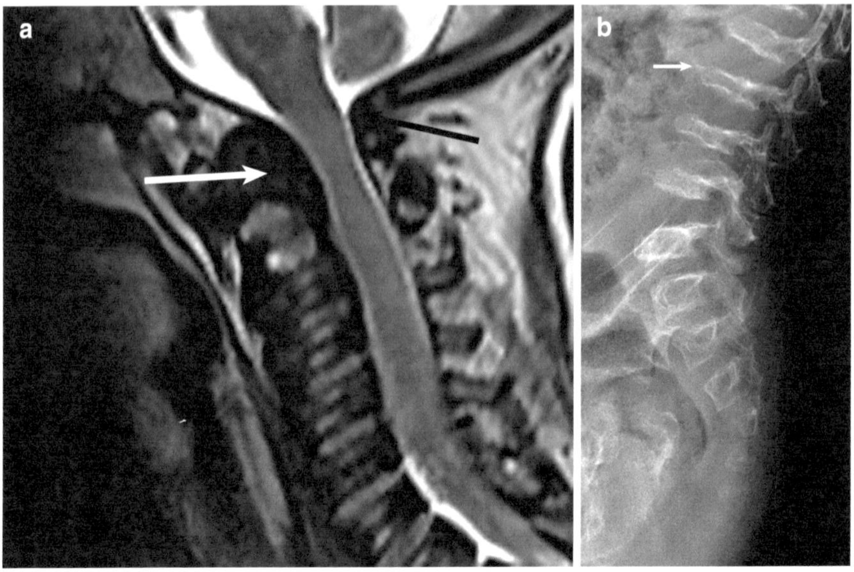

Fig. 10 Morquio syndrome. (**a**) Midsagittal T2 image of the craniovertebral junction shows dens hypoplasia with T2 hypointense soft tissue surrounding the dens (*grey arrow*) and anterior displacement of the posterior C1 arch (*black arrow*). (**b**) Lumbosacral spine radiographs in the same patient show classic anterior mid-vertebral body beaking

The Mucopolysaccharidoses

The craniovertebral junction is almost always affected in Morquio disease (mucopolysaccharidosis type IV) which is due to a defect of one of the two enzymes *N*-acetylgalactosamine-6-sulfatase (MPS IVA) or beta-galactosidase (MPS IVB) and results in accumulation of keratan sulfate and chondroitin-6 sulfate [79]. Atlantoaxial instability results from the dens hypoplasia which is often associated with a soft tissue mass posterior to the dens and results in a narrowed spinal canal (Fig. 10). This soft tissue mass generally shows low to intermediate T1 signal and low signal on T2-weighted MR images [50]. The etiology of this mass has been postulated to be the accumulation of glycosaminoglycans posterior to the dens [59, 106]. However several authors favor that it instead represents fibrous granulation tissue, possibly due to repetitive microtrauma in the region [50, 117].

Abnormalities of the craniocervical junction can also occur in other MPS such as Hurler disease (mucopolysaccharidosis I) and Maroteaux-Lamy syndrome (mucopolysaccharidosis VI), although to a lesser extent than in MPS IV [67, 117] (Fig. 11). Interestingly, hypoplasia of the odontoid has been shown to be reversible following bone marrow transplantation in patients with Hurler disease [48]. Yet there is no effect on the soft tissue mass posterior to the dens in these children.

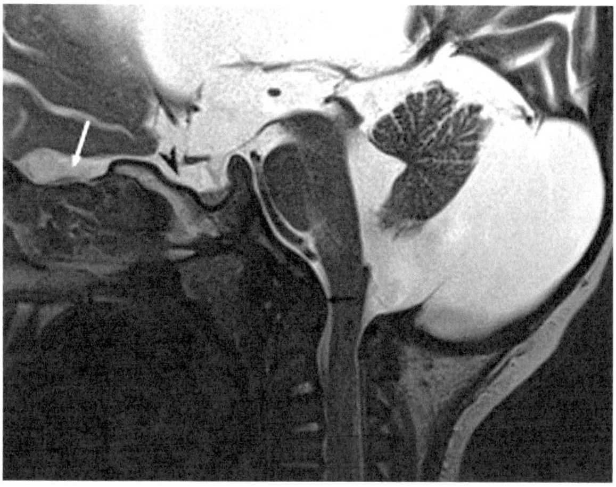

Fig. 11 Mucopolysaccharidosis type II. Midsagittal T2 image of MPS II shows an almost normal dens. There is retrodental T2 hypointense soft tissue (*black arrow*), a J-shaped sella (*black arrowhead*), and evidence of mucopolysaccharide deposition along the dural margins (*white arrow*). The patient also has hydrocephalus, a large CSF-filled posterior fossa with a deformity of the vermis, a deformity of the occipital bone, and a relative stenosis of the foramen magnum

Klippel-Feil Syndrome

Classically the triad of Klippel-Feil syndrome, first described in 1912, involves a short neck, a low hairline, and limited neck mobility [57]. However, fewer than 50 % of patients of congenital cervical fusion show all three signs [110] and today the term now refers to any congenital fusion of the cervical spine, of at least two cervical vertebral bodies [55]. The incidence of Klippel-Feil is estimated to be about 1:40,000–1:42,000 births. Other abnormalities associated with the syndrome include congenital scoliosis, rib anomalies, deafness, genitourinary abnormalities, Sprengel deformity, synkinesia, cervical ribs, and cardiovascular abnormalities [17, 46, 110]. The etiology of the syndrome is complex, and at least three genetic forms have been identified in the literature [110]. One association has been ascribed to a mutation in the fibroblast growth factor receptor 3 gene (*FGFR3*) which resulted in a coronal synostosis, dysmorphic vertebrae, and Sprengel deformity [60]. Another has been with a paracentric inversion of chromosome 8q leading to KFS and vocal cord impairment [13]. In addition, it is postulated that there is likely involvement of the genes associated with sclerotomal segmentation, *PAX*, and genes involved with the Notch signaling pathway, with questionable involvement of the *HOX* genes [13, 14, 110].

Although many classification systems have been suggested (the first one in 1919), they have been mainly concerned with an anatomic classification [55]. The most recent, put forth by Clarke and colleagues, classifies the disorder into four

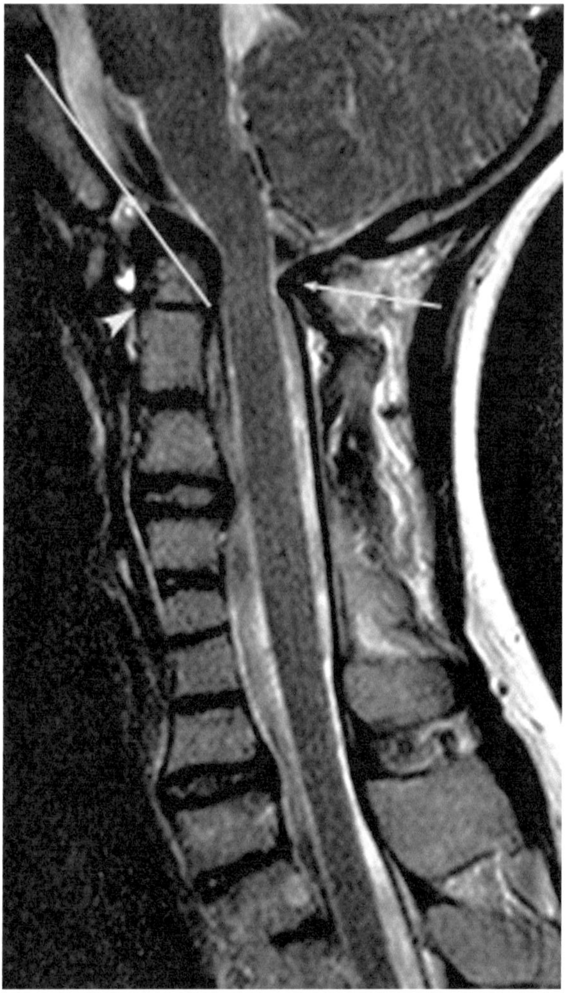

Fig. 12 A 11-year-old male with Klippel-Feil. Midsagittal T2-weighted MR image demonstrates protrusion of the dens beyond Wackenheim's line, persisting ossiculum terminale (*arrowhead*), and hypoplasia of the C1 arch (*arrow*) resulting in anterior-posterior narrowing of the spinal canal and crowding of structures at the cervicomedullary junction. There are multiple fusion anomalies of the lower cervical spine including "wasting" and rudimentary discs most prominent at C3–C4, C4–C5, and C5–C6

types [15]. *Klippel-Feil 1* (*KF1*) has fusions at C1 with or without more caudal fusions; KF1 has an autosomal recessive inheritance and is most frequently associated with other severe anomalies. *Klippel-Feil 2* (*KF2*) presents with the most rostral fusion at C2–C3 (as with KF1, more caudal fusions may be present); Klippel-Feil 2 has an autosomal dominant inheritance pattern with 100 % penetrance of the C2–C3 fusion. *Klippel-Feil 3* (*KF3*) is defined by isolated fusions of the cervical spine caudal to C1 and C2–C3 and shows reduced penetrance and either autosomal dominant or autosomal recessive inheritance (Fig. 12). *Klippel-Feil 4* (*KF4*) is considered synonymous with Wildervanck syndrome (congenital cervical synostosis, congenital hearing loss, and the Duane anomaly); this syndrome was thought to have an X-linked dominant inheritance pattern with hemizygous lethality [15].

Other abnormalities pertinent to the neuroradiologic evaluation of patients with Klippel-Feil syndrome involve the reported presence of diastematomyelia [20] and accelerated spondylosis at levels adjacent to non-segmented vertebrae increasing susceptibility to cervical cord insults and vertebral artery injury [42, 82].

22q11.2 Deletion Syndrome

The 22q11.2 deletion is present in patients with velocardiofacial syndrome, DiGeorge syndrome, conotruncal face anomaly syndrome, CHARGE syndrome, and numerous others [67]. One study showed the presence of cervical spine anomalies in all 79 patients studied, ranging from the occiput through the cervical spine. Characteristic findings include platybasia (91 %), open posterior C1 arch (59 %), a dysmorphic dens (58 %), and fusion of C2 and C3 (34 %) [97]. These findings can predispose to neurologic compromise, and therefore at some institutions, radiographic imaging of the cervical spine is routine in the assessment of these children [67].

Goldenhar Syndrome

This is a rare congenital disorder that results from abnormal development of the first and second branchial arches [35]. Cervical spine fusion has been reported in 8–61 % of cases and occipitalization of the atlas in 4.4–30 % [35, 44]. There have also been reports of odontoid hypoplasia and basilar impression, possibly resulting in cervical spine instability [1, 36]. The odontoid may be posteriorly inclined. Given these abnormalities at the craniocervical junction, imaging with flexion and extension views in asymptomatic patients every 6 months is recommended.

Spondyloepiphyseal Dysplasia Congenita (SEDC)

Spondyloepiphyseal dysplasia is a short-trunk disproportionate dwarfism with epiphyseal and vertebral anomalies. Forty percent of patients show atlantoaxial instability that can result in a myelopathy. Instability is usually due to odontoid hypoplasia, os odontoideum, or laxity of ligaments and can result in a myelopathy [77]. Patients at particular risk for myelopathy are those with coxa vara and short stature [77, 83]. These patients should be followed to adulthood, as many will require surgical correction beyond the pediatric years.

Osteogenesis Imperfecta

Osteogenesis imperfecta is a spectrum of conditions related to abnormalities in genes related to collagen formation. Sillence suggested a classification based on

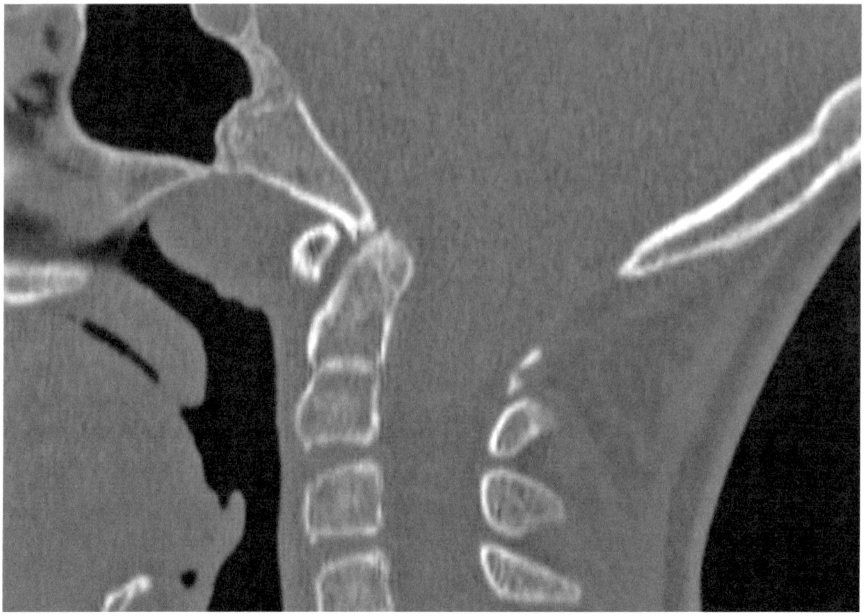

Fig. 13 A 11-year-old female with juvenile idiopathic arthritis. There is borderline-acquired basilar impression with the dens projecting 5 mm beyond Chamberlain's line. Erosive changes were noted at the atlanto-occipital joints

genetic analysis. About 25 % of all osteogenesis imperfecta and about 70 % of osteogenesis imperfecta type IV patients present with basilar impression [103]. This condition develops due to the softening of the skull base and may eventually result in spinal cord compression. While symptoms have been seen in children as young as 5 years old, they become significant in the second to fourth decades, reflecting the acquired etiology of the process [103].

Juvenile Idiopathic Arthritis

While involvement of the craniovertebral junction in adult rheumatoid arthritis is a well-known complication, its incidence in childhood arthritides was not as clear. A recent study found that the most frequent structural lesions in polyarthritic juvenile idiopathic arthritis, which encompasses both the seropositive juvenile form of RA and the seronegative more heterogenous group of diseases, were anterior atlantoaxial subluxation (33 %), erosion of the odontoid process (19 %), C1–C2 arthritis (17 %), and apophyseal joint arthritis (16 %) [27] (Fig. 13). In addition lesions of the cervical spine in pJIA were similar to those in RA except for the presence of ankylosis and hypertrophy of the vertebrae. The presence of cervical lesions correlated with a more severe disease [27].

Craniovertebral Junction Neoplasms

In a recent retrospective study of 38 children requiring surgery for neoplasms of the craniovertebral junction, Menezes found the most common neoplasm requiring surgery to be the chordoma (21 %), followed by meningioma (13 %), fibrous dysplasia (11 %), aneurismal bone cyst (11 %), eosinophilic granuloma (11 %), neurenteric cyst (11 %), plexiform neurofibroma (8 %), Ewing's sarcoma (5 %), osteoblastoma (5 %), and schwannoma (5 %) [72]. Chordomas are assumed to originate from remnants of the notochord which at this level in the embryo, after running in the middle of the vertebral centra, exits at the tip of the dens and runs within the perineural connective tissue before reentering the dorsal aspect of the cartilaginous clivus [85]. They are rare in children, and more commonly located at the craniovertebral junction than in adults, in which they are more typically sacral. A literature review up to 1996 found 79 cases of chordomas in children below the age of 19 with about a 1:1 distribution between males and females [8]. While in adults these tumors usually have a benign histology, atypical histologic findings with aggressive behavior have been reported with greater frequency in children younger than 5 years of age [31]. The tumors can be locally aggressive and destructive and are characteristically isointense (75 %) or hypointense (25 %) on T1-weighted MR images, with moderate to extreme hyperintensity on T2-weighted images [108], with variable enhancement. MRI is better at delineating the relationship of these tumors to adjacent vascular structures and their extent into the epidural space.

References

1. Anderson PJ, David DJ (2005) Spinal anomalies in Goldenhar syndrome. Cleft Palate Craniofac J 42:477–480
2. Bailey DK (1952) The normal cervical spine in infants and children. Radiology 59:712–719
3. Bharucha EP, Dastur HM (1964) Craniovertebral anomalies (a report on 40 cases). Brain 87:469–480
4. Bhatnagar M, Sponseller PD, Carroll C 4th, Tolo VT (1991) Pediatric atlantoaxial instability presenting as cerebral and cerebellar infarcts. J Pediatr Orthop 11:103–107
5. Bollo RJ, Riva-Cambrin J, Brockmeyer MM, Brockmeyer DL (2012) Complex Chiari malformations in children: an analysis of preoperative risk factors for occipitocervical fusion. J Neurosurg Pediatr 10:134–141
6. Bonadio WA (1993) Cervical spine trauma in children: part I. General concepts, normal anatomy, radiographic evaluation. Am J Emerg Med 11:158–165
7. Bonadio WA (1993) Cervical spine trauma in children: part II. Mechanisms and manifestations of injury, therapeutic considerations. Am J Emerg Med 11:256–278
8. Borba LA, Al-Mefty O, Mrak RE, Suen J (1996) Cranial chordomas in children and adolescents. J Neurosurg 84:584–591
9. Browd S, Healy LJ, Dobie G et al (2006) Morphometric and qualitative analysis of congenital occipitocervical instability in children: implications for patients with Down syndrome. J Neurosurg 105(Suppl 1):50–54
10. Caird MS, Wills BP, Dormans JP (2006) Down syndrome in children: the role of the orthopaedic surgeon. J Am Acad Orthop Surg 14:610–619

11. Chamberlain WE (1939) Basilar impression (platybasia): a bizarre developmental anomaly of the occipital bone and upper cervical spine with striking and misleading neurologic manifestations. Yale J Biol Med 11:487–496
12. Chevrel JP (1965) Occipitalization of the atlas. Arch Anat Pathol (Paris) 13:104–108
13. Clarke RA, Singh S, McKenzie H et al (1995) Familial Klippel-Feil syndrome and paracentric inversion inv(8)(q22.2q23.3). Am J Hum Genet 57:1364–1370
14. Clarke RA, Kearsley JH, Walsh DA (1996) Patterned expression in familial Klippel-Feil syndrome. Teratology 53:152–157
15. Clarke RA, Catalan G, Diwan AD, Kearsley JH (1998) Heterogeneity in Klippel-Feil syndrome: a new classification. Pediatr Radiol 28:967–974
16. Connolly B, Emery D, Armstrong D (1995) The odontoid synchondrotic slip: an injury unique to young children. Pediatr Radiol 25(Suppl 1):S129–S133
17. Copley LA, Dormans JP (1998) Cervical spine disorders in infants and children. J Am Acad Orthop Surg 6:204–214
18. Crockard HA, Stevens JM (1995) Craniovertebral junction anomalies in inherited disorders: part of the syndrome or caused by the disorder? Eur J Pediatr 154:504–512
19. Currarino G, Rollins N, Diehl JT (1994) Congenital defects of the posterior arch of the atlas: a report of seven cases including an affected mother and son. AJNR Am J Neuroradiol 15:249–254
20. David KM, Copp AJ, Stevens JM et al (1996) Split cervical spinal cord with Klippel-Feil syndrome: seven cases. Brain 119(Pt 6):1859–1872
21. David KM, Thorogood P, Stevens JM et al (1997) The one bone spine: a failure of notochord/sclerotome signalling? Clin Dysmorphol 6:303–314
22. David KM, Thorogood PV, Stevens JM, Crockard HA (1999) The dysmorphic cervical spine in Klippel-Feil syndrome: interpretations from developmental biology. Neurosurg Focus 6:e1
23. Debernardi A, D'Aliberti G, Talamonti G et al (2011) The craniovertebral junction area and the role of the ligaments and membranes. Neurosurgery 68:291–301
24. Dickman CA, Greene KA, Sonntag VK (1996) Injuries involving the transverse atlantal ligament: classification and treatment guidelines based upon experience with 39 injuries. Neurosurgery 38:44–50
25. Doyle JS, Lauerman WC, Wood KB, Krause DR (1996) Complications and long-term outcome of upper cervical spine arthrodesis in patients with Down syndrome. Spine (Phials Pa 1976) 21:1223–1231
26. Effendi B, Roy D, Cornish B et al (1981) Fractures of the ring of the axis. A classification based on the analysis of 131 cases. J Bone Joint Surg Br 63-B:319–327
27. Elhai M, Wipff J, Bazeli R et al (2013) Radiological cervical spine involvement in young adults with polyarticular juvenile idiopathic arthritis. Rheumatology (Oxford) 52(2):267–275
28. Erbengi A, Oge HK (1994) Congenital malformations of the craniovertebral junction: classification and surgical treatment. Acta Neurochir (Wien) 127:180–185
29. Fassett DR, McCall T, Brockmeyer DL (2006) Odontoid synchondrosis fractures in children. Neurosurg Focus 20:E7
30. Ferguson RL, Putney ME, Allen BL Jr (1997) Comparison of neurologic deficits with atlanto-dens intervals in patients with Down syndrome. J Spinal Disord 10:246–252
31. Forsyth PA, Cascino TL, Shaw EG et al (1993) Intracranial chordomas: a clinicopathological and prognostic study of 51 cases. J Neurosurg 78:741–747
32. Frank JB, Lim CK, Flynn JM, Dormans JP (2002) The efficacy of magnetic resonance imaging in pediatric cervical spine clearance. Spine (Phila Pa 1976) 27:1176–1179
33. Geipel P (1955) Studies on the fissure formation of the atlas and epistropheus. IV. Zentralbl Allg Pathol 94:19–84
34. Gholve PA, Hosalkar HS, Ricchetti ET et al (2007) Occipitalization of the atlas in children. Morphologic classification, associations, and clinical relevance. J Bone Joint Surg Am 89:571–578
35. Goldenhar M (1952) Associations malformatives de l'oeil et de l'oreille, en particulier le syndrome dermoide epibulbaire-appendices auriculaires-fistula auris congenitale et ses relations avec la dysostose mandibulofaciale. J Genet Hum 1:243–282

36. Gosain AK, McCarthy JG, Pinto RS (1994) Cervicovertebral anomalies and basilar impression in Goldenhar syndrome. Plast Reconstr Surg 93:498–506
37. Grabb PA, Mapstone TB, Oakes WJ (1999) Ventral brain stem compression in pediatric and young adult patients with Chiari I malformations. Neurosurgery 44:520–527; discussion 527–528
38. Grisoni NE, Ballock RT, Thompson GH (2003) Second cervical vertebrae pedicle fractures versus synchondrosis in a child. Clin Orthop Relat Res 413:238–242
39. Hankinson TC, Klimo P Jr, Feldstein NA et al (2007) Chiari malformations, syringohydromyelia and scoliosis. Neurosurg Clin N Am 18:549–568
40. Harris JH Jr, Carson GC, Wagner LK (1994) Radiologic diagnosis of traumatic occipitovertebral dissociation: 1. Normal occipitovertebral relationships on lateral radiographs of supine subjects. AJR Am J Roentgenol 162:881–886
41. Harris JH Jr, Carson GC, Wagner LK, Kerr N (1994) Radiologic diagnosis of traumatic occipitovertebral dissociation: 2. Comparison of three methods of detecting occipitovertebral relationships on lateral radiographs of supine subjects. AJR Am J Roentgenol 162:887–892
42. Hasan I, Wapnick S, Kutscher ML, Couldwell WT (2002) Vertebral arterial dissection associated with Klippel-Feil syndrome in a child. Childs Nerv Syst 18:67–70
43. Hawkins RJ, Fielding JW, Thompson WJ (1976) Os odontoideum: congenital or acquired. A case report. J Bone Joint Surg Am 58:413–414
44. Healey D, Letts M, Jarvis JG (2002) Cervical spine instability in children with Goldenhar's syndrome. Can J Surg 45:341–344
45. Hensinger RN (1986) Osseous anomalies of the craniovertebral junction. Spine (Phila Pa 1976) 11:323–333
46. Hensinger RN, Lang JE, MacEwen GD (1974) Klippel-Feil syndrome: a constellation of associated anomalies. J Bone Joint Surg Am 56:1246–1253
47. Hensinger RN, Fielding JW, Hawkins RJ (1978) Congenital anomalies of the odontoid process. Orthop Clin North Am 9:901–912
48. Hite SH, Peters C, Krivit W (2000) Correction of odontoid dysplasia following bone-marrow transplantation and engraftment (in Hurler syndrome MPS 1H). Pediatr Radiol 30:464–470
49. Horton WA, Lunstrum GP (2002) Fibroblast growth factor receptor 3 mutations in achondroplasia and related forms of dwarfism. Rev Endocr Metab Disord 3:381–385
50. Hughes DG, Chadderton RD, Cowie RA et al (1997) MRI of the brain and craniocervical junction in Morquio's disease. Neuroradiology 39:381–385
51. Jones K (1997) Chromosomal abnormality syndromes. In: Jones K (ed) Smith's recognizable patterns of human malformation. Saunders, Philadelphia, pp 8–10
52. Kao SC, Waziri MH, Smith WL et al (1989) MR imaging of the craniovertebral junction, cranium, and brain in children with achondroplasia. AJR Am J Roentgenol 153:565–569
53. Kirlew KA, Hathout GM, Reiter SD, Gold RH (1993) Os odontoideum in identical twins: perspectives on etiology. Skeletal Radiol 22:525–527
54. Klimo P Jr, Blumenthal DT, Couldwell WT (2003) Congenital partial aplasia of the posterior arch of the atlas causing myelopathy: case report and review of the literature. Spine (Phila Pa 1976) 28:E224–E228
55. Klimo P Jr, Rao G, Brockmeyer D (2007) Congenital anomalies of the cervical spine. Neurosurg Clin N Am 18:463–478
56. Klimo P Jr, Ware ML, Gupta N, Brockmeyer D (2007) Cervical spine trauma in the pediatric patient. Neurosurg Clin N Am 18:599–620
57. Klippel M, Feil A (1912) Un cas d'absence des vertebres cervicales. Avec cage thoracique remontant jusqu'a la base du crane (cage thoracique cervicale). Nouv Iconog Salpetriere 25:223–250; (1975 translation: "The classic: a case of absence of cervical vertebrae with the thoracic cage rising to the base of the cranium (cervical thoracic cage)". Clin Orthop Relat Res 109:3–8)
58. Kotil K, Kalayci M (2005) Ventral cervicomedullary junction compression secondary to condylus occipitalis (median occipital condyle), a rare entity. J Spinal Disord Tech 18:382–384
59. Kulkarni MV, Williams JC, Yeakley JW et al (1987) Magnetic resonance imaging in the diagnosis of the cranio-cervical manifestations of the mucopolysaccharidoses. Magn Reson Imaging 5:317–323

60. Larson AR, Josephson KD, Pauli RM et al (2001) Klippel-Feil anomaly with Sprengel anomaly, omovertebral bone, thumb abnormalities, and flexion-crease changes: novel association or syndrome? Am J Med Genet 101:158–162
61. MacAlister A (1893) Notes on the development and variations of the atlas. J Anat Physiol 27:519–542
62. Maiman DJ, Cusick JF (1982) Traumatic atlantoaxial dislocation. Surg Neurol 18:388–392
63. Matsuda Y, Sano N, Watanabe S et al (1995) Atlanto-occipital hypermobility in subjects with Down's syndrome. Spine (Phila Pa 1976) 20:2283–2286
64. Matsunaga S, Imakiire T, Koga H et al (2007) Occult spinal canal stenosis due to C-1 hypoplasia in children with Down syndrome. J Neurosurg 107(6 Suppl):457–459
65. Matthews LS, Vetter WL, Tolo VT (1982) Cervical anomaly simulating hangman's fracture in a child. Case report. J Bone Joint Surg Am 64:299–300
66. McGregor M (1948) The significance of certain measurements of the skull in the diagnosis of basilar impression. Br J Radiol 21(244):171–181
67. McKay SD, Al-Omari A, Tomlinson LA, Dormans JP (2012) Review of cervical spine anomalies in genetic syndromes. Spine (Phila Pa 1976) 37:E269–E277
68. McRae DL (1953) Bony abnormalities in the region of the foramen magnum: correlation of the anatomic and neurologic findings. Acta Radiol 40:335–354
69. McRae DL, Barnum AS (1953) Occipitalization of the atlas. Am J Roentgenol Radium Ther Nucl Med 70:23–46
70. Menezes AH (2004) Evaluation and treatment of congenital and developmental anomalies of the cervical spine. Invited submission from the joint section meeting on disorders of the spine and peripheral nerves, March 2004. J Neurosurg Spine 1:188–197
71. Menezes AH (2008) Craniocervical developmental anatomy and its implications. Childs Nerv Syst 24:1109–1122
72. Menezes AH (2008) Craniovertebral junction neoplasms in the pediatric population. Childs Nerv Syst 24:1173–1186
73. Menezes AH, Fenoy KA (2009) Remnants of occipital vertebrae: proatlas segmentation abnormalities. Neurosurgery 64:945–953; discussion 954
74. Meyer PG, Meyer F, Orliaguet G et al (2005) Combined high cervical spine and brain stem injuries: a complex and devastating injury in children. J Pediatr Surg 40:1637–1642
75. Mikulis DJ, Diaz O, Egglin TK, Sanchez R (1992) Variance of the position of the cerebellar tonsils with age: preliminary report. Radiology 183:725–728
76. Miyata I, Imaoka T, Masaoka T et al (1994) Pediatric cerebellar infarction caused by atlantoaxial subluxation – case report. Neurol Med Chir (Tokyo) 34:241–245
77. Miyoshi K, Nakamura K, Haga N, Mikami Y (2004) Surgical treatment for atlantoaxial subluxation with myelopathy in spondyloepiphyseal dysplasia congenita. Spine (Phila Pa 1976) 29:E488–E491
78. Mondschein J, Karasick D (1999) Spondylolysis of the axis vertebra: a rare anomaly simulating hangman's fracture. AJR Am J Roentgenol 172:556–557
79. Montano AM, Tomatsu S, Gottesman GS et al (2007) International Morquio A registry: clinical manifestation and natural course of Morquio A disease. J Inherit Metab Dis 30:165–174
80. Morgan MK, Onofrio BM, Bender CE (1989) Familial os odontoideum. Case report. J Neurosurg 70:636–639
81. Naderi S, Korman E, Citak G et al (2005) Morphometric analysis of human occipital condyle. Clin Neurol Neurosurg 107:191–199
82. Nagib MG, Maxwell RE, Chou SN (1984) Identification and management of high-risk patients with Klippel-Feil syndrome. J Neurosurg 61:523–530
83. Nakamura K, Miyoshi K, Haga N, Kurokawa T (1998) Risk factors of myelopathy at the atlantoaxial level in spondyloepiphyseal dysplasia congenita. Arch Orthop Trauma Surg 117:468–470
84. Nishikawa M, Sakamoto H, Hakuba A et al (1997) Pathogenesis of Chiari malformation: a morphometric study of the posterior cranial fossa. J Neurosurg 86:40–47

85. O'Rahilly R, Müller F, Meyer DB (1983) The human vertebral column at the end of the embryonic period proper. 2. The occipito-cervical region. J Anat 136:181–195
86. Pang D (2010) Atlantoaxial rotatory fixation. Neurosurgery 66(3 Suppl):161–183
87. Pang D, Li V (2005) Atlantoaxial rotatory fixation: part 2. New diagnostic paradigm and a new classification based on motion analysis using computed tomographic imaging. Neurosurgery 57:941–953
88. Pang D, Li V (2005) Atlantoaxial rotatory fixation: part 3. A prospective study of the clinical manifestation, diagnosis, management, and outcome of children with atlantoaxial rotatory fixation. Neurosurgery 57:954–972
89. Pang D, Thompson DN (2011) Embryology and bony malformations of the craniovertebral junction. Childs Nerv Syst 27:523–564
90. Pang D, Nemzek WR, Zovickian J (2007) Atlanto-occipital dislocation: part 1. Normal occipital condyle-C1 interval in 89 children. Neurosurgery 61:514–521; discussion 521
91. Pang D, Nemzek WR, Zovickian J (2007) Atlanto-occipital dislocation: part 2. The clinical use of (occipital) condyle-C1 interval, comparison with other diagnostic methods, and the manifestation, management, and outcome of atlanto-occipital dislocation in children. Neurosurgery 61:995–1015; discussion 1015
92. Powers B, Miller MD, Kramer RS et al (1979) Traumatic anterior atlanto-occipital dislocation. Neurosurgery 4:12–17
93. Pueschel SM, Scola FH, Tupper TB, Pezzullo JC (1990) Skeletal anomalies of the upper cervical spine in children with Down syndrome. J Pediatr Orthop 10:607–611
94. Raybaud C (2011) Anatomy and development of the craniovertebral junction. Neurol Sci 32(Suppl 3):S267–S270
95. Reed CM, Campbell SE, Beall DP et al (2005) Atlanto-occipital dislocation with traumatic pseudomeningocele formation and post-traumatic syringomyelia. Spine (Phila Pa 1976) 30:E128–E133
96. Rhoton AL Jr (2000) The posterior fossa cisterns. Neurosurgery 47(3 Suppl):S287–S297
97. Ricchetti ET, States L, Hosalkar HS et al (2004) Radiographic study of the upper cervical spine in the 22q11.2 deletion syndrome. J Bone Joint Surg Am 86-A(8):1751–1760
98. Richardson EG, Boone SC, Reid RL (1975) Intermittent quadriparesis associated with a congenital anomaly of the posterior arch of the atlas. Case report. J Bone Joint Surg Am 57:853–854
99. Ryken TC, Menezes AH (1994) Cervicomedullary compression in achondroplasia. J sNeurosurg 81:43–48
100. Sagiuchi T, Tachibana S, Sato K et al (2006) Lhermitte sign during yawning associated with congenital partial aplasia of the posterior arch of the atlas. AJNR Am J Neuroradiol 27:258–260
101. Segal LS, Drummond DS, Zanotti RM et al (1991) Complications of posterior arthrodesis of the cervical spine in patients who have Down syndrome. J Bone Joint Surg Am 73:1547–1554
102. Sharma A, Gaikwad SB, Deol PS et al (2000) Partial aplasia of the posterior arch of the atlas with an isolated posterior arch remnant: findings in three cases. AJNR Am J Neuroradiol 21:1167–1171
103. Sillence DO (1994) Craniocervical abnormalities in osteogenesis imperfecta: genetic and molecular correlation. Pediatr Radiol 24:427–430
104. Smoker WR (1994) Craniovertebral junction: normal anatomy, craniometry, and congenital anomalies. Radiographics 14:255–277
105. Smoker WR, Khanna G (2008) Imaging the craniocervical junction. Childs Nerv Syst 24:1123–1145
106. Stevens JM, Kendall BE, Crockard HA, Ransford A (1991) The odontoid process in Morquio-Brailsford's disease. The effects of occipitocervical fusion. J Bone Joint Surg Br 73: 851–858
107. Swischuk LE, Hayden CK Jr, Sarwar M (1979) The dens-arch synchondrosis versus the hangman's fracture. Pediatr Radiol 8:100–102

108. Sze G, Uichanco LS 3rd, Brant-Zawadzki MN et al (1988) Chordomas: MR imaging. Radiology 166(1 Pt 1):187–191
109. Thomason M, Young JW (1984) Case report 261: Os odontoideum (OO). Skeletal Radiol 11:144–146
110. Tracy MR, Dormans JP, Kusumi K (2004) Klippel-Feil syndrome: clinical features and current understanding of etiology. Clin Orthop Relat Res 424:183–190
111. Tubbs RS, Elton S, Grabb P et al (2001) Analysis of the posterior fossa in children with the Chiari 0 malformation. Neurosurgery 48:1050–1055
112. Tubbs RS, Iskandar BJ, Bartolucci AA, Oakes WJ (2004) A critical analysis of the Chiari 1.5 malformation. J Neurosurg 101(2 Suppl):179–183
113. von Torklus D, Gehle W (1972) Anomalies and malformations. In: The upper cervical spine. Thieme, Stuttgart, pp 14–53
114. Wackenheim A (1974) Roentgen diagnosis of the craniovertebral region. Springer, New York
115. Wang H, Rosenbaum AE, Reid CS, Zinreich SJ, Pyeritz RE (1987) Pediatric patients with achondroplasia: CT evaluation of the craniocervical junction. Radiology 164(2):515–519
116. Wellborn CC, Sturm PF, Hatch RS, Bomze SR, Jablonski K (2000) Intraobserver reproducibility and interobserver reliability of cervical spine measurements. J Pediatr Orthop 20(1):66–70
117. White KK (2011) Orthopaedic aspects of mucopolysaccharidoses. Rheumatology (Oxford) 50(Suppl 5):v26–v33
118. Wiesel SW, Rothman RH (1979) Occipitoatlantal hypermobility. Spine (Phila Pa 1976) 4(3):187–191
119. Woodring JH, Lee C (1993) Limitations of cervical radiography in the evaluation of acute cervical trauma. J Trauma 34(1):32–39

Anaesthesiological and Intensive Care Management in Craniovertebral Junction Surgery

Orazio Genovese, Federica Tosi, Marco Piastra, Antonio Chiaretti, Giorgio Conti, Concezio Di Rocco, and Massimiliano Visocchi

Contents

O. Genovese, MD (✉) • F. Tosi, MD • M. Piastra, MD • A. Chiaretti, MD • G. Conti, MD
Pediatric Intensive Care Unit, Institute of Anesthesiology and Intensive Care,
Università Cattolica del Sacro Cuore, Largo A. Gemelli 8, Rome 00168, Italy
e-mail: hor6505@yahoo.com

C. Di Rocco, MD
Department of Pediatric Neurosurgery, Università Cattolica del Sacro Cuore, Rome, Italy

M. Visocchi, MD
Institute of Neurosurgery, Università Cattolica del Sacro Cuore,
Rome, Italy

C. Di Rocco, N. Akalan (eds.), *Pediatric Craniovertebral Junction Diseases*,
Advances and Technical Standards in Neurosurgery 40,
DOI 10.1007/978-3-319-01065-6_5,

Abstract The main factors of modern perioperative care of the craniovertebral junction surgery include a comprehensive approach to the patients, including a thorough cardiorespiratory, neurophysiological, and metabolic assessment, intraoperative monitoring of spinal cord function, safe airway management, and judicious use of fluids and blood transfusions. Admission in PICU shortly after the CVJ surgery is mandatory to ensure haemodynamic and respiratory stability and to recognize postoperative complications. Anticipating complications in order to achieve an early treatment and adverse event prophylaxis can contribute to reduced morbidity and mortality and increased patients' safety. Multidisciplinary management of perioperative patient care and careful pain control is mandatory in order to improve the outcomes.

Keywords Cervical spine surgery • Paediatric intensive care • Postoperative pain • Difficult airway • Craniovertebral junction anomalies

Introduction

Anaesthesia and intensive care for the surgical treatment of craniovertebral junction (CVJ) anomalies are particularly challenging. Indeed, the anaesthetist is faced with a variety of pathological conditions ranging from congenital bone, neurological and vascular malformations to acquired disorders, such as those due to metabolic diseases, traumas, infections and tumours (Table 1). Age is an important factor to be taken into account for the potential blood loss associated to the surgical procedure [45]. The presence of a vascular compromise at the level of the cervical spinal cord as well as atlanto-axial instability complicates the manoeuvres of patient's intubation and positioning. Kyphoscoliosis can lead to pulmonary hypertension and cor pulmonale. Finally, in several instances, further limitations may be related to the necessity of repeating anaesthesia induction and maintenance in patients who have already undergone multiple operations. Therefore, a comprehensive approach to the

Table 1 American Society of Anesthesiologists (ASA) classification

Class	Description
I	The patient is normal and healthy
II	The patient has mild systemic disease that does not limit their activities (e.g., controlled hypertension or controlled diabetes without systemic sequelae)
III	The patient has moderate or severe systemic disease, which does limit their activities (e.g., stable angina or diabetes with systemic sequelae).
IV	The patient has severe systemic disease that is a constant potential threat to life (e.g., severe congestive heart failure, end-stage renal failure).
V	The patient is morbid and is at substantial risk of death within 24 h, with or
E	Emergency status: In addition to indicating underlying ASA status (1–5), any patient undergoing an emergency procedure is indicated by the suffix "E". For example, a fundamentally healthy patient undergoing an emergency procedure is classified as I–E. If the patient is undergoing an elective procedure, the "E" designation is not used.

patients, including a thorough cardiorespiratory, neurophysiological and metabolic assessment, is recommended before proceeding to CVJ surgery [44].

Preoperative Anaesthesiological Assessment

Besides the general assessment of the physical status of the patient, as established by the American Society of Anesthesiologists (Table 1), the evaluation of a child who is undergoing a surgical procedure on the CVJ should take into account the possible coexistence of malformations or physiological problems associated to pathogenic conditions to be dealt with. Anaesthesiologists should also not underestimate the importance of the psychological background of the patients and the family, especially in case of repeated surgical procedures and hospitalizations.

Intubation Versus Tracheostomy

The choice whether intubation or tracheostomy would assure the best airway management requires a full agreement between the anaesthesiologist and the surgeon. Such a common decision should be based on the precise preoperative knowledge of the 'syndromic' pattern of a given malformation, that is, all the possible anatomical features limiting the manoeuvres of intubation and/or a thorough evaluation of the risk of performing the surgical procedure itself as well as postoperative complications, namely, postoperative upper airway oedema [5]. A further aspect to be taken into account is the choice of the anterior or posterior surgical approach [64].

Micrognathia and mandibular hypo-dysplasia as well as macroglossia constitute an absolute cause of difficult intubation due to reduced anatomical space between the basihyoid bone and the mandible which limits the displacement of the soft parts from the laryngoscopes (during laryngoscopy). Difficult intubation may be encountered also in Goldenhar syndrome and Klippel-Feil syndrome due to the reduced mobility between atlanto-occipital and the cervical vertebrae [52]. Anaesthesia and surgery were associated with worsening of previously unrecognized abnormalities in children with Down syndrome, abnormalities that probably reflected some degree of pre-existing cord compression. Therefore, if there is any suspicion of signs or symptoms consistent with cervical cord compression, a thorough history and physical examination should be conducted [36]. In mucopolysaccharidosis, mainly in type IV (i.e. Morquio syndrome), the macroglossia and the reduction of the upper airway volume play a role in favouring alternatives to classic orotracheal intubation. Airway management in this patients can be complicated by macroglossia, prognathism, and hypertrophy of pharyngeal and laryngeal tissues, which make mask fit, mask ventilation, laryngoscopy, and correct tracheal tube placement difficult [42]. In this and similar pathological conditions, no method of airway assessment is foolproof for predicting the difficult airway; nevertheless, commonly accepted

Table 2 Mallampati score

Class	Anatomy of the oral cavity
Class I	Full visibility of soft palate, tonsils, and uvula
Class II	Visibility of soft palate but only the upper portion of the tonsils and uvula
Class III	Soft and hard palate and base of the uvula are visible
Class IV	Only hard palate is visible

Table 3 Upper lip bite test

Grade	Description
Grade 1	Ability of lower incisors to fully cover the upper lip and extend superior to the vermillion border
Grade 2	Lower incisors can bite the upper lip but only inferior to the vermillion border
Grade 3	Lower incisors are not able to bite the upper lip at all

Table 4 Cormack and Lehane grades

Grade	Anatomy of the oral cavity
Grade 1	Most of glottis visualized
Grade 2	Only posterior portion of the glottis is visualized
Grade 3	Only epiglottis but no glottic structures are visualized
Grade 4	Neither epiglottis nor the glottis is visualized

preoperative assessment evaluation does exist, such as the Mallampati classification, which is based on the anatomical structures visualized when patients open their mouths (Table 2).

A Mallampati class of III or IV is predictive of airway management difficulty in acromegalics [59]. In older children, an alternate airway assessment modality is the upper lip bite test (ULBT) in which a patient is asked to cover the vermillion of the upper lip with the lower incisors (Table 3). A higher grade can be predictive of airway management difficulty [27]. The Cormack and Lehane grade, at the time of laryngoscopy, is used to define difficulty with laryngoscopy (Table 4). Patients with a Cormack and Lehane grade 3 or 4 are considered to pose difficulty with laryngoscopy.

In general, tracheal intubation is considered difficult if more than two failed attempts occur in requiring rescue anaesthesiological techniques, e.g. laryngoscope blade change, bougie, video laryngoscopy, and fibre-optic bronchoscope [55]. In this case awake fibre-optic intubation can be strongly advocated in case of surgical procedures on the CVJ but also tracheostomy must be taken into consideration.

Modern fibre-optic technology offers a safe and effective method of airway management. However, it requires great skills and acquired experience and is very difficult to perform with uncooperative patients, especially children [59]. Moreover, this technique may be particularly difficult in relation with retropharyngeal swelling and adenoidal hypertrophy in children.

It is worth to note that in the last 15 years, adequate instruments for fibre-optic bronchoscopy have been introduced in the anaesthesiological armamentarium, thus making easier the application of this technique in the paediatric population, including infants and small children [6], consequently overcoming the difficulties encountered in the past when only 'adult' fibre-optic apparatus, 6 mm in diameter, were available. Failure to intubate may necessitate alternative airway control devices such as video-assisted intubation devices or intubation through laryngeal mask airways (LMA). LMA may be particularly useful in this setting, and endotracheal tube placement can be achieved using the fibrescope through the LMA/iLMA as a guide [38]. However, till more evidence is available, there are not strong recommendations for standardized procedures in children with difficult or failed intubation. This is the reason why for a continuous search of better intubating devices such as, for example, the video laryngoscopes, are able to provide a better laryngeal view as compared to direct laryngoscopy [69].

The decision to intubate or perform a tracheostomy is essentially made by estimating the risk of upper airway oedema that may occur postoperatively. If excessive oedema is expected, a tracheostomy should be taken into consideration to assure a controlled and stable airway in the postoperative period. This would permit while allowing an early wake-up, useful to obtain an immediate neurological postoperative evaluation and prevent from harmful consequences of a prolonged tracheal intubation [58].

Although tracheostomy and tracheotomy are used interchangeably, it should be reminded that tracheostomy from the Greek word *stomoun* refers to the act of providing an opening, whereas tracheotomy, from the Greek word *tome*, to cut, means specifically the result of surgical cut. The need of cervical external orthosis, that is, a Halo Vest system, should suggest to proceed to the intervention of tracheostomy in order to prevent the necessity of performing an emergency procedure in the postoperative phase due to overwhelming respiratory distress.

The Choice of the Surgical Route

Two surgical routes can be chosen by the paediatric neurosurgeon, the anterior dealing with direct decompression of the cervical spinal cord and the posterior dealing with both neurological decompression and instrumentation and fusion of the cervical spine [67].

The Anterior Route

Orotracheal intubation can be chosen in case of endoscopic transnasal approach since no conflict with the surgeon activity is provoked. The choice of orotracheal intubation can be more debatable in case of transoral, transmandibular, or transmaxillary approaches as some surgeons do not mind about the possible conflict of pharyngeal spreaders of the oral distractor with the orotracheal tube; others prefer a nasotracheal intubation performed by the anaesthesiologist, so reducing the possible conflict with the oral distractor, while others prefer to keep the surgical channel free of any foreign body by using tracheostomy (Figs. 1 and 2).

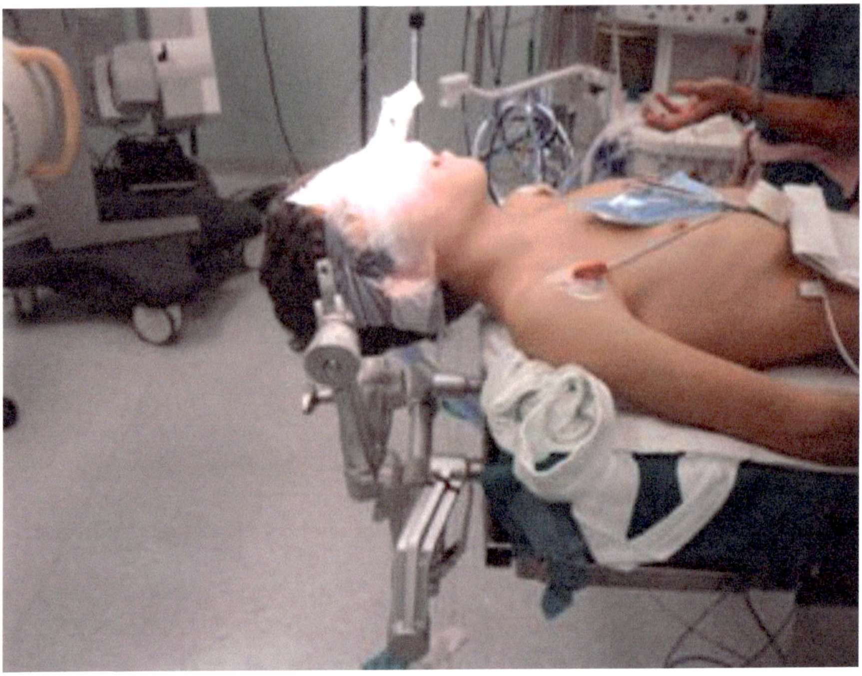

Fig. 1 Endonasal intubation, head fixation with Mayfield head holder, and oral distraction with Crockard distractor (Codman J&J) for anterior transoral decompression

The Posterior Route

In case of posterior surgical approach (decompressive and instrumentation and fusion techniques), tracheostomy is not obtained for surgical requirements, since the airways are far from the surgical target. Nevertheless, in case of pre-existing brainstem damage which could suggest an occurrence of postoperative respiratory disturbances, along with the need of a Halo Vest system, tracheostomy could be advocated (Figs. 3 and 4) [64, 65, 66].

Sedation and Drug Delivering

Sedation is necessary to evaluate spontaneous breathing and ventilation. When the oxygenation and ventilation are adequate, it is possible to proceed to laryngoscopy after induction with administration of not irritating inhalational agents (sevoflurane) or intravenous drugs (propofol and remifentanil). In cases where difficult intubation is anticipated, it is useful to consider the use of a fibre-optic bronchoscope. Indeed, fibre-optic techniques have gained greater use in selected paediatric patients following a combination of topical anaesthesia, local airway blocks and IV sedation, or under general anaesthesia by mask with maintenance of spontaneous ventilation [44]. The ideal size of fibrescope depends on the diameter of the endotracheal tube to be passed through. Intubation requires an ETT size that is only slightly larger than

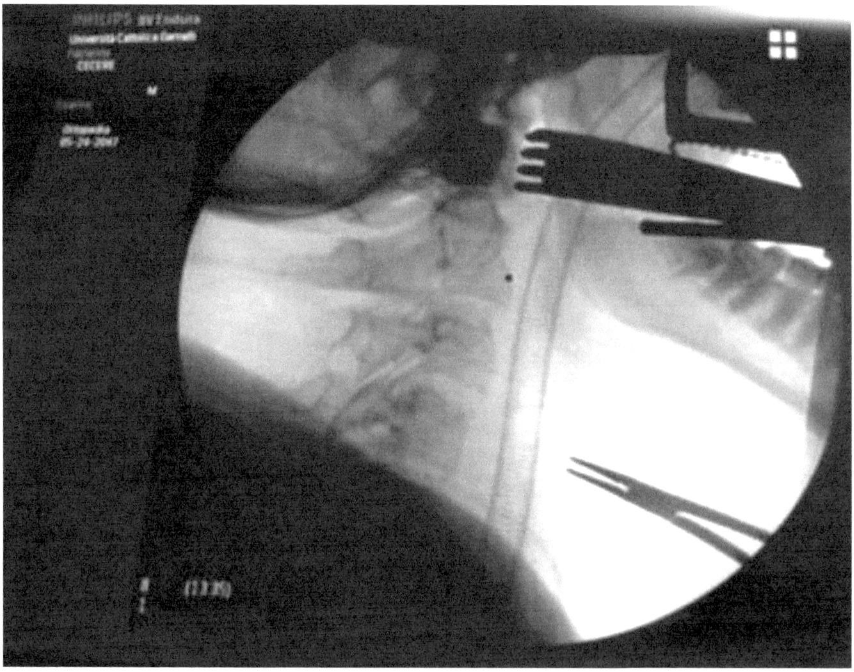

Fig. 2 Intraoperative assessment of Crockard distractor visualizing the nasotracheal tube (the *black square* is the operative 'minus' filled of contrast medium (Iopamiro) to visualize the decompression

the diameter of the fibrescope. The modern flexible fibrescopes arrive to a diameter of 2 Fr and allow the passage of endotracheal tube inside diameter of 2.5 Fr.

Providing moderate levels of sedation without causing respiratory distress or haemodynamic instability, dexmedetomidine could be successfully used in patients requiring awake fibre-optic intubation for cervical spine surgery [3, 33]. In all patients, electrocardiography pulse oximetry and blood pressure recordings must be monitored throughout the procedure. The maintenance of anaesthesia is obtained with Sevorane (MAC 1, 1.5) in O2 plus air with a paCO2 target level of 32–35 mmHg. Muscle relaxation is obtained with cisatracurium besylate.

Intraoperative Neurophysiological Monitoring

Intraoperative monitoring of spinal cord function is considered a standard of care in spinal surgery [54]. The methods of monitoring the integrity of the spinal cord function intraoperatively include:

1. The wake-up test
2. Somatosensory evoked potentials (SSEP)
3. Motor evoked potentials (MEPs)
4. Dermatomal responses

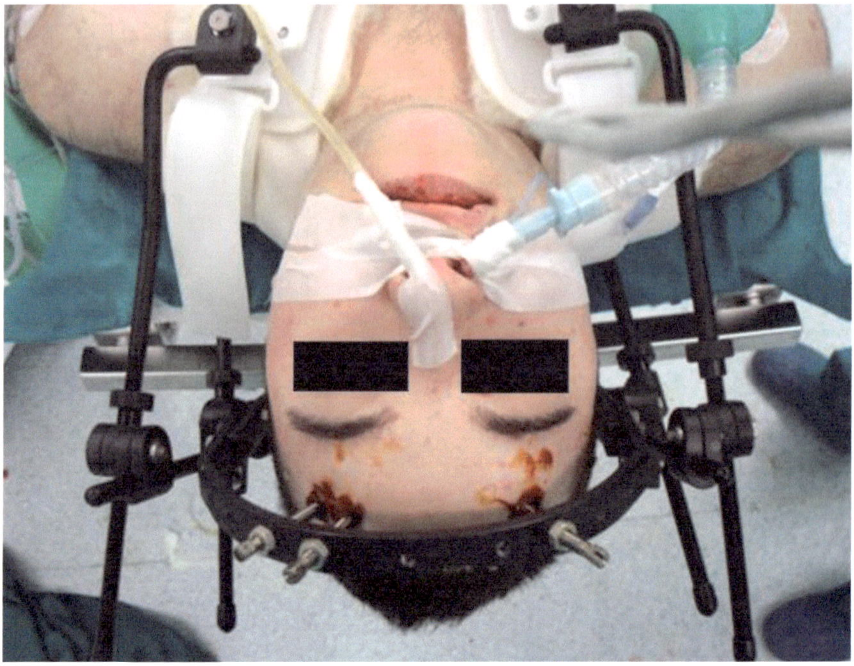

Fig. 3 After operation, the patient is fixed with a paediatric external orthosis Halo Vest (De Puy Spine Bremer). Nasogastric tube in the left nostril and nasotracheal tube in the right nostril are shown

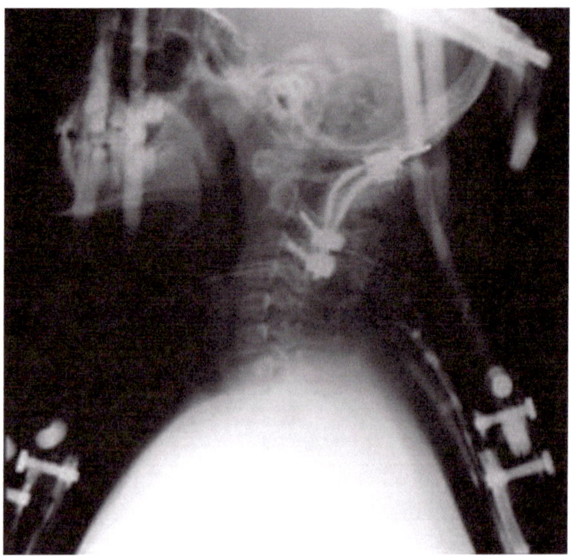

Fig. 4 Postoperative X-ray control of external orthosis after double-staged instrumentation and fusion procedure. Note the airway's patency and chest expansion with the vest

The Wake-Up Test

Before the use of electrical monitoring, this test was a method of assessing spinal cord function during corrective procedures of the spine. The hazards of this test include accidental extubation, dislodgement of fixators and air embolism on deep inspiration. Its major limitation is that spinal cord function is evaluated only at one specific time (i.e. during the wake-up test) and not continuously during the procedure. Both inhalation and i.v. anaesthetic techniques are suitable for the 'wake-up' test. Furthermore, a standard wake-up test cannot be performed in infants and small children. Alternatives such as tetanic stimulation of the lower legs and observation of the clinical response can be tried in this age subgroup.

SSEP and MEPs

Somatosensory evoked responses represent the more widespread method of electrical monitoring of the spinal cord [30]. The response of constant current stimulation of the median, tibial, and, rarely, the sural nerve is recorded at the level of the cortex using surface scalp electrodes or a bipolar electrode placed epidurally. Baseline SSEPs are recorded in order to exclude neurological dysfunction and also to determine the feasibility of the operative monitoring. Neurophysiology technicians monitor the latency and amplitude of the recordings continuously during anaesthesia and surgery. A 0.50 % decrease in SSEP amplitude is deemed significant. Numerous anaesthetic agents interfere with the latency and amplitude of the SSEP. Surgical stimulation level and hypothermia also interfere with SSEP. Volatile agents, cold, hypoxia, hypercarbia, and spinal ischaemia suppress both SSEPs and MEPs. Responses recorded from the cerebral cortex are more sensitive to the effects of anaesthetic agents than epidurally recorded responses. Neuromuscular block reduces muscle artefact on the recorded SSEPs. SSEP monitoring is a pathway-specific method; an injury not involving the sensory pathway will not be detected. In cervical spine surgery, SSEPs and MEPs should be used. Although MEPs are still not available in many intraoperative neurophysiological departments, their use should be encouraged since MEPs represent the most appropriate and reliable tool to assess the functional integrity of descending motor tracts [53].

Dermatomal Potentials

Dermatomal somatosensory evoked potentials (DSEPs) involve recording cerebral evoked responses from cutaneous stimulation of areas of known dermatomal innervation providing a pure sensory input to any level of the spinal cord. However, given the lack of evidence in the literature, current evidence is insufficient to determine appropriateness.

Perioperative Fluid and Blood Volume Management

Intraoperative fluid therapy may start at the time of the surgical treatment as simply as replacing the deficits of the preoperative fasting status and maintenance of normal fluid condition or as complex therapy need at correcting preoperative abnormal deficits. During the surgery, care should be given to compensate intraoperative translocated fluids and variable blood loss.

Because of their high metabolic rate and water turnover, significant hypoglycaemia and dehydration may occur in infants who are required to fast preoperatively for prolonged periods of time. If not provided previously, the fluid deficit occurred during fasting should be replaced during anaesthesia. Assuming that a healthy child is in water and electrolyte balance at the time oral feedings are discontinued, the fluid deficit at the start of anaesthesia can be estimated by multiplying the child's hourly maintenance fluid requirement by the number of hours that have elapsed since the last feeding. This deficit may be replaced by giving half of the calculated volume during the first hour of anaesthesia and the other half over the next 2 h, in addition to intraoperative maintenance fluids. Five percent dextrose in quarter-normal saline (5 % dextrose/0.25 NS) is frequently used for fluid maintenance.

Conflicting data do exist in the literature about the intraoperative use of glucose. The metabolic need for glucose in the infant age group is 5 g/kg/day. Infants under 4 years of age who are kept fasting for over 6 h may become hypoglycaemic and irritable. Since the metabolic rate and oxygen consumption of infants and small children is significantly greater than older children and adults, it has been recommended to provide 5 % dextrose for all infants at risk of hypoglycaemia (serum glucose <40 mg/dl) from preoperative starvation. It must be remembered, however, that preterm infants receiving glucose infusions should be monitored carefully for hyperglycaemia, since their kidneys are unable to hyperfiltrate in the presence of hyperglycaemia. Hyperglycaemia (glucose >200 mg/dl) has also been noted in older infants and children given 5 % dextrose in lactated Ringer's as an intraoperative maintenance fluid. Elevated blood glucose concentrations may lead to an osmotic diuresis and may exacerbate neurological injury associated with a cardiac arrest or other cerebral insults (i.e. cerebral ischaemia and asphyxia). The clinical significance of postoperative hyperglycaemia in otherwise healthy children would seem to be minimal. However, in major surgical cases, such hyperglycaemia and osmotic diuresis may complicate or confuse ongoing fluid therapy. Therefore, we can consider blood glucose control as a reasonable goal for the majority of the cases and a critical goal in a few children. Blood glucose control can be achieved in several ways. Most children receiving glucose-free intravenous fluids during surgical procedures demonstrate an increase in their blood glucose concentration. Physiological factors accounting for the hyperglycaemic response to anaesthesia and surgery include increased sympathoadrenal activity leading to a decrease in glucose tolerance, decreased glucose utilization, and increased gluconeogenesis. However, about 12 % of patients who receive glucose-free solutions fail to increase their blood glucose concentrations. Since hypoglycaemia may be undetected during anaesthesia, it would seem prudent to measure intraoperative glucose concentrations if glucose-free solutions are used and to treat hypoglycaemia if diagnosed. It seems paradoxical, however, to be depending on the stress of surgery to increase glucose at a time when 'stress-free' anaesthetics are being advocated. Therefore, in general, we advocate the use of glucose-containing solutions. One way to avoid hyperglycaemia with a 5 % dextrose solution is to decrease the infusion rate, but this may contribute to hypotension in fluid-depleted children. A less concentrated glucose solution (e.g. 2.5 % dextrose in lactated Ringer's) given at recommended infusion rates provides adequate glucose for healthy children (300 mg/kg/h) and adequate volume replacement while avoiding hyperglycaemia and hypoglycaemia. Since 2.5 % dextrose in lactated Ringer's is not commercially available, it can easily be made by the individual practitioner with 50 % dextrose solution.

Intraoperative Third-Space Losses

Surgical traumas are associated with the isotonic transfer of fluids from the extracellular fluid compartment (and to a lesser extent from the intracellular compartment) to a nonfunctional interstitial compartment. This acute sequestration of fluid to a nonfunctional compartment has been called third-space loss and should be replaced. In neurosurgery, it is negligible (1–2 ml/kg/h) [16]. Generally, lactated Ringer's solution or normal saline is used to restore third-space losses.

Blood and Blood Component Therapy

Paediatric patients undergoing major procedures (e.g. tumour resection, reconstructive surgery, cardiac surgery, organ transplantation, trauma surgery, or surgery for burns) will invariably require some form of blood volume replacement. Indications for blood or blood component therapy are not always clear-cut; hence, the anaesthesiologist should formulate a preoperative plan of management utilizing scientific rationale for a decision on blood therapy. Factors on which this decision is based include the patient's blood volume estimates, preoperative haematocrit, general medical condition, and ability to provide adequate oxygen transport to the tissues, as well as the nature of the surgical procedure and the risks vs. benefits of transfusion [49, 62]. All blood loss in neonates, infants, and children should somehow be replaced. An accurate measurement of blood loss and an accurate assessment of acceptable blood loss in the child are vital to any replacement regimen. Calculation of sponge weight, the use of calibrated miniaturized suction bottles, and a visual estimation (combined with a 'guess factor') make it possible to define the magnitude of the blood loss. The transfusion practice guidelines of the American Society of Anesthesiologists Task Force on Blood Component Therapy [3] are largely applicable to paediatric patients without cardiopulmonary disease. The concept of allowable red-cell loss or allowable blood loss, preferable as a guide to blood replacement normovolemic haemodilution to a predetermined haematocrit, can be achieved with crystalloid or colloid solutions. Blood volume is age-related: The neonatal blood volume has been reported to vary widely from 65 to 129 ml/kg, depending on the magnitude of the placental transfusion [17].

Estimating Allowable Blood Loss

Several methods have been proposed for estimating allowable blood loss from the blood volume, weight, and haematocrit. The formulas range from the simple to the complex, but all involve an estimate of blood volume. The safest haemoglobin or haematocrit that is allowed during surgery is debatable and clearly depends on the type of surgery, the patient's postoperative activity, and his/her underlying medical condition. As a general rule, we accept haematocrits of 28–30 as the lowest acceptable haematocrit. In the newborn, 40 % is the lowest acceptable haematocrit. A simple method of calculating allowable blood loss (ABL) uses the original haematocrit (Ho), the lowest acceptable haematocrit (H1), and the average of the two haematocrits $(\mathrm{Ho}+\mathrm{H1})/2$ as follows [9]:

$$\mathrm{ABL} = \mathrm{Wt} \times \mathrm{EBV} \times \left[\mathrm{Ho} - \mathrm{H1}\right] / \left[\mathrm{H}\right]$$

In this equation, all haematocrits are decimal values (i.e. 0.6, 0.5). There is controversy as to whether the blood volume should be supported with crystalloid or colloid, while the haematocrit is being allowed to decrease. If colloid (i.e. albumin, fresh frozen plasma) is used, then ongoing blood loss is replaced millilitre for millilitre. If isotonic crystalloid is administered, Furhman et al. recommend replacing ongoing blood loss with an equal volume of lactated Ringer's solution until the serum protein concentration approaches 5 g/dl; after this point, blood volume is maintained with 5 % albumin until the allowable blood loss has been exceeded [56]. Others replace blood loss with 2–4 times the volume of lactated Ringer's solution. However, with these large volumes of crystalloid replacement, hypoproteinaemia may result. We replace blood loss with volumes of crystalloid 2 times the measured or calculated loss. In major surgery involving 1–2 body cavities, intravascular albumin may be transiently depleted or translocated. Consequently, we follow serum protein levels and begin replacing with 5 % albumin when serum protein levels approach 5.0 g/dl.

Blood Component Therapy

Blood component therapy depends on the clinical setting and the availability of various blood products. Bleeding from thrombocytopaenia is rare with a platelet count of more than 50,000; serious bleeding is usual below 20,000. Normal adult values for clotting factors are attained between 1 and 12 months of age, depending on the specific factor. Fresh whole blood (less than 4 h old) has a limited availability. If predicted blood loss is greater than or equal to 40 % of blood volume, it is helpful to supply platelets and clotting factors. Packed red blood cells have a haematocrit of between 70 and 80 %. An average of 1 ml/kg packed cells increases the haematocrit by 1.5 %. The units of packed cells can be subdivided into paediatric packs of 80–100 ml. The fluid of these cells is relatively hyperkalaemic (K+, 15–20 mEq/l), acidotic (pH<7.0), and low in ionized Ca++. When the maximum allowable blood loss is approached, consider transfusion with packed fresh red blood cells (PRBC) to adjust the haematocrit to about 30 %. When the amount of blood lost approaches one blood volume, labile clotting factors are greatly reduced; normal clotting requires 5–20 % of factor V and 30 % of factor VIII. All of the coagulation factors except platelets are present in normal quantities in fresh frozen plasma.

We prefer to give 2:1 volumes of lactated Ringer's solution and packed cells (haematocrit 35–40 %) to patients with massive blood loss (i.e. >1 blood volume). This ratio of cells and crystalloid can be varied to produce any desired haematocrit. In patients with clinical signs of bleeding or documented abnormal clotting studies, crystalloid is replaced with fresh frozen plasma. The FFP is then administered with equal volumes of packed cells. The therapeutic value of FFP is related to volume expansion and provision of procoagulants. FFP contains 70 % or more of the procoagulant factors of fresh plasma [57] and is best utilized to replace depleted clotting factors in patients with von Willebrand's disease, haemophilia A, and liver disease. It is also used in association with massive blood transfusion and perhaps DIC. The latter two conditions do not always represent clear-cut indications for FFP transfusion. Guidelines for FFP administration include reversal of oral anticoagulant, replacement of factor deficiencies as determined by the laboratory, treatment of immunodeficiencies, treatment of thrombotic thrombocytopaenia purpura, treatment in antithrombin III deficiency, and massive blood transfusion (when factors V and VIII are less than 25 % of normal) [41]. The use of FFP carries with it risks of transfusion transmitted diseases, as is the case with any blood product [3]. The need for platelets intraoperatively may be predicted from the preoperative platelet count. Platelets can be mobilized from the spleen and bone marrow as bleeding occurs. An infant with a high preoperative count (>250,000) may not need a platelet transfusion until 2–3 blood volumes are lost, whereas an infant with a low count (<150,000) may need platelets after only 1 blood volume is lost. One platelet pack per 10 kg is usually adequate.

Postoperative Care

Admission in PICU shortly after the CVJ surgery is mandatory to ensure haemodynamic and respiratory stability and for prompt recognition of postoperative complications and management of airways.

Postoperative Fluid Management

Fluid management is carefully monitored, avoiding fluid overload as well as hypovolaemia. It is advisable to give crystalloids (normal saline 0.9 % NaCl or Ringer's lactate) in order to allow an adequate glycaemic level. It has been documented that hyperglycaemia is common in critically ill children and is associated with mortality and morbidity in PICU [1, 39]. However, the actual relevance of strict glycaemic control is particularly controversial in the context of neurocritical care. In the first 24 h after neurosurgery, hyperglycaemia is observed in many children, even in the absence of glucose infusion. After traumatic brain injury (TBI), hyperglycaemia has been associated with poor outcome, explained either by a more severe TBI or by the neurotoxicity of glucose [7, 60]. Hyperglycaemia increases oxidative stress and inflammation, augments excitotoxicity mediated by NMDA receptors, and alters microcirculatory perfusion. On the other hand, brain metabolism depends on a constant supply of glucose, and hypoglycaemia also favours excitotoxicity, apoptosis, and oxygen free-radical accumulation. Neuroglycopaenia and metabolic crisis can occur with even mild hypoglycaemia. It is therefore advisable to keep blood glucose levels less than 150 mg/dl through insulin infusion and, at the same time, prevent hypoglycaemia by adding glucose solution when serum glucose falls below 70 mg/dl [25].

Prophylactic and Supportive Measures

Short course antibiotic prophylaxis is initiated just before the operation. Guidelines recommend that antibiotic prophylaxis should be given only at premedication, but in clinical practice, antibiotic prophylaxis is often unnecessarily prolonged through the next few days. Prophylaxis against stress ulcers should be recommended for the prevention of upper gastrointestinal bleeding in these patients. A systematic review and meta-analysis found limited high-quality data to recommend routine use of stress ulcer prophylaxis [47]. At the present time, stress ulcer prophylaxis using ranitidine, sucralfate, or proton-pump inhibitors (PPIs) is instituted in children with risk factors for development of stress ulcers.

Cold fluid is allowed starting from the third postoperative day. CT scans are usually performed 3–7 days after surgery, and at the same time, patients start mobilization. After 24–48 h (i.e. when haemodynamic parameters, metabolic conditions, and neurological status are stable at least for 8 h), the patient is transferred to the surgical ward.

Respiratory Support and Mechanical Ventilation

If the patient is admitted to PICU yet with an endotracheal tube, rapid awakening is recommended in order to evaluate the neurological condition as soon as possible. Prolonged invasive ventilation is associated with numerous complications, including airway injury, higher risk for gastrointestinal bleeding, thromboembolism, barotrauma, and ventilator-associated pneumonia [12]. However, the need to protract sedation and mechanical ventilation is determined by the surgical procedure itself and the general patient's condition. In case of spinal cord traumatic injury (SCI), the control of intracranial hypertension, appropriate sedation, careful management of haemodynamic instability, and metabolic issues all represent the core of the intervention and should drive treatment decisions. These patients often require to maintain intubation and mechanical ventilation due to decreased levels of consciousness, impaired airway protection, neuromuscular weakness, or pulmonary complications. A Glasgow Coma Scale ≤8 is usually taken as a cutoff to secure the airway, although in some patients with a lower score, successful extubation has been performed. The routine use of sedation and neuromuscular blockade in severe paediatric traumatic brain injury is not supported by scientific evidence, but their use may be necessary to prevent intracranial hypertension raised by coughing, bucking on the tube and suctioning manoeuvres.

Patients with cervical SCI have significantly reduced vital capacity and ventilatory reserve because of interruption of the neural pathways to the diaphragm and respiratory muscles of chest and abdomen, resulting in a restrictive ventilatory impairment. The ensuing respiratory insufficiency directly correlates with the level of the injury and the degree of motor severity damage. Patients with acute cervical SCI frequently need prolonged mechanical ventilation (MV) due to paresis or paralysis of the respiratory muscles, worsening pulmonary vital capacity and severe impairment of peak cough flow, which is ineffective to clear tracheobronchial secretions. If prolonged mechanical respiration is needed, tracheostomy may improve respiration and facilitate weaning by reducing airway resistance, as well as preventing complications from prolonged orotracheal intubation.

The basic tenets of postoperative ventilator support for CVJ patient are the same as for all patients in the OR. These include the provision of adequate oxygenation and ventilation while limiting the potentially deleterious effects of mechanical ventilation on cardiovascular function. The goal of oxygenation is to maintain the PaO2 ≥60 mmHg (PaO2 ≥8 kPa). If adequate oxygenation cannot be maintained at inspired oxygen concentrations (FiO2) of 0.5–0.6, the usual practice is to increase positive end-expiratory pressure (PEEP). In patients with associated traumatic brain injury (TBI), however, it must be remembered that as PEEP increases, it may impact the overall cerebral perfusion pressure (CPP) [35]. Therefore, in patients with TBI, it may be better to attempt to increase mean airway pressure and augment oxygenation by first increasing the inspiratory time, FiO2, and peak inflation pressure rather than PEEP. Although practised routinely in the past for patients with TBI, hyperventilation is generally avoided unless there is a precipitous increase in ICP with impending herniation.

Weaning from Mechanical Ventilation

The ability to sustain spontaneous respiration after mechanical ventilation depends on achieving a balance between the work required for effective ventilation and the capacity of the respiratory muscles. Neuromuscular drive to breathe can potentially be impaired at any level; the respiratory upper airway and swallowing muscles may contribute directly or indirectly to a failure of independent breathing. Failure to breathe after artificial ventilation following CVJ surgery may be due to several different clinical situations. The patient may have a diagnosed pre-existing neurological disability affecting swallowing, breathing capacity, or airway control such as the central sleep apnoea syndrome associated with Chiari I malformation.

Prolonged mechanical ventilation is not the rule after elective CVJ surgery in the absence of significative compression of spinal cord. Respiratory function can be slightly impaired in patients with chronic atlanto-axial subluxation before surgery, and, in some cases, a postoperative compromise of lung capacity and forced expiratory flow persisting for some day after extubation can be expected [45, 46]. Respiratory mechanics may be affected by airway obstruction, pectus deformities, and mechanical distortion of the thorax in some clinical syndromes such as Morquio or Klippel-Feil syndrome. However, chest wall abnormalities severe enough to cause weaning failure are uncommon. Knowledge of factors associated with successful early extubation and those associated with prolonged mechanical ventilation in patients undergoing surgery for CVJ disease may help with patient selection and planning perioperative care that is crucial to successful early extubation. A high mortality rate has been documented in both paediatric and adult patients who have required re-intubation after extubation failure. Extubation failure is independently associated with a fivefold increased risk of death in paediatric patients [13, 15]. Avoiding re-intubation is therefore an important goal in weaning mechanically ventilated patients.

When the indications that were met for provision of mechanical ventilation are no longer present, then the patient can be weaned from mechanical ventilation. Weaning should start when (a) gas exchange is adequate; (b) no conditions exist that impose an undue burden on the respiratory muscles, such as severe hyperinflation, severe malnutrition, and multiple organ system failure; and (c) the patient is capable of sustaining spontaneous ventilation, keeping airway protected, and clearing tracheobronchial secretions. A reliable method of assessing readiness for weaning and predicting extubation success is not evident from the paediatric literature. The criteria for assessing readiness to wean have neither been validated nor adapted to the paediatric population. A spontaneous breathing test (SBT), the reference screening test for weaning, precedes extubation; it can be achieved and carried out in three ways: (1) T-piece trials, the patient is removed from the ventilator but does not undergo extubation, (2) CPAP trial with a low level (e.g. 5 cm H2O) of CPAP (superimposed pressure), or (3) with a low level of PSV. The duration of the trial can range from 30 min to 2 h.

When SBT is successful, the patient can undergo extubation. Before extubation, the child is given nothing by mouth for 4–6 h. The patient must be awake, be alert, and have airway protective reflexes. The patient must be breathing effectively, without undue exertion. Adequate gas exchange with a relatively low FiO2 must be established. The tube and pharynx are suctioned thoroughly, and the child is ventilated with 100 % oxygen to provide a reservoir of oxygen as a buffer against laryngospasm at extubation. With the lungs fully inflated, the endotracheal tube is removed, and the child is provided with humidified oxygen and observed closely. After endotracheal tube removal, a trial of non-invasive mechanical ventilation (NIV) or CPAP support can be successfully taken into account in spontaneously breathing patients showing a progressive respiratory distress detected by pulse oximetry, in order to improve gas exchange and reduce the rate of re-intubation [26]. NIV use in weaning right after planned extubation following tolerance of an SBT is applied in order to prevent post-extubation respiratory failure, which some patients might develop, and by extension re-intubation, with its associated risks. Several randomized controlled trials have been conducted in adults, but its place in weaning protocols for children needs yet to be determined [14]. NIV to facilitate extubation should be carried out only if the patient is awake, alert and able to breathe spontaneously, has intact bulbar function with a preserved cough reflex, has stable haemodynamic status, and has a low requirement for supplemental oxygen ($FiO2 \leq 40$ %).

Ineffective cough (especially in the presence of excess respiratory secretions and/or poor mental status) predisposes to extubation failure. This raises the question of whether cough-enhancement techniques could improve extubation outcome. A strategy combining NIV with manual and mechanical cough assistance techniques may prevent re-intubation after episodes of acute respiratory failure. However, in children with bulbar dysfunction, significative compression of spinal cord, or severe mechanical distortion of the thorax, respiratory mechanics may be significantly compromised and can predict failure of the non-invasive strategy.

Postoperative Airway Management

The main challenge of the postoperative care in patients after craniovertebral surgery is the airway management. Post-extubation stridor is common and may range from mild to life-threatening. Children younger than 4 years are most frequently affected by post-extubation stridor. Cool mist or humidified oxygen is sufficient treatment for children with mild symptoms. Nebulized epinephrine relieves more severe upper airway obstruction in most children, probably by local vasoconstriction. Following its use, oedema may recur, so close observation must continue. The value of corticosteroids in post-extubation stridor is more controversial, although dexamethasone (0.3–0.5 mg/kg every 6 h for 1 or 2 days) does appear beneficial in high-risk patients (e.g. those with multiple intubation attempts) [4, 28, 31].

Patients undergoing prolonged procedures in the prone position may develop airway and glottic swelling. In addition, CVJ disease and surgery can predispose to lower cranial nerve dysfunction that can further compromise the airway. This phenomenon occurs particularly after surgical repair as well as the lateral extrapharyngeal transcervical approach [36] and may place them at risk for postoperative airway compromise Though rare, upper airway compromise and frank obstruction represent a potentially catastrophic complication because the difficulty relates to re-intubation. Potential causes of airway obstruction include postoperative reactive swelling, hematoma, cerebrospinal fluid leak, angioedema, and graft or plate dislodgment. Pharyngeal oedema in cases of anterior fusion and anterior-posterior fusion and postoperative fixed neck in cases of posterior fusion make the emergency re-intubation challenging [51]. In the case where re-intubation is needed, the use of intubating devices or endotracheal intubation via awake fibre-optic bronchoscopy can be a safe way of airway control [58, 63, 69]. Approaching patients undergoing upper cervical spine surgery may involve fixation with a rigid collar or placement of a halo traction system. These devices, alongside other anatomical conditions such as mandibular hypoplasia or limited mouth opening, can be expected to increase significantly the difficulty of airway management. Therefore, when considering extubation of a patient with previous difficult intubation, a more cautious approach has to be taken. For patients deemed to be at high risk for excessive airway oedema, e.g. prolonged anaesthetic time in prone position or large fluid and blood replacement, the endotracheal tube should be left in place overnight and the awakening delayed for 12–24 h, although this practice does not rule out the risk completely. Only when haemodynamic and respiratory parameters are stable over a 4–6 h period of postoperative observation and the patient has a satisfactory gag reflex, an air leak after tracheal tube cuff deflation and minimal facial oedema, the endotracheal tube is removed. Most clinicians often use dexamethasone in order to reduce airway oedema in children; although widely used, it is unclear whether it can help to reduce oedema in patients having major anterior cervical spine surgery [11].

Postoperative Pain Management

Pain Assessment

Postoperative pain treatment has become a major concern in paediatric anaesthesia. Postoperative pain is common after CVJ surgery and can limit activity increasing the risk for medical complications, such as pneumonia, venous stasis, and thromboembolism increase in morbidity, resulting in longer hospital stays, a slower recovery time, and a delay in resumption of normal life activities. Additionally, ineffective management of acute pain may also increase the risk for chronic pain later in life. Although effective analgesics and age-specific pain evaluation tools are available, postoperative pain is still undertreated in children. Differently from the adult patients in paediatric age, it is more difficult to assess and treat efficaciously the pain. Paediatric guidelines have been issued in order to focus the attention on an interdisciplinary therapeutic approach, including pharmacologic, cognitive-behavioural, psychological, and physical treatments [43]. Some principles can be extended to all forms of acute pain, but some of them are particularly decisive in postoperative pain management. The need of a multidisciplinary team and of a pre- and postoperative pain management programme represents an important goal in order to obtain effective pain relief and optimize medical care and rapid recovery after postoperative procedures. Pain assessment should be performed regularly by using a scale appropriate to the age of the patient and routinely documented. Observational and behavioural measures consider child's reaction to pain. Self-report measures rely on the child's description of his experience of pain. Biological measures consider some physiological parameters that may be modified by the presence of pain, such as heart and respiratory rates and blood pressure. In infants and non-verbal children, self-report measures are unavailable, but behavioural indices (motor responses, vocalization, facial expressions, crying, body movements and complex behavioural responses such as the sleep-wake patterns) can be easily evaluated to assess pain. Different behavioural scales have been validated by several studies that enrolled infants and neonates. The most appropriate are the Crying, Requires oxygen, Increased vital signs, Expression, and Sleepless (CRIES) score for newborns and the revised Face, Legs, Activity, Cry, and Consolability (FLACC) pain tool for children who have difficulty verbalizing pain or children with neurocognitive impairment (Grunau et al. 1990; Hadjistavropoulos et al. 1994; Voepel-Lewis et al. 2002). Composite measures of pain have been developed combining behavioural and biological items, such as the Objective Pain Scale. The COMFORT scale, which relies on the measurement of five behavioural variables (alertness, facial tension, muscle tone, agitation, and movement) and three physiological variables (heart rate, respiration and blood pressure), is a validated tool for the assessment of grade of sedation [2, 24]. The Children's Hospital of Eastern Ontario Pain Scale (CHEOPS) is largely used for postoperative pain management [32]. Self-report measures of pain represent the gold standard in older children who can describe the subjective pain experience. These methods include different strategies such as routine and direct questioning, verbal and non-verbal methods (i.e. pictorial scales) and self-rating scales. In patients between 3 and 8 years of age, self-reporting techniques such as 'faces scales' using either photographs or drawings of faces may be used, although their application in the critical care environment is often difficult and only partially validated. Visual Analogue Scale (VAS) and Faces Pain Scale-Revised [21] are two of the commonest self-rating scales to assess pain intensity in children. The Oucher scale is a variant of the faces scale and is designed to measure pain intensity in children aged 3–12 years [18, 23].

Pain Therapy

Despite the enormous strides made in this field over the last 30 years, children continue to experience unrelieved pain postoperatively or during procedures. These pains in principle should be easy to manage using multimodal analgesics and non-drug interventions. Perioperative pain management therefore begins during the preoperative visit by preparing both the parent and the child about the upcoming surgery and information about the type of pain that is associated with it. Currently, the best approach is a combination of multiple analgesics, including acetaminophen (paracetamol), NSAIDs, opioids, and local/regional anaesthesia, with additive or synergistic effects yet with different side-effect profiles so that adequate analgesia can be provided with the least amount of side effects (Table 5).

Table 5 Criteria to meet before initiating weaning

1	Alert mental status
2	Good cough and gag reflexes
3	Core temperature below 38.5 °C
4	Spontaneous respiratory effort
5	pH 7.32–7.47
6	PaO2 >60 mm Hg or pulse oximetry reading >95 % PaCO2 <50 mm Hg – Fio2 <0.50
7	PEEP <7 cm H2O
8	No further need for vasoactive agents
9	No clinical need for increased ventilator support in the past 24 h
10	No planned operative procedures requiring heavy sedation in the next 12 h

Despite the increasing use of a variety of different analgesic strategies, opioids continue as the mainstay for management of moderate to severe acute pain after CVJ and spine surgery because of their high efficacy. All opioids are associated with tolerance, resulting in increasing requirements to maintain adequate analgesia/sedation. However, concerns remain about their potential adverse effects on ventilation. The most commonly used term 'respiratory depression' only describes part of that risk. Opioid-induced ventilatory impairment (OIVI) is a more complete term encompassing opioid-induced central respiratory depression (decreased respiratory drive), decreased level of consciousness (sedation) and upper airway obstruction, all of which, alone or in combination, may result in decreased alveolar ventilation and increased arterial carbon dioxide levels. Risks are often said to be higher in patients with obstructive sleep apnoea. Therefore, children with neurological or respiratory disturbances need careful cardiorespiratory monitoring and the availability of supportive therapy when first exposed to intense analgesia. Other side effects such as urinary retention, constipation and postoperative nausea and vomiting (PONV) may represent a major source of discomfort for patients. As the majority of opioid-related adverse effects are dose related, modalities that decrease total opioid consumption play a significant role in decreasing or preventing opioid-associated adverse effects [40, 22]. Drugs such as paracetamol and NSAIDs (e.g. ibuprofen, naproxen, diclofenac, and ketorolac) act through the inhibition of the enzyme cyclooxygenase, thereby blocking the synthesis of prostaglandins. When used alone, they are adequate to treat mild pain, although they need to be combined with other agents for treating moderate to severe pain. In distinction to opioids, these agents demonstrate a ceiling effect so that once a specific plasma concentration is achieved, no further analgesia is provided by increasing the dose. Paracetamol is an antipyretic with weak analgesic properties. It exerts the antipyretic effect at the hypothalamus and the analgesic effects by blocking central prostaglandin synthesis, reducing substance P-induced hyperalgesia and modulating the production of hyperalgesic nitric oxide in the spinal cord. The initial dose is up to 45 mg/kg administered rectally before awakening from anaesthesia. Additional doses can be given orally (10–15 mg/kg) or rectally (20 mg/kg) every 4–6 h (and not as needed) to produce analgesia. The total daily dose of acetaminophen should not exceed 100 mg/kg for children and 75 mg/kg for infants. NSAIDs are combined with weak opioids (codeine or oxycodone) for oral administration to control moderate pain or added to parenteral opioids and regional anaesthetic techniques for severe pain [61]. NSAIDs do not replace opioids but rather provide adjunctive analgesia, thereby lowering the total amount of opioids required. When used for this purpose, NSAIDs are administered around-the-clock and not on an as-needed basis. Adverse effects of NSAIDs are uncommon, but they may be serious when they occur. They include gastritis bleeding, decreased renal blood flow, hepatic dysfunction and inhibition of platelet function. Although the overall incidence of bleeding is very low, NSAIDs should not be used in the child with a bleeding diathesis or at risk for bleeding or when surgical haemostasis is a prominent concern. NSAIDs have been shown to decrease osteoblast activity in animal studies; thus, they may slow bone healing, particularly following bone grafting [29, 32]. Given the lack of evidence in the literature, care should be taken regarding the risk of bleeding, particularly in the postoperative period and in the highly stressed patient in whom gastric bleeding is more likely (Table 6).

Ketamine is a nonopioid analgesic that can be used in addition, or as a supplement, to opioids for pain control in the perioperative period [8]. Patients with subacute or chronic spine disease often have subacute or chronic pain treated with multiple analgesics, and little is known about the use of ketamine in opioid tolerant patients with chronic pain who undergo surgery. If analgesia is inadequate, a 0.5–1 mg/kg bolus of ketamine can be given i.v. followed by a continuous infusion at 10–50 mcg/min. Ketamine generally increases heart rate and blood pressure as well as provides bronchodilatation because of the release of endogenous catecholamines. Its main feature is to result in minimal respiratory depression in clinically relevant doses and may preserve airway protective reflexes. Ketamine is an alternative when pain is poorly controlled in postoperative paediatric neurosurgical patients and is able to prevent the potential adverse consequences of inadequate analgesia and opioid adverse effects.

In the multimodal approach, sedative agents, such as benzodiazepines, play a key role in the postoperative care after cervical spine surgery in children. Midazolam, a drug commonly employed for the sedation in children, has specific activity at GABA receptors and has the shortest elimination half-time among the benzodiazepines. The main adverse events include the development of the tolerance, dependence and withdrawal after subsequent discontinuation. Given by continuous infusion, midazolam allows an adequate level of sedation in critically ill children. The level of sedation should be regularly assessed and documented using a sedation assessment scale, wherever possible using a validated scoring system such as the COMFORT scale. The desired level of sedation should be identified for each patient and should be regularly reassessed. From a practical point of view, pain after cervical spine surgery usually requires the use of an opioid-based technique (morphine sulphate or fentanyl or remifentanil) supplemented with scheduled paracetamol administration and, wherever required, mild sedation [48]. Remifentanil combined with low-dose midazolam provides very reliable analgesia and sedation for early extubation. Dose of opioids and benzodiazepines should be titrated in order to produce the desired sedative effect. Before withdrawal of

Table 6 Opioid analgesia

Drug	Indications	Dose	Elimination	Comments
Fentanyl Infusion	Analgesia	1–5 mcg/Kg/min	Hepatic metabolism	Large bolus doses can cause hypotension
	Intense analgesia/anesthesia in ventilatedpatients	10–15 mcg/Kg/min		Respiratory depression
Bolus Fentanyl Pulmonary hypertension		10–50 mcg/k	Neonates may have long elimination half-lives, with delayed recovery	
Morphine	Analgesia with sedation	Loading dose 0.05 –0.2 mg/Kg	Hepatic followed by renal excretion of active metabolite (morphine-6-glucuronide)	Delayed recovery in neonates
	Controlled analgesia in the extubated patient Infusion	5–30 mcg/Kg/h Neonates: lower infusion rates 5–20 mcg/k/h	Reduced doses may be needed with renal impairment because of accumulation of morphine-6-glucuronide	Nausea and vomiting can be problematic in older children
Oral morphine	Longer term analgesia once absorption has recovered	200–500 mcg/Kg 4-hourly	Oral doses need to be larger than IV doses because of reduced bioavailability and first pass metabolism	
Alfentanil Infusion	Rapid offset, useful for fast-track surgery	Loading dose: 50–100 mcg/Kg/min	Hepatic metabolism Small volume of distribution and short elimination half-life make its Infusion: offset very rapid 0.5–4 mcg/k/min Highly protein bound with a small volume of distribution.	

Remifentanil Infusion in ventilated patients	Analgesia	0.1–0.5 mcg/Kg /min	Metabolized rapidly by plasma and tissue cholinesterases.	Alternative analgesia is required before the infusion is stopped Intense, rapid onset/offset (largely independent of age or infusion duration)
	Anesthesia	0.5–1.5 mcg/kg/min		Unsuitable for the extubated, spontaneously breathing patient
Codeine phosphate	Oral medication 4–6 hourly	Neonate: 0.5–[illegible] mg/Kg Child up to 12 years: 0.5–1 mg/kg Adult max dose: 240 mg >12 years: 30–50 m	Hepatic and renal clearance	Also used for treatment of diarrhea because of constipating effects
Tramadol	Oral medication 8 hourly	>12 years: 50–100 mg 4–6: hourly Adult max dose: 400 mg	Hepatic and renal clearance	Only patients >12 years Nausea, vomiting, constipation Respiratory depression in large doses

remifentanil, a loading dose of opioid, usually morphine, is needed to avoid hyperalgesia. After extubation, a combination therapy with scheduled paracetamol plus an opioid (morphine sulphate) represents an adequate strategy for moderate to severe pain management. Gabapentin, when given preoperatively and for 5 days postoperatively, will reduce morphine requirements for up to 2 days and pain score immediately after paediatric spinal fusion [50]. For extensive spine surgery, severe pain may be prevented by bupivacaine 0.5 % infusion through an epidural catheter placed intraoperatively into the subfascial paravertebral space [10]. Infiltration of the wound at the end of surgery with local anaesthetic will improve pain relief in the immediate postoperative period.

References

1. Agus MS, Steil GM, Wypij D, Costello JM, Laussen PC, Langer M, Alexander JL, Scoppettuolo LA, Pigula FA, Charpie JR, Ohye RG, Gaies MG, SPECS Study Investigators (2012) Tight glycemic control versus standard care after pediatric cardiac surgery. N Engl J Med 367:1208–1219
2. Ambuel B, Hamlett KW, Marx CM, Blumer JL (1992) Assessing distress in pediatric intensive care environments: the COMFORT scale. J Pediatr Psychology 17:95–109
3. American Society of Anesthesiologists Task Force on Blood Component Therapy (1996) Practice guidelines for blood component therapy. Anesthesiology 84:732–747
4. Anene O, Meert KL, Uy H, Simpson P, Sarnaik AP (1996) Dexamethasone for the prevention of postextubation airway obstruction: a prospective, randomized, double-blind, placebo-controlled trial. Crit Care Med 24:1666–1669
5. Auden SM (1999) Cervical Spine Instability and dwarfism: fibreoptic intubation for all. Anaesthesiology 91:580
6. Bergese SD, Patrick Bender S, McSweeney TD, Fernandez S, Dzwonczyk R, Sage K (2010) A comparative study of dexmedetomidine with midazolam and midazolam alone for sedation during elective awake fiberoptic intubation. J Clin Anesth 22:35–40
7. Chiaretti A, Piastra M, Pulitanò S, Pietrini D, De Rosa G, Barbaro R, Di Rocco C (2002) Prognostic factors and outcome of children with severe head injury: an 8-year experience. Childs Nerv Syst 18:129–136
8. Dahmani S, Michelet D, Abback PS, Wood C, Brasher C, Nivoche Y, Mantz J (2011) Ketamine for perioperative pain management in children: a meta-analysis of published studies. Paediatr Anaesth 21:636–652
9. Desmet L, Lacroix J (2004) Transfusion in pediatrics. Crit Care Clin 20:299–311
10. Elder JB, Hoh DJ, Liu CY, Wang MY (2010) Postoperative continuous paravertebral anesthetic infusion for pain control in posterior cervical spine surgery: a case-control study. Neurosurgery 66:99–106
11. Emery SE, Akhavan S, Miller P, Furey CG, Yoo JU, Rowbottom JR, Bohlman HH (2009) Steroids and risk factors for airway compromise in multilevel cervical corpectomy patients: a prospective, randomized, double-blind study. Spine 34:229–232
12. Epstein S, Tobin M (2006) Complications in ventilator supported patients. In: Tobin M (ed) Principles and practice of mechanical ventilation. McGraw Hill, New York, pp 877–902
13. Epstein SK, Ciubotaru RL, Wong JB (1997) Effect of failed extubation on the outcome of mechanical ventilation. Chest 112:186–192
14. Esteban A, Frutos-Vivar F, Ferguson ND, Arabi Y, Apezteguía C, González M, Epstein SK, Hill NS, Nava S, Soares MA, D'Empaire G, Alía I, Anzueto A (2004) Noninvasive positive-pressure ventilation for respiratory failure after extubation. N Engl J Med 350:2452–2460

15. Farias JA, Retta A, Alía I, Olazarri F, Esteban A, Golubicki A, Allende D, Maliarchuk O, Peltzer C, Ratto ME, Zalazar R, Garea M, Moreno EG (2001) A comparison of two methods to perform a breathing trial before extubation in pediatric intensive care patients. Intensive Care Med 27:1649–1654
16. Filston HC (1992) Fluid and electrolyte management in the pediatric surgical patient. Surg Clin North Am 72:1189–1205
17. Furman EB, Roman DG, Lemmer LA, Hairabet J, Jasinska M, Laver MB (1975) Specific therapy in water, electrolyte, and blood-volume replacement during pediatric surgery. Anesthesiology 42:187–193
18. Goodenough B, Addicoat L, Champion G, McInerney M, Young B, Juniper K, Ziegler JB (1997) Pain in 4- to 6-year-old children receiving intramuscular injections: a comparison of the Faces Pain Scale with other self-report and behavioral measures. Clin J Pain 13:60–73
19. Grunau RV, Johnston CC, Craig KD (1990) Neonatal facial and cry responses to invasive and non-invasive procedures. Pain 42(3):295–305
20. Hadjistavropoulos HD, Ross MA, von Baeyer C (1990) Are physicians' ratings of pain affected by patients' physical attractiveness? Soc Sci Med 31:69–72
21. Hicks C, von Baeyer C, Spafford P, van Korlaar I, Goodenough B (2001) The Faces Pain Scale-Revised: toward a common metric in pediatric pain measurement. Pain 93:173–183
22. Hiller A, Helenius I, Nurmi E, Neuvonen PJ, Kaukonen M, Hartikainen T, Korpela R, Taivainen T, Meretoja OA (2012) Acetaminophen improves analgesia but does not reduce opioid requirement after major spine surgery in children and adolescents. Spine (Phila Pa 1976) 37:1225–1231
23. Hunter M, McDowell L, Hennessy R, Cassey J (2000) An evaluation of the Faces Pain Scale with young children. J Pain Symptom Manag 20:122–129
24. Ista E, van Dijk M, Tibboel D, de Hoog M (2005) Assessment of sedation in pediatric intensive care patients can be improved by using the COMFORT 'behavior' scale. Pediatr Crit Care Med 6:58–63
25. Jacobi J, Bircher N, Krinsley J, Agus M, Braithwaite SS, Deutschman C, Freire AX, Geehan D, Kohl B, Nasraway SA, Rigby M, Sands K, Schallom L, Taylor B, Umpierrez G, Mazuski J, Schunemann H (2012) Guidelines for the use of an insulin infusion for the management of hyperglycemia in critically ill patients. Crit Care Med 40:3251–3276
26. James CS, Hallewell CP, James DP, Wade A, Mok QQ (2011) Predicting the success of non-invasive ventilation in preventing intubation and re-intubation in the paediatric intensive care unit. Intensive Care Med 37:1994–2001
27. Khan ZH, Kashfi A, Ebrahimkhani E (2003) A comparison of the upper lip bite test (a simple new technique) with modified Mallampati classification in predicting difficulty in endotracheal intubation: a prospective blinded study. Anesth Analg 96:595–599
28. Khemani RG, Randolph A, Markovitz B (2009) Corticosteroids for the prevention and treatment of post-extubation stridor in neonates, children and adults. Cochrane Database Syst Rev 8(3):CD001000
29. Kokki H (2003) Nonsteroidal anti-inflammatory drugs for postoperative pain: a focus on children. Paediatr Drugs 5:103–123
30. Kombos T, Suess O, Da Silva C, Ciklatekerlio O, Nobis V, Brock M (2003) Impact of somatosensory evoked potential monitoring on cervical surgery. J Clin Neurophysiol 20(2):122–128
31. Lee CH, Peng MJ, Wu CL (2007) Dexamethasone to prevent postextubation airway obstruction in adults: a prospective, randomized, double-blind, placebo-controlled study. Crit Care 11:R72
32. Lönnqvist PA, Morton NS (2005) Postoperative analgesia in infants and children. Br J Anaesth 95:59–68
33. Mason KP, Lerman J (2011) Dexmedetomidine in children: current knowledge and future applications. Anesth Analg 113:1129–1142
34. McGrath PA (1987) An assessment of children's pain: a review of behavioral, physiological and direct scaling techniques. Pain 31:147–176
35. McGuire G, Crossley D, Richards J, Wong D (1997) Effects of varying levels of positive end-expiratory pressure on intracranial pressure and cerebral perfusion pressure. Crit Care Med 25:1059–1062

36. Menezes AH (2008) Surgical approaches: postoperative care and complications "posterolateral–far lateral transcondylar approach to the ventral foramen magnum and upper cervical spinal canal". Childs Nerv Syst 24:1203–1207
37. Menezes AH (2008) Specific entities affecting the craniocervical region: Down's syndrome. Childs Nerv Syst 24:1165–1168
38. Menezes AH (2012) Craniocervical fusions in children. J Neurosurg Pediatr 9:573–585
39. Mesotten D, Gielen M, Sterken C, Claessens K, Hermans G, Vlasselaers D, Lemiere J, Lagae L, Gewillig M, Eyskens B, Vanhorebeek I, Wouters PJ, Van den Berghe G (2012) Neurocognitive development of children 4 years after critical illness and treatment with tight glucose control: a randomized controlled trial. JAMA 308:1641–1650
40. Michelet D, Andreu-Gallien J, Bensalah T, Hilly J, Wood C, Nivoche Y, Mantz J, Dahmani S (2012) A meta-analysis of the use of nonsteroidal antiinflammatory drugs for pediatric postoperative pain. Anesth Analg 114:393–406
41. O'Shaughnessy DF, Atterbury C, Bolton Maggs P, Murphy M, Thomas D, Yates S, Williamson LM, British Committee for Standards in Haematology, Blood Transfusion Task Force (2004) Guidelines for the use of fresh-frozen plasma, cryoprecipitate and cryosupernatant. Br J Haematol 126:11–28
42. Petrini F, Accorsi A, Adrario E, Agrò F, Amicucci G, Antonelli M, Azzeri F, Baroncini S, Bettelli G, Cafaggi C, Cattano D, Chinelli E, Corbanese U, Corso R, Della Puppa A, Di Filippo A, Facco E, Favaro R, Favero R, Frova G, Giunta F, Giurati G, Giusti F, Guarino A, Iannuzzi E, Ivani G, Mazzon D, Menarini M, Merli G, Mondello E, Muttini S, Nardi G, Pigna A, Pittoni G, Ripamonti D, Rosa G, Rosi R, Salvo I, Sarti A, Serafini G, Servadio G, Sgandurra A, Sorbello M, Tana F, Tufano R, Vesconi S, Villani A, Zauli M, G Task Force, SIAARTI Study Group Difficult Airway (2005) Recommendations for airway control and difficult airway management. Minerva Anestesiol 71:617–657
43. Playfor S, Jenkins I, Boyles C, Choonara I, Davies G, Haywood T, Hinson G, Mayer A, Morton N, Ralph T, Wolf A, United Kingdom Paediatric Intensive Care Society Sedation; Analgesia and Neuromuscular Blockade Working Group (2006) Consensus guidelines on sedation and analgesia in critically ill children. Intensive Care Med 32:1125–1136
44. American Society of Anesthesiologists Task Force on Management of the Difficult Airway (2003) Practice guidelines for management of the difficult airway: an updated report by the American Society of Anesthesiologists Task Force on Management of the Difficult Airway. Anesthesiology 98:1269–1277
45. Rath GP, Bithal PK, Guleria R, Chaturvedi A, Kale SS, Gupta V, Dash HH (2006) A comparative study between preoperative and postoperative pulmonary functions and diaphragmatic movements in congenital craniovertebral junction anomalies. J Neurosurg Anesthesiol 18:256–261
46. Reddy KR, Rao GS, Devi BI, Devi BI, Prasad PV, Ramesh VJ (2009) Pulmonary function after surgery for congenital atlantoaxial dislocation: a comparison with surgery for compressive cervical myelopathy and craniotomy. J Neurosurg Anesthesiol 21:196–201
47. Reveiz L, Guerrero-Lozano R, Camacho A, Yara L, Mosquera PA (2010) Stress ulcer, gastritis, and gastrointestinal bleeding prophylaxis in critically ill pediatric patients: a systematic review. Pediatr Crit Care Med 11:124–132
48. Rigby-Jones A, Priston MJ, Sneyd JR, McCabe AP, Davis GI, Tooley MA, Thorne GC, Wolf AR (2007) Remifentanil-midazolam sedation for pediatric patients receiving mechanical ventilation after cardiac surgery. Br J Anaesth 99:252–261
49. Roseff SD, Luban NL, Manno CS (2002) Guidelines for assessing appropriateness of pediatric transfusion. Transfusion 42:1398–1413
50. Rusy LM, Hainsworth KR, Nelson TJ (2010) Gabapentin use in pediatric spinal fusion patients: a randomized, double-blind, controlled trial. Anesth Analg 110:1393–1398
51. Sagi HC, Beutler W, Carroll E, Connolly PJ (2002) Airway complications associated with surgery on the anterior cervical spine. Spine 27:949–953

52. Sahin A, Salman MA, Erden IA, Aypar U (2004) Upper cervical vertebrae movement during intubating laryngeal mask, fibreoptic and direct laryngoscopy: a video-fluoroscopic study. Eur J Anaesthesiol 21:819–823
53. Sala F, Squintani G, Tramontano V, Coppola A, Gerosa M (2011) Intraoperative neurophysiological monitoring during surgery for Chiari malformations. Neurol Sci 32: S317–S319
54. Sala F, Krzan MJ, Deletis V (2002) Intraoperative neurophysiological monitoring in pediatric neurosurgery: why, when, how? Childs Nerv Syst 18:264–287
55. Samsoon GL, Young JR (1987) Difficult tracheal intubation: a retrospective study. Anaesthesia 42:487–490
56. Schmidt PJ (1982) Component therapy. In: Stehling LC (ed) Techniques of blood transfusion. Int Anesthesiol Clin 20:23–43
57. Schmitt H, Buchfelder M, Radespiel-Troger M et al (2000) Difficult intubation in acromegalic patients: incidence and predictability. Anesthesiology 93:110–114
58. Serocki G, Bein B, Scholz J, Dorges V (2010) Management of the predicted difficult airway: a comparison of conventional blade laryngoscopy with video-assisted blade laryngoscopy and the GlideScope. Eur J Anaesthesiol 27:24–30
59. Sharma D, Prabhakar H, Bithal PK, Ali Z, Singh GP, Rath GP, Dash HH (2010) Predicting difficult laryngoscopy in acromegaly: a comparison of upper lip bite test with modified Mallampati classification. J Neurosurg Anesthesiol 22:138–143
60. Smith RL, Lin JC, Adelson PD, Kochanek PM, Fink EL, Wisniewski SR, Bayir H, Tyler-Kabara EC, Clark RS, Brown SD, Bell MJ (2012) Relationship between hyperglycemia and outcome in children with severe traumatic brain injury. Pediatr Crit Care Med 13:85–91
61. Standing JF, Tibboel D, Korpela R, Olkkola KT (2011) Diclofenac pharmacokinetic meta-analysis and dose recommendations for surgical pain in children aged 1–12 years. Paediatr Anaesth 21(3):316–324
62. Stehling L, Luban NL, Anderson KC, Sayers MH, Long A, Attar S, Leitman SF, Gould SA, Kruskall MS, Goodnough LT (1994) Guidelines for blood utilization review. Transfusion 34:438–448
63. Weiss M, Engelhardt T (2010) Proposal for the management of the unexpected difficult pediatric airway. Paediatr Anaesth 20:454–464
64. Visocchi M, Fernandez EM, Ciampini A, Di Rocco C (2009) Reducible and irreducible os odontoideum treated with posterior wiring, instrumentation and fusion. Past or present? Acta Neuroch (Wien) 151:1265–1274
65. Visocchi M, Pietrini D, Tufo T, Fernandez E, Di Rocco C (2009) Preoperative irreducible C1–C2 dislocations: intraoperative reduction and posterior fixation. The always posterior strategy. Acta Neurochir 151:551–559
66. Visocchi M: Response to Wang et al., re Letter re Visocchi M, Pietrini D, Tufo T, Fernandez E, Di Rocco C (2009) Pre-operative irreducible C1-C2 dislocations: intra-operative reduction and posterior fixation. The "always posterior strategy". Acta Neurochir (Wien) 151:551–559; discussion 560
67. Visocchi M (2010) The craniovertebral junction: posterior and anterior approaches. State of art. Crit Rev Neurosurg WFNS 1:1–11
68. Voepel-Lewis T, Merkel S, Tait AR, Trzcinka A, Malviya S (2002) The reliability and validity of the Face, Legs, Activity, Cry, Consolability observational tool as a measure of pain in children with cognitive impairment. Anesth Analg 95:1224–9
69. White MC, Marsh CJ, Beringer RM, Nolan JA, Choi AY, Medlock KE, Mason DG (2012) A randomised, controlled trial comparing the Airtraq™ optical laryngoscope with conventional laryngoscopy in infants and children. Anaesthesia 67:226–231

Advances

Technical Advances in Pediatric Craniovertebral Junction Surgery

Mark E. Oppenlander, James Kalyvas, Volker K.H. Sonntag, and Nicholas Theodore

Contents

Abstract Surgery for conditions in the craniovertebral junction in the pediatric population poses unique challenges. The posterior approach has emerged as the gold standard for arthrodesis in this region. Anterior fixation or decompression also may be indicated. Intraoperative image guidance and neurophysiological monitoring improve the safety and efficacy of these procedures. The specific technical advances in surgery of the craniovertebral junction that have improved patient outcomes are reviewed.

Keywords Craniovertebral junction surgery • Pediatrics • Arthrodesis • Image guidance • Neurophysiological monitoring

M.E. Oppenlander, MD • J. Kalyvas, MD • V.K.H. Sonntag, MD • N. Theodore, MD (✉)
Division of Neurological Surgery, Barrow Neurological Institute,
St. Joseph's Hospital and Medical Center, 350 W Thomas Rd,
Phoenix, AZ 85013, USA
e-mail: neuropub@chw.edu

C. Di Rocco, N. Akalan (eds.), *Pediatric Craniovertebral Junction Diseases*,
Advances and Technical Standards in Neurosurgery 40,
DOI 10.1007/978-3-319-01065-6_6, © Springer International Publishing Switzerland 2014

Introduction

Conditions involving the craniovertebral junction in children include congenital disorders, inflammatory conditions, traumatic dislocation or fracture, and neoplastic etiologies. Unique challenges are associated with surgery for decompression and internal fixation of the pediatric craniovertebral junction, including the small osseous structures and variable anatomy of children. These issues complicate both the diagnosis and treatment of craniovertebral disorders in this age group.

Anterior and posterior approaches to the craniovertebral junction have been described in detail, reflecting a significant evolution in the surgical management of conditions affecting this region. Furthermore, techniques for intraoperative image guidance and neurophysiological monitoring continue to emerge for surgery of the craniovertebral junction. With these advances have come improvements in patient outcomes and rates of arthrodesis. This chapter outlines specific technical advances underlying this evolution.

Posterior Approaches

Posterior Fixation Techniques

The challenge of stabilizing the craniovertebral junction lies in the complex biomechanics and anatomy of the region. In the pediatric population, these issues are complicated by a skeletally immature spine and smaller bony landmarks. The posterior approach remains the standard for definitive arthrodesis of the craniovertebral junction, and several technical advances in instrumentation and techniques have led to a high rate of success in these patients [1, 2].

Early attempts to stabilize the craniovertebral junction utilized simple bone graft onlay techniques. Suboccipital and sublaminar wiring was introduced to secure the bone graft, but these methods still necessitated postoperative external rigid orthosis (Fig. 1) [21].Wiring techniques also often incorporated subaxial nonpathologic segments into the construct to ensure stability, thus necessitating increased surgical exposure while subsequently limiting the patient's range of motion.

Rod-and-wire fixation techniques, for example with the Steinmann pin, offer several advantages to earlier constructs. When used in combination with bone graft, this construct is associated with a higher rate of fusion [3, 15]. The use of a rod construct offers more rigid internal fixation, thus decreasing reliance on external orthosis. In the pediatric population, rod-and-wire may be an appropriate technique if anatomy limits the use of screws (Fig. 2) [21].

The rod-and-wire technique involves bending a rod into a U-shape and using sublaminar wires or braided cables to fixate the rod and bone graft to the occiput and cervical spine. As with graft-and-wire techniques, however, rod-and-wire may require incorporation of subaxial segments, further limiting range of motion.

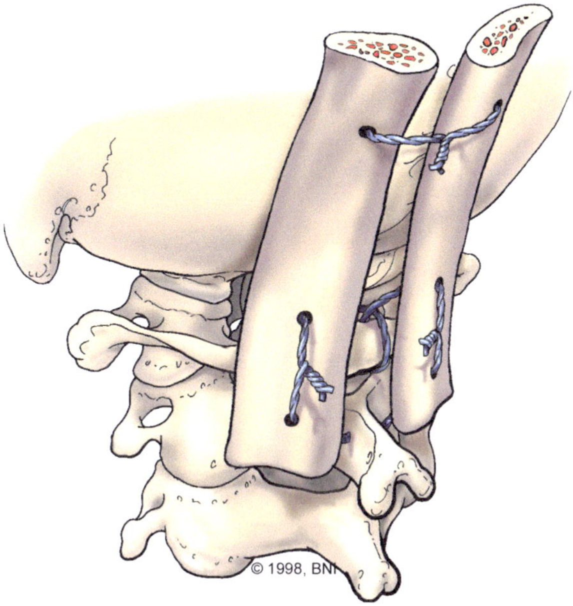

Fig. 1 Graft-and-wire technique. A rib graft is wired to the occiput and the cervical laminae for occipitocervical fusion (Used with permission from Barrow Neurological Institute)

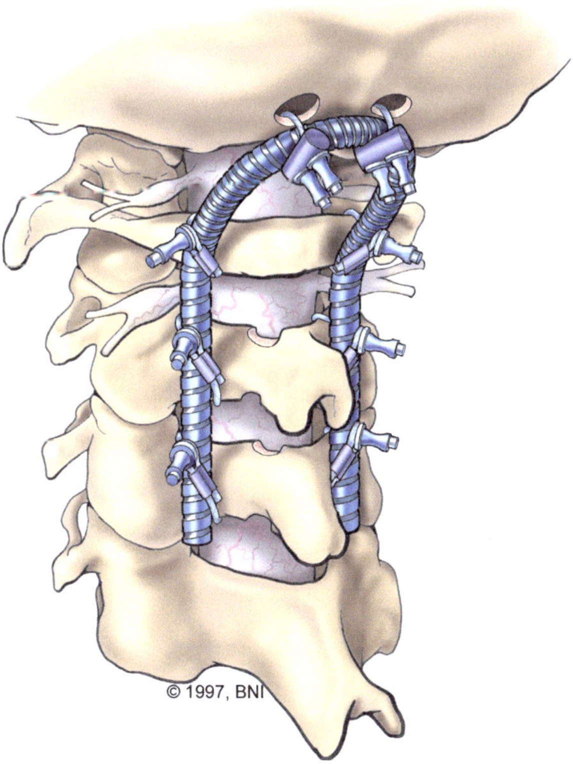

Fig. 2 Rod-and-wire technique. Occipitocervical fixation and fusion are accomplished by securing a threaded Steinmann pin to the craniovertebral junction with wire or braided cable (Used with permission from Barrow Neurological Institute)

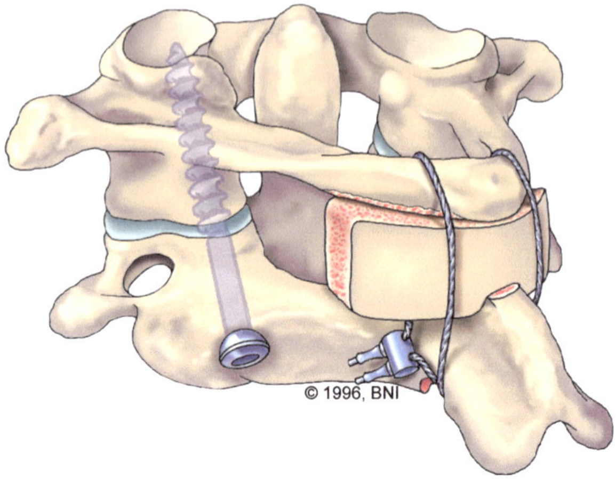

Fig. 3 Atlantoaxial fixation, combining the Dickman-Sonntag interspinous fusion technique with transarticular screws (Used with permission from Barrow Neurological Institute)

Biomechanically, both graft-and-wire as well as rod-and-wire techniques are inferior to rigid screw-based techniques [6].

Specific attention has focused on the interspinous methods of fixating the atlas to the axis. These methods place a bone graft between the spinous processes of C1 and C2. A braided cable then places the graft under compression, providing a posterior buttress to promote bony fusion. Specific examples include the Brooks fusion [5] or the Dickman-Sonntag technique [7]. As with other grafting techniques, the interspinous graft is made more biomechanically rigid when combined with screw fixation (Fig. 3).

The introduction of screw-based techniques for craniovertebral junction fixation offers superior biomechanical rigidity compared with previous constructs [7]. Furthermore, screw fixation is feasible in the pediatric population as long as the patient has no precluding anatomic constraints [21]. Early screw-based constructs utilized lateral mass plates, whereas new constructs use polyaxial screw heads and rods (Fig. 4).

The rods may be composed of a variety of metals, most commonly stainless steel, titanium, or Vitallium (cobalt chromium). Titanium is lighter weight and produces lower artifact on imaging when compared with stainless steel, whereas Vitallium has similar stiffness to stainless steel while still retaining the light weight and low imaging artifact of titanium [13].

Numerous options for screw fixation of the atlantoaxial complex have been described. Transarticular screw fixation, described by Magerl and Seeman [16], results in a stable and rigid construct (Fig. 3). Combining C1 lateral mass screws with C2 pars or C2 pedicle screws offers similar biomechanics to the transarticular construct [17]. C2 translaminar screws are an alternative if unsuitable anatomy excludes pars articularis or pedicle screws at the C2 level [27]. The choice of any particular screw option depends on the patient's anatomy and surgeon's preference. The transarticular screw, for example, is infeasible in as many as 23 % of cases because of unfavorable anatomy [18].

New screw-based techniques for the occiput have also evolved. Earlier constructs utilized bilateral plates or rods extending from the bilateral occipital regions.

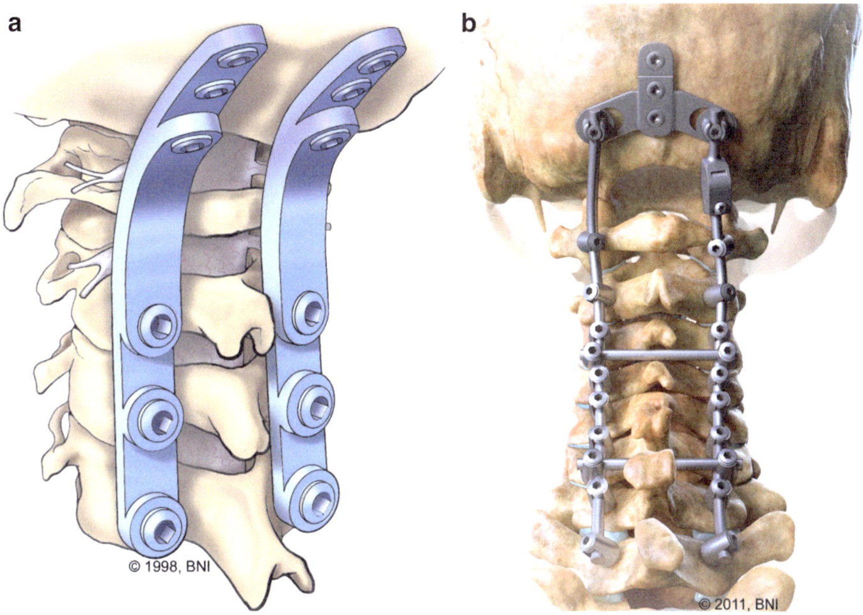

Fig. 4 Occipitocervical fusion with screw-based constructs. (**a**) Early screw-plate system. (**b**) Modern construct using polyaxial screw heads and rods (Used with permission from Barrow Neurological Institute)

This method has the disadvantage of fixating to a point lateral to midline on the occiput where the bone is thinner. Newer constructs fixate the occiput in the midline keel where bone is thickest and screw purchase is maximized. Combining screw-based rigid fixation with bone graft support maximizes stability and the likelihood of bony fusion (Fig. 5).

Considerations in the Very Young

Craniovertebral junction pathology and fixation techniques in the very young pediatric population (<10 years old) require special consideration. The degree of bony spine maturation in the pediatric population has a profound impact on the spine's response to trauma and its potential surgical management. Because ossification does not complete until the teenage years, fractures of the spine are rare and ligamentous injuries predominate in the younger age group. Furthermore, due to smaller bony structures, fixation techniques must be tailored to the individual child's anatomy. The pedicles, facets, and lateral masses of a young child are often too small to accommodate screw fixation, especially when considering potential danger to the closely approximated vertebral artery and spinal cord. In these cases, Steinmann pin and sublaminar wiring are preferred. Care is taken to avoid subperiosteal dissection of adjacent laminae and spinous processes so that creep fusion of the bystander vertebra can be avoided [8, 9].

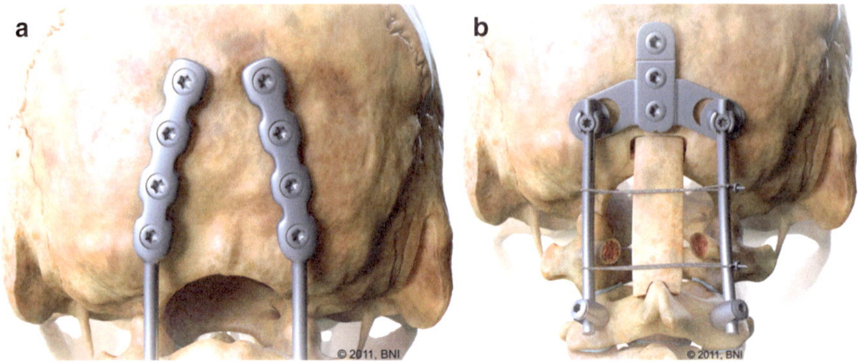

Fig. 5 Multiple options exist for screw fixation to the occiput. (**a**) Lateral fixation has the disadvantage of thinner bone. (**b**) A midline occipital plate utilizes thicker bone in the keel. This illustration depicts the posterior view of an occiput-to-C2 fusion construct with placement of a rib graft. In this case, the bone graft offers additional stability by its placement between the C2 spinous process and a shelf drilled at the base of the occipital bone (Used with permission from Barrow Neurological Institute)

The impact of successful arthrodesis on subsequent spinal column development at the fused levels remains controversial. In our experience (Theodore N and Sonntag VHK, unpublished data, 2008), intervertebral disc height of fused levels decreased significantly compared to unfused levels in younger patients undergoing occipitocervical posterior fixation. Presumably, the disuse of discs may lead to early degeneration, calcification, and ultimately fusion. We have also observed a significant decrease in the growth of the width of fused cervical vertebral bodies in patients younger than 10 years while vertebral body height is maintained. Therefore, axial loading may contribute to vertical growth while lateral motion in these patients is restricted and width growth is arrested. Comparatively, both fused and unfused cervical spines after age 10 behave like the adult growth pattern. Finally, children undergoing occipitocervical fusion show no significant change in the diameter of the spinal canal between fused and unfused levels over time, perhaps related to the pulsation of cerebrospinal fluid and growth of the spinal cord (Theodore N and Sonntag VHK, unpublished data, 2008).

Anterior Approaches

Transoral Decompression

The simplest and most direct access to the anterior craniovertebral junction is through the transoral approach. Transoral surgery in the pediatric patient is usually indicated in the setting of irreducible ventral midline extradural compression of the upper cervical spinal cord or lower brainstem. Ventral pathologies include congenital deformity, basilar impression, autoimmune inflammatory conditions, infectious

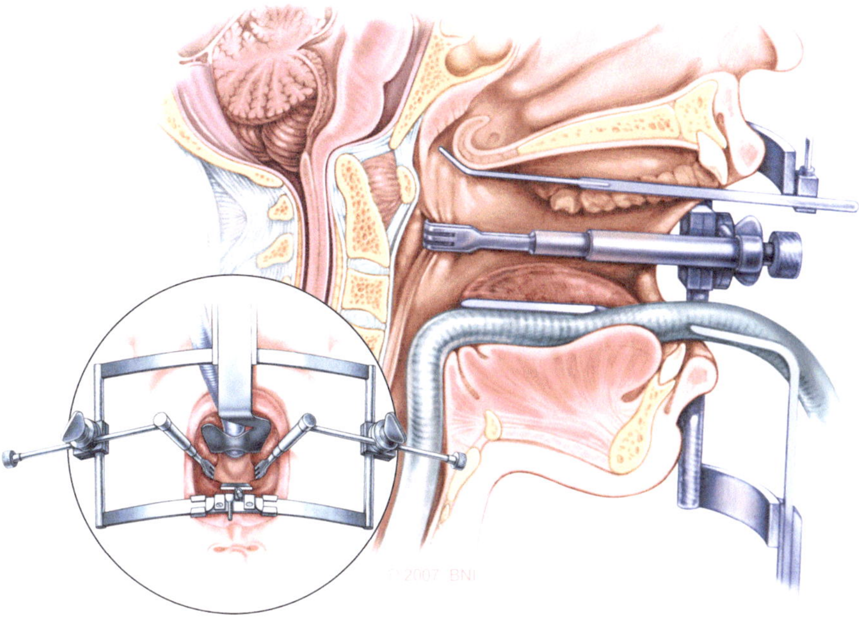

Fig. 6 Sagittal view illustrating the transoral retractor. *Inset*: Surgeon's view of the operative field (Used with permission from Barrow Neurological Institute)

processes, or neoplasms [24]. The goal of the transoral approach is decompression because options for transoral fixation techniques are limited [22]. Posterior stabilization is therefore usually subsequently indicated. Use of the operative microscope and intraoperative neuronavigation increase the safety and efficacy of the decompression.

Transoral surgery offers special challenges in the pediatric population. The surgical corridor is limited due to a child's small oropharynx. Adenoid and tonsillar hypertrophy further limits visualization and working space. Standard transoral retractor systems can often be used in a child, but less force should be applied to the retractor to avoid dislocation of the jaw (Fig. 6).

First described by Kanavel in 1919 [12], the transoral approach has been modified for use in children to circumvent the aforementioned pitfalls. Various modifications aimed at increasing exposure to the anterior craniovertebral junction include the mandibulotomy, mandibuloglossotomy, and/or the palatotomy [3, 28]. The simplest procedure that provides the necessary extent of exposure should be chosen, but children tend to require extensive modifications more often than adults [28].

Odontoid Screw Fixation

Acute odontoid fractures in the younger age group result from high-energy trauma [1]. Direct screw fixation of the odontoid can be performed via an anterior

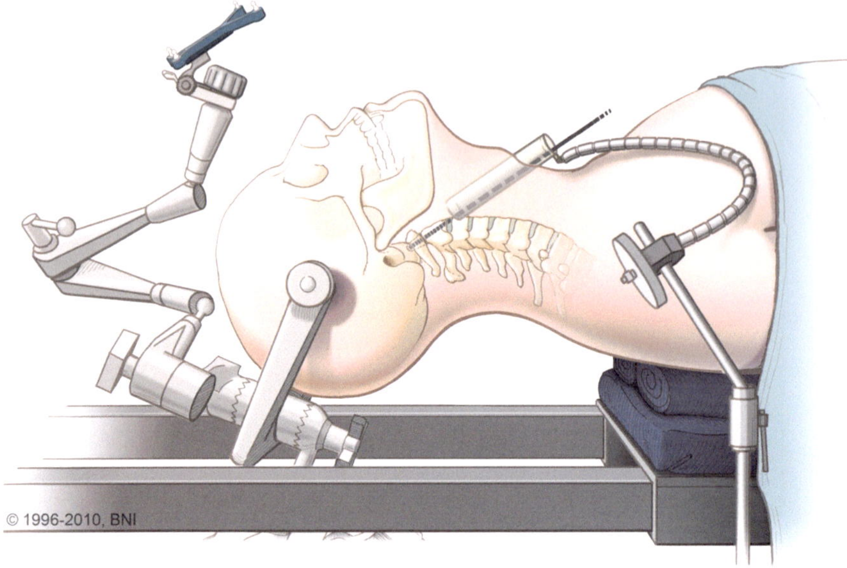

Fig. 7 Patient position during odontoid screw placement, with use of intraoperative image guidance to assess the entry point and trajectory of the screw (Used with permission from Barrow Neurological Institute)

transcervical approach. Intraoperative radiography or neuronavigation is needed to determine if the screw trajectory and anatomic alignment are appropriate (Fig. 7). The anterior odontoid screw method can only be used if the cruciate ligament is preserved [22]. Odontoid screw fixation has the advantages of maintaining normal C1 motion and avoiding a more extensive posterior approach. It should be avoided if there is significant displacement of the odontoid or with subacute and chronic fracture nonunions.

Image Guidance

Evolution within the field of intraoperative imaging has kept pace with advances in anterior and posterior surgical techniques for the treatment of pediatric diseases of the craniovertebral junction, improving their safety and efficacy and, in some instances, widening their application to a broader group of patients. Specifically, computed tomography (CT)-based three-dimensional neuronavigation, with its established efficacy in cranial-based surgery, is now being used in spinal surgery and is being tailored to meet the specific associated challenges.

The craniovertebral junction is an anatomically complex and variable region, particularly in children, with vital structures in proximity—including the brain stem, spinal cord, vertebral arteries, and nerve roots—making the surgical margin for error small. Yet in the case of spinal instrumentation, malpositioned hardware has been reported in as many as 31 % of cases even in the most experienced hands, with serious neurological consequences in up to 5 % of cases [11]. Risk of vertebral artery injury alone is reported in more than 2 % of C1-2 transarticular screws placed [10]. Use of traditional fluoroscopy with anteroposterior and lateral x-rays is beneficial but cumbersome and time-consuming, and it offers limited information about the anatomy of the soft tissues.

In contrast, CT neuronavigation provides almost real-time three-dimensional anatomic information that can guide placement and length of the incision: extent and adequacy of exposure and decompression and the entry point, trajectory, and screw morphometry (length and width) for occipital and cervical screw placement (Fig. 8). These features allow a tailored approach–of special importance in a region marked by prevalent anatomic anomalies. For example, despite the structural superiority of cervical pedicle screws, they are rarely placed in this region due to the risk of injuring neural structures and anomalous vertebral arteries. With the aid of CT neuronavigation, however, Rajasekaran et al. demonstrated that upper cervical pedicle screws could be placed safely in as many as 93 % of pediatric patients who were evaluated with preoperative CT, including those with otherwise preclusive anomalies [20]. Of 26 C1 or C2 pedicle screws placed, none were associated with a critical breach that threatened neurovascular structures or needed revision. Without neuronavigation, the rate of critical breach associated with cervical pedicle screw placement has been as high as 66 % [14]. Neuronavigation thus has the potential to more safely expand the application of procedures to a broader cohort of patients.

Many authors have demonstrated the accuracy and utility of neuronavigation in the pediatric craniovertebral junction across multiple disease entities, including congenital disorders, unstable fractures, and neoplastic lesions, as well as across multiple procedures, including transoral odontoid decompression, occipitocervical fusion, and minimally invasive percutaneous screw-based fusion. Veres et al., for example, reported superior anatomic awareness, improved surgical confidence, and reduced exposure to traditional fluoroscopy when neuronavigation is used in transoral decompressions, particularly when establishing midline for the pharyngeal incision and determining the adequacy of bony decompression of the C1 arch and dens [25]. Welch et al. touted the ability of neuronavigation to improve screw trajectories during placement of C1-2 transarticular screws and to reduce exposure during the resection of upper cervical nerve sheath tumors [26]. Multiple authors have commented on the utility of knowing the precise location of the vertebral arteries during surgery and on the ability to preserve C2 ganglia when placing C1 lateral mass screws, which otherwise may be sacrificed.

Neuronavigation correlates CT or magnetic resonance imaging to three-dimensional anatomy based on spatial relationships between a patient's anatomic landmarks and a fixed reference arc, which are established during a registration process. Current technology is primarily based on infrared light emission and detection from a source camera, which measures light returned from ball reflectors placed on the reference arc and on probes or surgical instruments. Accuracy of anatomic correlation to the imaging or "fit" is determined at a separate computer work station.

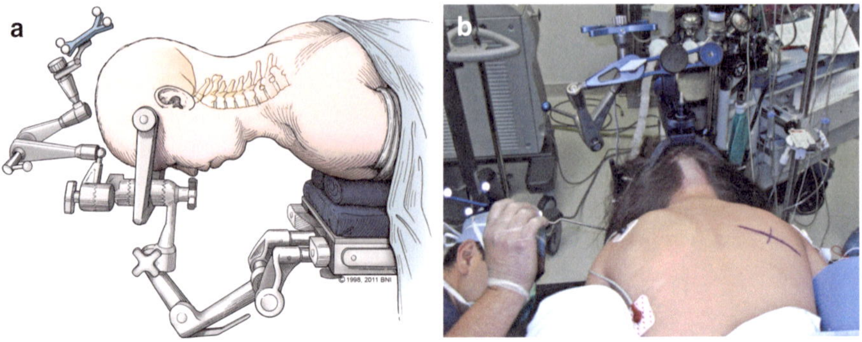

Fig. 8 Occipitocervical fusion utilizing stereotactic navigation. (**a**) The patient is placed in the prone position with the head secured in a Mayfield skull clamp. The reference frame for stereotactic navigation is attached to the Mayfield apparatus. (**b**) Note the minimal hair clip and the site for rib harvest (Used with permission from Barrow Neurological Institute)

Surgery can proceed if the margin of error is below an acceptable threshold. Accuracy of the system, however, is more challenging in spinal surgery compared to cranial surgery. The spine is relatively mobile and has fewer anatomic landmarks for registration. It therefore often requires intraoperative reassessment and reregistration, which can prolong surgical times [4]. One proposed solution has been to treat the upper cervical spine as an extension of the skull base [25]. Fiducials are placed lower on the skull base at the mastoids in addition to the usual locations for cranial surgery before a preoperative CT is obtained to increase registration accuracy of the skull base and upper cervical spine. This technique, however, is predicated on fixing the anatomic relationships of the craniovertebral junction with a halo vest, and accuracy may deteriorate at lower cervical levels.

Greater accuracy may await technological refinement of the available neuronavigation systems. The two primary infrared systems in use (BrainLAB Vector Vision system/Arcadis Orbic Isocentric C-arm and Stealth Treon System/O-arm) require fixed reference arcs, which cannot compensate for spinal mobility. Newer light-emitting diode arrays or ultrasonic emitters can detect localizers placed at each vertebral level, allowing for real-time information when spinal movement occurs [26]. Such systems are commercially available, but their assessment in the literature is limited.

Aside from accuracy, neuronavigation in the spine often requires intraoperative CT, in addition to pre- and postoperative CT, increasing the long-term radiation risks associated with exposure in a sensitive pediatric population. This risk must be weighed against potentially reduced radiation exposure from traditional fluoroscopy and the potential surgical risk to important neurovascular structures. Appropriate long-term follow-up and intraoperative shielding are indicated. Finally, significant up-front costs associated with neuronavigation may be offset by reduced surgical times and lower morbidity and mortality rates, but a cost-benefit analysis in the literature is needed.

Monitoring

Intraoperative electrophysiologic monitoring is routinely used to improve patient safety during surgery of the pediatric craniovertebral junction by providing the surgeon with real-time feedback about the integrity and function of the afferent and efferent tracts of the central and peripheral nervous systems. In concept, any warning signals regarding at-risk neural structures may guide surgical intervention, for example, by altering traction, degree of reduction, or screw placement.

Although now routine in spinal surgery, the use of monitoring has been somewhat undermined by the high rate of false-positive warning signals, which limit its utility and universal use. For example, false-positive rates associated with electromyography (EMG) can occur in 34 % of cases and can cloud surgical decision-making [19]. As a result, multimodality monitoring with somatosensory-evoked potentials (SSEPs), motor-evoked potentials (MEPs), and EMG are often used to improve sensitivity and specificity, so that a more complete electrophysiologic assessment of neural integrity can be achieved. In adult spinal surgery, for example, Quaraishi et al. reported that the sensitivity and specificity of multimodality monitoring for neurologic deficits were 100 and 84 %, respectively [19].

Recently, Thuet et al. demonstrated the accuracy of multimodality monitoring during pediatric spinal deformity surgery in 3,436 children over a 23-year experience at a single institution [23]. Over a broad range of spinal procedures for multiple diagnostic groups, monitoring correctly predicted permanent neurologic status in 99.6 % of patients. Although 74 patients had true-positive warning signals on monitoring, confirmed by intraoperative "wake-up" tests, this number was reduced to six patients with permanent deficits after modifying the surgical intervention, indicating the utility of such monitoring.

Tailoring monitoring technique to surgical context is key to reduce the rate of missed injury. When false-negative readings occur, they are often attributed to monitoring at incorrect dermatomal or myotomal levels. Therefore, pre- and intraoperative communication between the surgical and monitoring team is paramount. Nerve root damage can also be more difficult to assess than spinal cord injury due to the susceptibility of the nerve root to more indirect injury, such as prolonged compression or stretch related to positioning.

Even with limitations, multimodality monitoring is now widely used as another important source of information to help broaden the surgical context, to guide the surgeon toward appropriate intervention, and ultimately to increase safety for patients undergoing surgery at the craniovertebral junction.

Additional New Technologies

Other technologies, such as robotic systems and electrical conductivity monitoring systems for spinal screw placement, are on the horizon to address the shortcomings of both intraoperative imaging and monitoring. For example, Zellar et al. described early, qualified success placing pediatric cervical spine screws with a drill that measures electrical conductivity differences between various tissues such as bone and fat [29]. Using audible feedback, the surgeon can distinguish when cancellous bone interfaces with cortical bone, or when cortical bone is breached, and thus alters trajectory accordingly.

Along with novel monitoring systems, additional innovations in surgical tools are decreasing operative times while increasing patient safety. The Aquamantys (Salient Surgical Technologies, Portsmouth, NH), for example, is an irrigating bipolar device with the potential to decrease blood loss and to speed operative exposures. It offers simultaneous delivery of radiofrequency energy and saline to create a hemostatic sealing of soft tissue and bone at the operative site.

An additional advancement is the "bone scalpel" (ultrasonic harmonic scalpel, Ethicon Endo-surgery, Inc., Cincinnati, OH). This tool has the potential to replace the high-speed drill for laminectomies and other bone work. It utilizes an ultrasonic generator; the blades vibrate longitudinally to enhance bone cutting while maintaining tactile feel for the surgeon. The same vibration seals small vessels to aid hemostasis.

Conclusions

Indications for decompression and stabilization of the pediatric craniovertebral junction vary. While posterior surgical techniques have become the standard for definitive arthrodesis of this region, anterior approaches also may be indicated. The concomitant development of intraoperative image guidance and electrophysiological monitoring has increased patient safety while decreasing operative times. The expanding sphere of technological advances in surgery for the pediatric craniovertebral junction promises to continue improving safety and efficacy of procedures in this region.

References

1. Ahmed R, Traynelis VC, Menezes AH (2008) Fusions at the craniovertebral junction. Childs Nerv Syst 24:1209–1224
2. Anderson RC, Ragel BT, Mocco J et al (2007) Selection of a rigid internal fixation construct for stabilization at the craniovertebral junction in pediatric patients. J Neurosurg 107: 36–42
3. Apostolides PJ (1998) Technique of transoral odontoidectomy. Oper Tech Neurosurg 1:58–62
4. Braun V (2001) In vivo experiences with frameless stereotactically guided screw placement in the spine – results from 75 consecutive cases. Neurosurg Rev 24:74–79
5. Brooks AL, Jenkins EB (1978) Atlanto-axial arthrodesis by the wedge compression method. J Bone Joint Surg Am 60:279–284

6. Dickman CA, Lekovic GP (2005) Biomechanical considerations for stabilization of the craniovertebral junction. Clin Neurosurg 52:205–213
7. Dickman CA, Sonntag VK, Papadopoulos SM et al (1991) The interspinous method of posterior atlantoaxial arthrodesis. J Neurosurg 74:190–198
8. Dogan S, Safavi-Abbasi S, Theodore N et al (2006) Pediatric subaxial cervical spine injuries: origins, management, and outcome in 51 patients. Neurosurg Focus 20:E1
9. Eleraky MA, Theodore N, Adams M et al (2000) Pediatric cervical spine injuries: report of 102 cases and review of the literature. J Neurosurg 92:12–17
10. Haque A, Price AV, Sklar FH et al (2009) Screw fixation of the upper cervical spine in the pediatric population. Clinical article. J Neurosurg Pediatr 3:529–533
11. Hedequist D, Proctor M (2009) Screw fixation to C2 in children: a case series and technical report. J Pediatr Orthop 29:21–25
12. Kanavel AB (1919) Bullet locked between atlas and the base of the skull: technique for removal through the mouth. Surg Clin 1:361–6
13. Knott PT, Mardjetko SM, Kim RH et al (2010) A comparison of magnetic and radiographic imaging artifact after using three types of metal rods: stainless steel, titanium, and vitallium. Spine J 10:789–794
14. Ludwig SC, Kramer DL, Vaccaro AR et al (1999) Transpedicle screw fixation of the cervical spine. Clin Orthop Relat Res 359:77–88
15. MacKenzie AI, Uttley D, Marsh HT et al (1990) Craniocervical stabilization using Luque/Hartshill rectangles. Neurosurgery 26:32–36
16. Magerl F, Seemann PS (1987) Stable posterior fusion of the atlas and axis by transarticular screw fixation. In: Kehr WA, Weidner A (eds) Cervical spine I, vol 1. Springer, New York, pp 322–327
17. Melcher RP, Puttlitz CM, Kleinstueck FS et al (2002) Biomechanical testing of posterior atlantoaxial fixation techniques. Spine (Phila Pa 1976) 27:2435–2440
18. Paramore CG, Dickman CA, Sonntag VK (1996) The anatomical suitability of the C1-2 complex for transarticular screw fixation. J Neurosurg 85:221–224
19. Quraishi NA, Lewis SJ, Kelleher MO et al (2009) Intraoperative multimodality monitoring in adult spinal deformity: analysis of a prospective series of one hundred two cases with independent evaluation. Spine (Phila Pa 1976) 34:1504–1512
20. Rajasekaran S, Kanna PR, Shetty AP (2012) Safety of cervical pedicle screw insertion in children – a clinico-radiological evaluation of computer assisted insertion of 51 cervical pedicle screws including 28 Sub-axial pedicle screws in sixteen children. Spine (Phila Pa 1976) 37:E216–E223
21. Schultz KD Jr, Petronio J, Haid RW et al (2000) Pediatric occipitocervical arthrodesis. A review of current options and early evaluation of rigid internal fixation techniques. Pediatr Neurosurg 33:169–181
22. Sonntag VK, Dickman CA (1993) Craniocervical stabilization. Clin Neurosurg 40:243–272
23. Thuet ED, Winscher JC, Padberg AM et al (2010) Validity and reliability of intraoperative monitoring in pediatric spinal deformity surgery: a 23-year experience of 3436 surgical cases. Spine (Phila Pa 1976) 35:1880–1886
24. Tuite GF, Veres R, Crockard HA et al (1996) Pediatric transoral surgery: indications, complications, and long-term outcome. J Neurosurg 84:573–583
25. Veres R, Bago A, Fedorcsak I (2001) Early experiences with image-guided transoral surgery for the pathologies of the upper cervical spine. Spine (Phila Pa 1976) 26:1385–1388
26. Welch WC, Subach BR, Pollack IF et al (1997) Frameless stereotactic guidance for surgery of the upper cervical spine. Neurosurgery 40:958–963
27. Wright NM (2004) Posterior C2 fixation using bilateral, crossing C2 laminar screws: case series and technical note. J Spinal Disord Tech 17:158–162
28. Youssef AS, Guiot B, Black K et al (2008) Modifications of the transoral approach to the craniovertebral junction: anatomic study and clinical correlations. Neurosurgery 62:145–154
29. Zeller R, Canavese F, Kulkarni AV et al (2009) Technique for drilling instrument monitoring electrical conductivity in pediatric cervical spine screw insertion: a preliminary report. J Pediatr Orthop 29:760–764

Craniovertebral Junction Instability: Special Reference to Paediatric Age Group

Atul Goel

Contents

A. Goel, MCh Neurosurgery
Department of Neurosurgery,
K.E.M Hospital and Seth G.S. Medical College, Parel, Mumbai 400012, India
e-mail: atulgoel62@hotmail.com

C. Di Rocco, N. Akalan (eds.), *Pediatric Craniovertebral Junction Diseases*,
Advances and Technical Standards in Neurosurgery 40,
DOI 10.1007/978-3-319-01065-6_7, © Springer International Publishing Switzerland 2014

Abstract Craniovertebral junction is the centre for stability and of mobility of the spine. The region is ingeniously designed and structured to permit a complex array of movements whilst preserving the stability. The occipitoatlantal joint is the centre for stability, whilst atlantoaxial joint is the centre for mobility. Despite the flawless architecture, a range of factors can influence the stability of the region. Majority of instability is related to affection of the atlantoaxial joint. Special issues confront the surgeon whilst dealing with instability of the craniovertebral junction in paediatric age group. Authors will discuss the issue of instability of craniovertebral junction, more particularly as it relates to paediatric patients, and discuss the methods of stabilisation.

Keywords Atlantoaxial dislocation • basilar invagination • craniovertebral anomaly

Craniovertebral Junction Instability: Special Reference to Paediatric Age Group

The craniovertebral junction is the centre for stability and of mobility of the spine. The region is anatomically and biomechanically complex. The embryological development of the region is intricate and ill-understood. The pathogenesis of a number of anomalies of the region is still debated. The region is strong, supple and 'fluid' in paediatric age group, and traumatic affections to both bone and soft tissues are relatively uncommon. The 'new' and 'fresh' ligaments and muscles of the region in children permit free and wider range movements. Although trauma may less commonly be a cause, majority of clinical conditions that lead to instability at the craniovertebral junction in paediatric age group are related to developmental defects or genetic syndromes that lead to abnormal ligamentous laxity. Developmental craniovertebral anomalies as a result of defects in segmentation or of formation of the structure that are identified in this age group are relatively more complex than those identified in older age group. It is crucial to be vigilant of spinal abnormalities in children with specific genetic abnormalities.

The surgical management of craniovertebral anomalies is complex due to the relative difficulty in accessing the region, critical relationships of neurovascular structures and the intricate biomechanical issues involved. The subject of craniovertebral junction anomalies is under discussion and evaluation for over a century. A number of classical reviews have attempted to clarify a variety of complex associated issues. Despite the volumes of publications on the subject, it appears that the last word has not yet been said. A large array of complex bony and neural anomalies has been described in this region. The issues in the management include consideration for decompression of the region and provision of firm and stable fixation which is able to bear the stresses and strains of movements, distraction and compression. If correct and timely treatment is provided to these patients, a satisfying long-term outcome can be obtained. As the malformation is basically mechanical in nature, a successful treatment may lead to improvement in a child who will otherwise have a full life.

The surgical treatment of instability of the craniovertebral junction in paediatric age group has special consideration. The issues are discrete for infants, children up to age of 10 years and for young adults (age 10–20 years). The treatment consideration will vary with age: younger the patient more complex is the treatment.

Special Issues That Pertain to Surgical Treatment in Paediatric Age Group

1. The affected patient may be investigated for systemic disease and generalised muscle-ligament affection due to genetic syndrome.
2. Elaborate imaging is necessary to evaluate the bone malformations, abnormal segmentations and abnormal fusions.
3. The bones, particularly the arch of atlas, may be ill-formed, bifid or cartilaginous making midline surgical procedures difficult and sometimes impossible.
4. The degree of atlantoaxial dislocation is generally more pronounced as the instability is due to unusually supple or lax ligaments.
5. The clinical presenting symptoms are relatively subtle and long-standing and can be missed.
6. There are relatively large venous plexuses in the region of the lateral masses making the dissection relatively complex on occasions. The venous plexuses are generally larger than those encountered in adults.
7. The articular cartilage is well formed and 'slippery', much more than in adults.
8. Blood loss during surgery is relatively poorly tolerated.
9. The facets of atlas and axis are relatively well formed even when the midline structures are weak or poorly developed, making the lateral mass fixation procedures ideal.
10. The interfacetal distance is usually large, making transarticular screw fixation surgery relatively difficult.

11. Manipulation and distraction of the facets and their realignment are relatively easier in paediatric age group.
12. The tissues, including the C2 ganglion, are remarkably flexible and elastic, making retraction of this structure safer when exposure and joint treatment is contemplated.
13. The fixation needs to be segmental as including a number of spinal segments may affect the growth of neck. Also there is a potential for the development of secondary abnormalities.
14. Recovery following a successful surgical procedure is more remarkable, pronounced and quick when compared to that seen in adults.
15. External arthrosis before and after surgery is poorly tolerated.
16. Rotatory dislocation or facetal locking is usually seen more often in children.

Craniovertebral junction is elegantly designed and structured to provide strength and free movements to the most mobile and stable region of the body. Anatomical studies of craniovertebral junction of animals depict the remarkable features of structural formations related to functional needs [32]. The function of stability of the region is inversely related to the extent of mobility of the region. More the stability less is the mobility and vice versa. The occipitoaxial joint is the centre for stability and the atlantoaxial joint is the centre for mobility. More stable the craniovertebral junction (like in lions, horse) stronger is the occipitoatlantal joint and more mobile is the region the joint is proportionately weaker (like in birds). The size and suppleness of the atlantoaxial joint determine the extent of neck movements.

A direct inspection of the joints in a human cadaver will reveal that the ligaments in the region of occipitoatlantal joint are so strong and 'steel-like' that it will take considerable effort and heavy and sharp instruments to dislodge the joint, the effort being significantly more than any other joint of the body. The human spine mimics a pillar that bifurcates in its upper part to support the roof. The facets of atlas and axis and the occipital condyles form the superior bifurcation of the vertical pillar formed by the vertebral bodies of the spine, giving the 'human spinal pillar' a 'Y-shaped' design. Craniovertebral instability is more often a result of affection of the pillar and manifests by abnormalities in the alignment of atlantoaxial facetal articulation. The majority of craniovertebral instability is related to the affection of the atlantoaxial joint, whilst a small minority of cases have instability related to the affection of the occipitoatlantal joint.

Generalised ligamentous laxity due to genetic syndromes can lead to multiple joint affection in paediatric age group. The affection of C0–C1 joint is more frequently encountered in children, particularly with genetic syndromes, than in adults. Laxity of the ligaments also results in 'rotatory' dislocation encountered essentially in young children [30].

Craniovertebral instability has been associated with following known syndromes: Larsen syndrome, diastrophic dysplasia, Goldenhar syndrome, Down syndrome, pseudoachondroplasia, Morquio's syndrome, Kniest dysplasia, spondyloepiphyseal dysplasia congenita, 22q11.2 deletion syndrome and fibrodysplasia ossificans progressiva.

Of these, instability related to Down syndrome is more frequent and is a result of ligamentous laxity at C1–2 and rarely at C0–1 levels. There can be cervical spine instability at other cervical levels in this syndrome. Morquio's syndrome is the other more common type of genetic disorder that is associated with atlantoaxial dislocation. Pseudoachondroplasia and Morquio's syndrome have C1–2 instability due to generalised ligamentous laxity and frequently identified odontoid dysplasia (hypoplasia and os odontoideum). Morquio's patients also have soft tissue glycosaminoglycan deposits that can cause stenosis of the canal and lead to myelopathy. Severely affected patients with spondyloepiphyseal dysplasia congenita can be at risk of myelopathy due to atlantoaxial instability in addition to underlying stenosis. Kniest syndrome can be associated with AAD.

Cervical spine anomalies in Goldenhar syndrome are varied and can be severe. Fibrodysplasia ossificans progressiva features severe deforming heterotopic ossifications that can become life-threatening.

Bone deformities in infants can be due to failure of vertebral segmentation in cervical spine or failure of vertebral formation.

It is important to be vigilant in the diagnosis and treatment of spinal abnormalities in patients with genetic syndromes.

Anatomy of the Lateral Masses of Atlas and Axis and of Vertebral Artery in Relationship to the Craniovertebral Junction

The C1 and C2 vertebrae are called 'atypical vertebrae', having a unique shape and architecture and a characteristic vertebral artery relationship [4, 39]. Injury to the artery during surgery can lead to catastrophic intraoperative bleeding. Vertebral artery compromise is tolerated better by patients in paediatric age group. Injury and sacrifice of both vertebral arteries can also be tolerated well by children. However, the effects of compromise are unpredictable and will depend on adequacy of blood flow from other arteries of the brain.

The vertebral artery adopts a serpentine course in relationship to the craniovertebral region. The artery has multiple loops and an intimate relationship with the atlas and axis bones. We observed a wide variability of the course of the artery in our specimens. The shape, size and location of the vertebral artery groove on the inferior aspect of the superior articular facet of the C2 and over the posterior arch of the atlas have wide variations. The vertebral artery during its entire course is covered with a large plexus of veins. The venous plexuses are the largest in the region lateral to the C1–2 joint.

After a relatively linear ascent of the vertebral artery in the foramen transversarium of C6 to C3, the artery makes a loop medially towards an anteriorly placed superior articular facet of the C2 vertebra, making a deep groove on its inferior surface. The vertebral artery loops away from the midline underneath the superior articular facet of the C2.

Techniques for Craniovertebral Stabilisation

Operative Technique for Lateral Mass Plate (or Rod) and Screw (Mono-Axial or Polyaxial) Fixation [14, 18]

Cervical traction is set up prior to induction of anaesthesia, and the weights are progressively increased to approximately 3–5 kg depending on the weight and age of the patient. The patient is placed prone with the head end of the table elevated to about 35°. Cervical traction stabilises the head in an optimally reduced extension position and prevents any rotation. The traction also ensures that the weight of the head is directed superiorly towards the direction of the traction and the pressure over the face or eyeball by the headrest is avoided. The head is in 'hanging' position, headrest being placed only for additional or minimal support. Elevation of the head end of the table, which acts as a countertraction, helps in reducing venous engorgement in the operative field. The suboccipital region and the upper cervical spine are exposed through an approximately 8-cm longitudinal midline skin incision centred on the spinous process of the axis. The spinous process of the axis is identified, and the attachment of paraspinal muscles to it is sharply sectioned. The large second cervical ganglion is closely related to the vertebral artery on its lateral aspect. It is first exposed widely and then sectioned sharply. In children, the ganglion is relatively elastic and supple and can be retracted rather than cut to expose the joint. This procedure provides a wide exposure of the lateral masses of the atlas and axis [33]. Bleeding from the large venous sinuses in the region and in the extradural space can be troublesome. Packing of the region with *Surgicel* and Gelfoam can assist in the control of venous bleeding. Blood loss can be significant in children due to the presence of larger venous plexuses. The joint capsule is cut sharply, and the articular surfaces of the joint are exposed. The adjacent synovial articular surfaces of the atlantoaxial joint are decorticated widely with a microdrill, and pieces of bone harvested from the iliac crest are stuffed into the joint space. The synovial or articular surface of the joint is significantly smoother and slippery in children than in adults. The lateral aspect of the lamina and a part of the pars of the axis are drilled to make the posterior surface of the lateral mass of the axis relatively flat so that the metal plate can be placed snugly and parallel to the bone. Drilling also helps in reducing the length of the plate and in placing the screw more superiorly and almost directly into the pedicle and facet of the axis. Actual vertebral artery exposure is unnecessary either lateral to the pars of the axis or superior to the arch of the atlas.

Screws are implanted into the previously created guide holes in the lateral mass of the atlas and axis through a two-holed (approximately 2 cm in length) metal (stainless steel or titanium) plate. First, a screw is placed into the atlas. It is directed at an angle of approximately 15° medial to the sagittal plane and 15° superior to the axial plane. The preferred site of screw insertion is at the centre of the posterior surface of the lateral mass, 1–2 mm above the articular surface. Whenever necessary, careful drilling of the inferior surface of the lateral aspect of the posterior arch of the atlas in relation to its lateral mass can provide additional space for the placement of the plate and screw implantation. The screw may even be implanted by choosing an insertion point on the articular surface of the lateral mass of the atlas. Such a site is useful more frequently in children than in adult patients. Screws can also be implanted into the facet of atlas through the lateral aspect of the posterior arch of the atlas.

Due to the intimacy of vertebral artery relationships, screw implantation in the axis is relatively unsafe and needs to be precise. It was observed that the screw implantation in the superior facet of the C2 vertebra has to be sharply medial and directed towards the anterior tubercle of the C1 for transarticular fixation and towards the vertebral body of C2 for C1–2 lateral mass fixation. The pars interarticularis can be divided into nine quadrants [39]; the superior and medial compartments can be used for C1–C2 lateral mass technique of plate–screw implantation. Neuronavigation can be of assistance in identifying the best and the safest trajectory of screw. The direction of screw implantation must be sharply medial and superior and should be towards the superior aspect of the body of the axis vertebra towards the midline. The medial surface of the pedicle of the axis is identified before the implantation of the screw. The screw is directed at an angle approximately 25° medial to the sagittal plane and 15° superior to the axial plane. The angle of screw insertion varies, depending on the local anatomy and the size of the bones. The quality of cancellous bone in the lateral masses of the atlas and axis in the proposed trajectory of screw implantation is generally good, providing an excellent purchase of the screw, and avoids the vertebral artery.

The screws used are 2.9 mm in diameter in the adult patients and 2.7 mm in diameter in the paediatric patients. The length of the required screw is calculated on the basis of the size of the lateral masses observed on the preoperative radiological studies. The approximate lengths of the atlas screws are 26–28 mm in adults and 22–26 mm in children. The screws in the atlas and axis were almost similar in their length. *Thicker screws are used by some, particularly when polyaxial screws are employed.* The lateral masses of the atlas and axis are firm and cortical in nature, and although preferable, it is not mandatory that the screws engage both the posterior and anterior cortices. If the screw traverses beyond the anterior cortex, it will lie harmlessly in the anteriorly displaced soft tissue. Injury to critical neurovascular and pharyngeal wall is possible in such a situation but is extremely rare. Intraoperative fluoroscopic control was found to be helpful but not essential in determining the state of the screws. Large pieces of corticocancellous bone graft from the iliac bone are then placed over the adequately prepared posterior elements of atlas and axis. After the wound is closed, cervical traction is discontinued. The patients are mobilised as soon as possible and advised to wear hard cervical collar for 3 months. Lateral mass plate and screw fixation technique can provide an opportunity of manipulating atlas and axis independently by obtaining fixation points in their strongest elements and hence has very versatile applications.

Magerl's Technique

Magerl's technique of fixation involves use of transarticular lateral mass screws [38]. This technique also involves stabilisation of the joints and is a popular and satisfactory method of stabilisation. Transarticular method of stabilisation is relatively difficult in children when compared to adults due to the usually encountered increased interfacetal distance.

Double Insurance Fixation (*Fig. 6*)

An alternative method of atlantoaxial fixation that combines transarticular method of fixation and the interarticular fixation technique can be used [24]. The technique combines the biomechanical strengths of both the more commonly used techniques of fixation and provides maximal stability to the implants.

Joint Jamming Technique

Jamming of spiked spacers within the atlantoaxial joints can provide a satisfactory method of atlantoaxial fixation [25]. Joint jamming technique can be suitable in cases where the atlantoaxial dislocation is not remarkably mobile as is usually encountered in cases with congenital atlantoaxial dislocations. Such a method of fixation can usually be employed as a supplement to other techniques of fixation. However, in children, due to the excessive mobility of the joints, placement of a spacer is usually not indicated.

Use of Spinous Process and Lamina for Insertion of Axial Screws

Placement of screws in the large and stubby spinous process of the axis can be a useful method [20]. Insertion of the screw in the spinolaminar junction or in the lamina has been described to provide a stable fixation point. Such a screw can be used to stabilise the axial end of the occipitocervical plate or atlantoaxial plate or rods.

Atlantoaxial Dislocation (Figs. 1, 2, 3, 4, 5, and 6)

Atlantoaxial dislocation can be due to a number of etiological factors. The dislocation can be of mobile and reducible type or of a 'fixed' or irreducible type. In the more common form of AAD, the atlas dislocates over the axis. In cases with occipitalisation of the atlas, the head and atlas form one unit, and the axis and the rest of the spine form the other unit. The odontoid process of the axis is normally in close approximation with the anterior arch of the atlas. In AAD, the head and atlas dislocate ventrally on the axis on flexion of the head, markedly widening the atlantodental interval and reducing the diameter of the spinal canal, with consequent pressure on the cervicomedullary junction cord. The dislocation increases on flexion of the head and reduces in extension in the mobile variety of AAD. In the fixed or irreducible variety, the dislocation persists entirely or at least partially on full extension of the head. In our recent analysis we identified that atlantoaxial dislocation is very rarely of fixed or irreducible variety and can almost always be reduced by direct manipulation and distraction of the facets [14, 18].

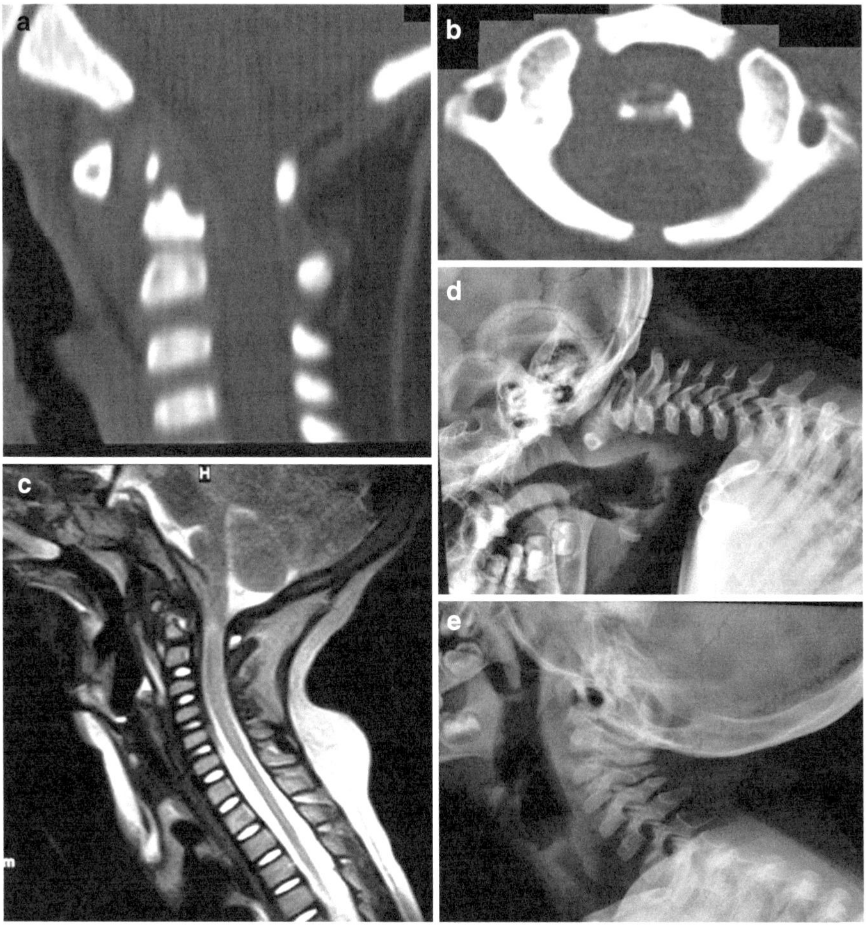

Fig. 1 Images of a 2.5 year old boy. (**a**) Sagittal view of CT scan showing craniovertebral instability. (**b**) Axial view of arch of atlas showing its trifid nature. (**c**) T2-weighted MRI in neutral position showing cord changes suggesting evidence of injury. (**d**) Lateral X-ray with the head in flexion showing atlantoaxial dislocation. (**e**) X-ray with the head in extension showing reduction of the dislocation. (**f**) Postoperative scan showing fixation in reduced position. (**g**) Axial images showing screws in the lateral mass of the axis. (**h**) Sagittal image showing lateral mass plate and screw fixation. Images of 6-year-old boy

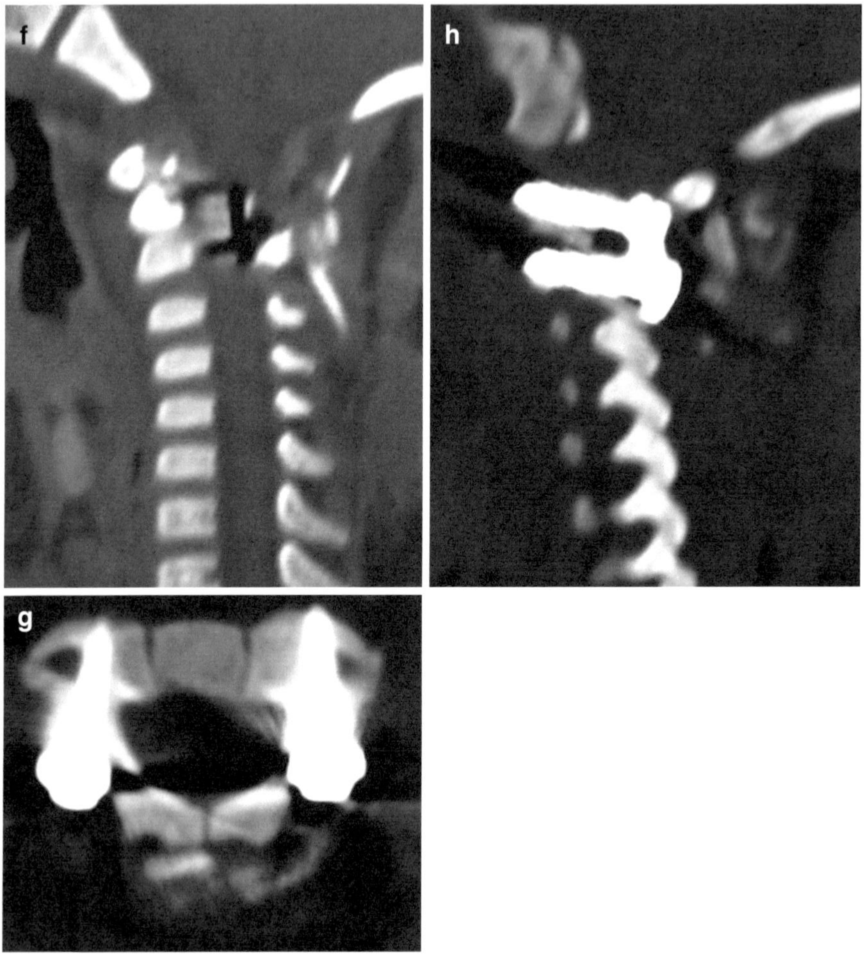

Fig. 1 (continued)

Mobile and Reducible Atlantoaxial Dislocation

In the year 2001, we analysed 160 cases with mobile and reducible atlantoaxial dislocation treated in our department [18]. Whilst trauma leads to mechanical disruption of ligaments of the region, in 'congenital' dislocation, laxity or incompetence of the ligaments is more often the cause. In several cases, the exact differentiation between a congenital and acquired cause is difficult to decipher. The range of mobility of the dislocation is in general significantly higher in cases with congenital dislocation than in cases with trauma-related dislocation. Children usually tolerate dislocation better and symptoms may be subtle and long-standing. In children, the dislocation is usually reducible.

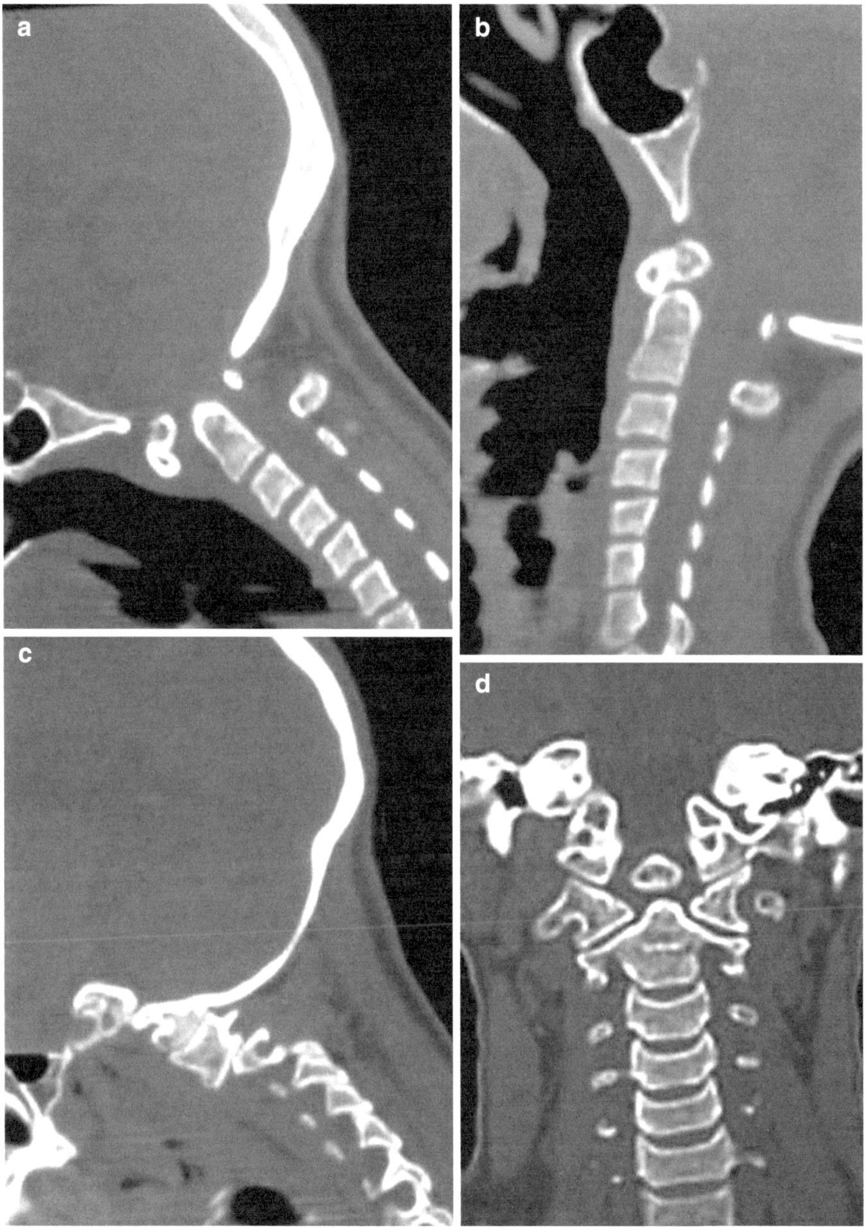

Fig. 2 (**a**) Sagittal image showing atlantoaxial dislocation. There is os odontoideum. (**b**) CT scan with head in extension showing reduction of dislocation. (**c**) Lateral view of sagittal image showing listhesis of facet of C1 over facet of C2. (**d**) Coronal image showing the craniovertebral junction. Os odontoideum is distinctly seen. (**e**) T2-weighted MRI showing the compression of the cord. (**f**) Postoperative scan showing reduction of dislocation. (**g**) Image showing plate and screw fixation of the facets

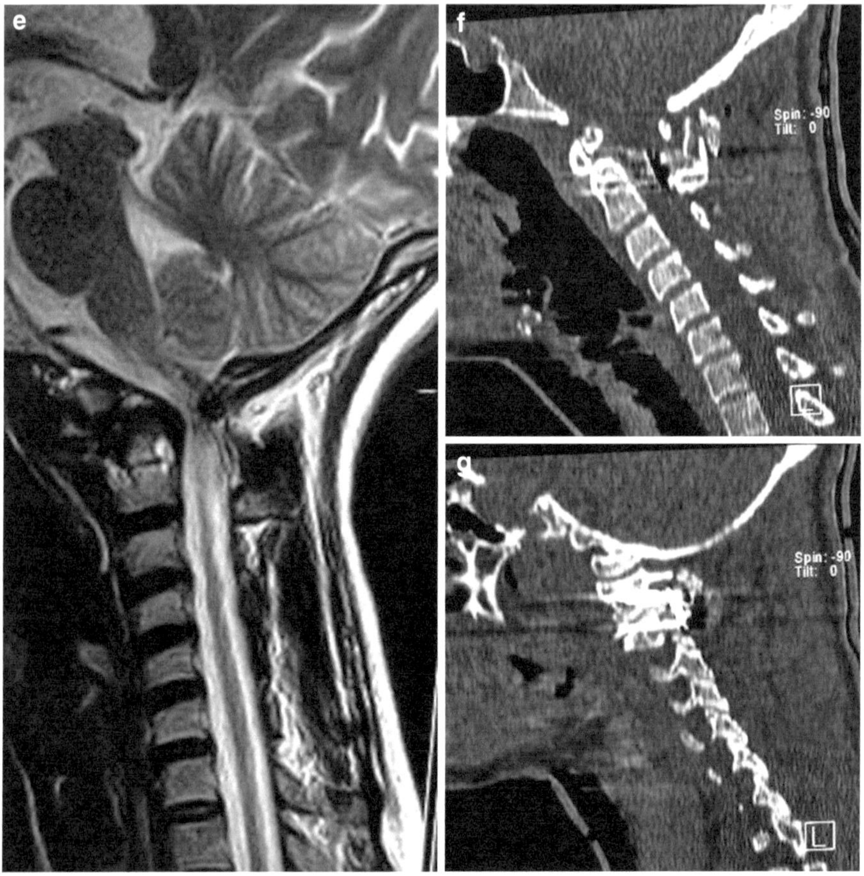

Fig. 2 (continued)

Symptoms

Pain in the upper part of the neck and restriction of neck movements are common symptoms. The patient may give a history of an injury that flexed the head and neck (as when he is hit on the back of the head) as the precipitating factor. Weakness and spasticity of all limbs can follow the event of trauma. A range of motor and sensory deficits can occur. The sensory deficits are relatively less severe. Severe injuries to the cervicomedullary cord may produce respiratory paralysis, coma and even death. The tissues are more supple and stronger in children and traumatic dislocations are relatively uncommon. However, pre-existing muscle/ligament disorder can lead to atlantoaxial dislocation.

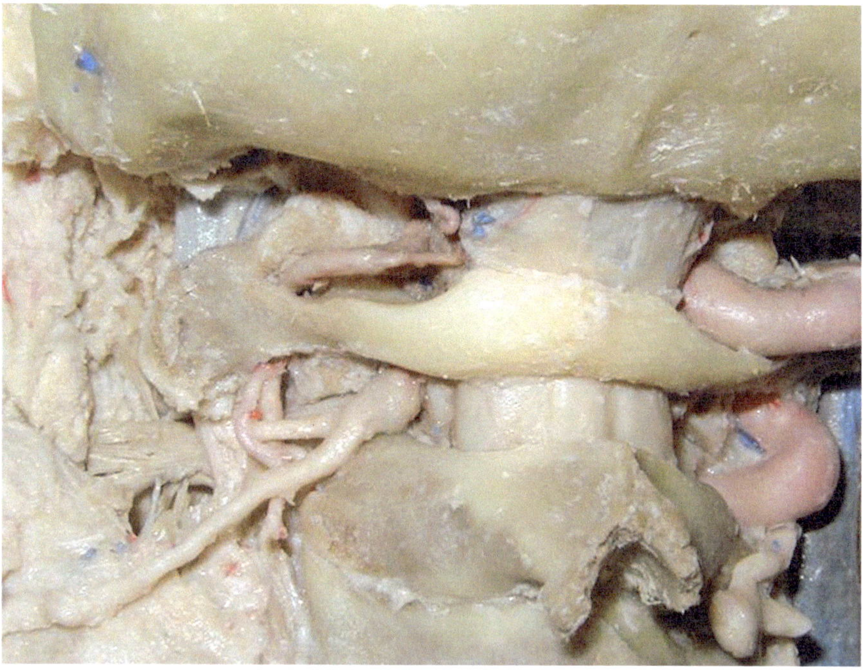

Fig. 3 Cadaver dissection picture is shown. Note the relationship of the C2 ganglion with the atlantoaxial joint. Also note the hypoplastic vertebral artery on the left side and the dominant vertebral artery on the right side

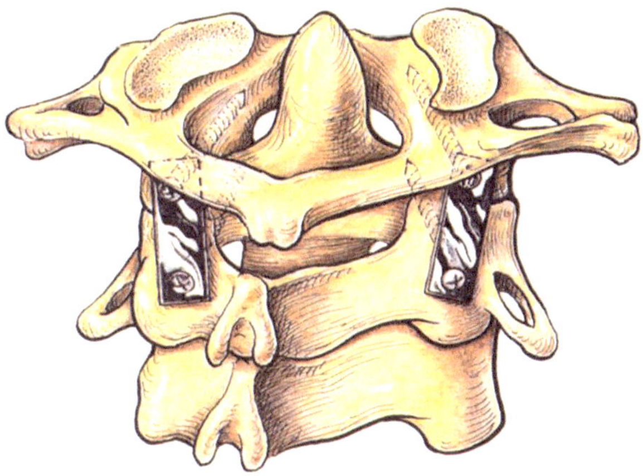

Fig. 4 Line drawing showing plate and screw fixation of the atlantoaxial joint. Screws are inserted into the facets of the atlas and facets of axis. The C2 ganglion is sectioned, joint cavity is opened, articular surface is denuded, bone graft is inserted into the cavity, and subsequently plate and screw fixation is done

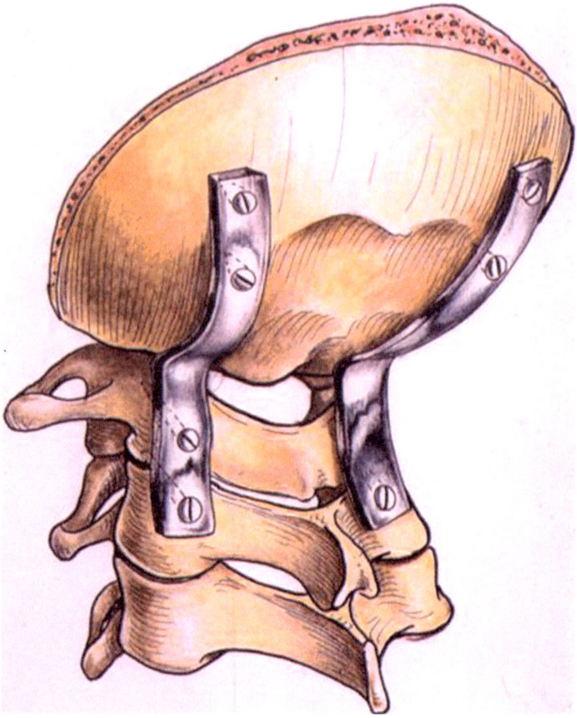

Fig. 5 Line drawing showing occipitocervical fixation. The occipital end of the plate is fixed with occipital screws, and the cervical end of the plate is fixed with screws inserted into facets of C2 alone and into facets of C1 and C2

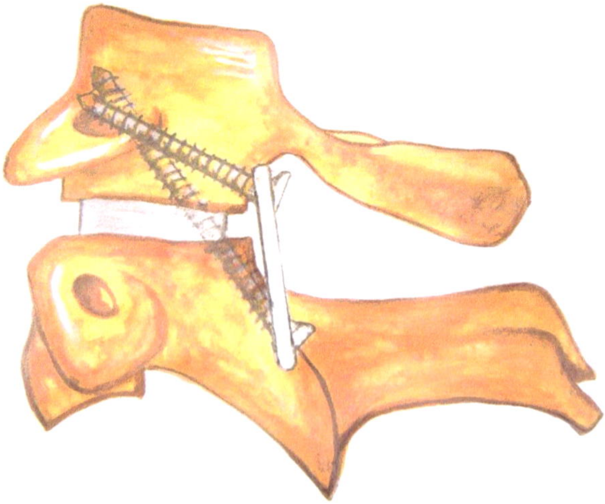

Fig. 6 Line drawing showing 'double insurance' atlantoaxial fixation. The C1 screw is inserted directly into the facet of atlas, whilst C2 screw is inserted in a transarticular fashion

Investigations

Radiographs showing the lateral views of the atlantoaxial region with the head and neck flexed and extended are always done. The atlantodental interval of less than 3 mm is generally considered within the normal range in infants and children in Group A and Group B. The atlantodental interval of more than 3 mm usually confirms the diagnosis. Dynamic CT scan with appropriate reconstruction images shows the dislocation clearly. MR showing signal alterations are important and frequently confirmatory evidence indicating compression of the cervicomedullary cord. MR and CT angiography can show the relationship of the vertebral artery to the facets of C2 and C1. Such information is crucial when lateral mass fixation techniques are employed for surgery. MRI provides useful information regarding the nature of soft tissue alterations. The status of bones in general and of facets in particular should be elaborately evaluated on investigations.

Treatment

The treatment of patients with atlantoaxial instability is a surgical challenge, and achieving a successful outcome for these patients is gratifying. The complications of surgery, however, are potentially lethal. Various methods of fixation have been described and used successfully in the treatment of patients with atlantoaxial instability. The techniques of craniovertebral fixation evolved during the twentieth century as the anatomy and biomechanics of the craniovertebral region became clearer. The aim of surgery in general is to restore normal or the best possible alignment and to achieve stability of the atlantoaxial joint. The techniques of fixation for atlantoaxial dislocation can be divided into midline procedures that involve the fixation of arch of the atlas with the lamina of axis and lateral mass fixation procedures. Midline methods of fixation include sublaminar wire fixation and metal loop fixation. Metal implants and fixation methods provide an initial period of fixation of the region facilitating bony fusion. Bony fusion takes about 3 months, and the metal implants should be strong enough to hold the region for that period. It ultimately depends on bony fusion to provide stability to the region. Bone harvested from the patient's own iliac crest has been identified by several authors to be superior to any other form of bone graft or artificial material [34]. Compromise on using the type of bone graft can lead to inadequate fusion, a phenomenon that can mar the entire operative procedure. Multiple pieces of corticocancellous bone graft should be placed in the craniovertebral region after elaborately preparing the host bone. The movements in the atlantoaxial region occur in atlantoaxial joint. Any method of stabilisation that directly fixes the joint and the fixation is segmental in nature, having superiority over methods that employ fixation remote to the site of maximum movements and those that attempt to fix multiple bone segments [29]. The lateral mass fixation techniques have been identified to be philosophically superior and biomechanically stronger to the techniques that involve fixation of the midline structures like lamina and arch of atlas (Fig. 4). In children with multiple joint ligamental laxity, occipitocervical fixation may sometimes be necessary. Methods incorporating screw fixation of the occipital end of the implant and inclusion of C1 and C2 facets by screw fixation were first described by us [14] (Fig. 5).

Irreducible or Fixed Atlantoaxial Dislocation

The issue of 'irreducible' or 'fixed' atlantoaxial dislocation has been under discussion for a long time. On the basis of our analysis we have concluded that atlantoaxial dislocation is only rarely fixed and can be manually distracted and reduced [23]. The joint is usually active and functional when a joint space is evident of CT scanning and the articular surfaces are smooth and well defined even when they are not in alignment. Direct distraction of facets of atlas and axis and placement of bone graft within it, with or without additional support of metallic spacers, can result in significant or complete reduction of dislocation. Subsequent atlantoaxial fixation that can sustain the reduction is then carried out. The mechanism of the screw tightening can also be modified and can simulate the technique used in the treatment of spondylolisthesis [23, 42]. The C2 screw is tightened first completely and subsequently the C1 screw is tightened. Such a technique assists in pulling the C1 back into alignment. Transoral decompression of the odontoid process followed by posterior fixation is also a useful method of treatment, particularly when the surgeon is not familiar with lateral mass fixation and distraction procedures.

Basilar Invagination (Figs. 7, 8, 9, and 10)

Basilar invagination forms a prominent component of the craniovertebral anomalies. Chiari malformation and syringomyelia are common associates of basilar invagination and are the soft tissue components of the dysgenesis. Plain radiological and tomographic parameters have been principally used to diagnose basilar invagination for many years. There has been a renewed interest in the normal anatomy and pathologic lesions of the craniovertebral junction with the development of imaging by high-resolution CT scan and MRI. Dynamic MRI and CT scan have helped in the evaluation of the pathology of basilar invagination, in the assessment of biomechanics of the joints and in the formulation of a rationale surgical strategy. Despite the clarity of imaging, controversy regarding the management of basilar invagination continues. Even the natural history has not been clearly elucidated in the literature. The surgical indications for a given approach together with the timing of the surgical stages are still under discussion.

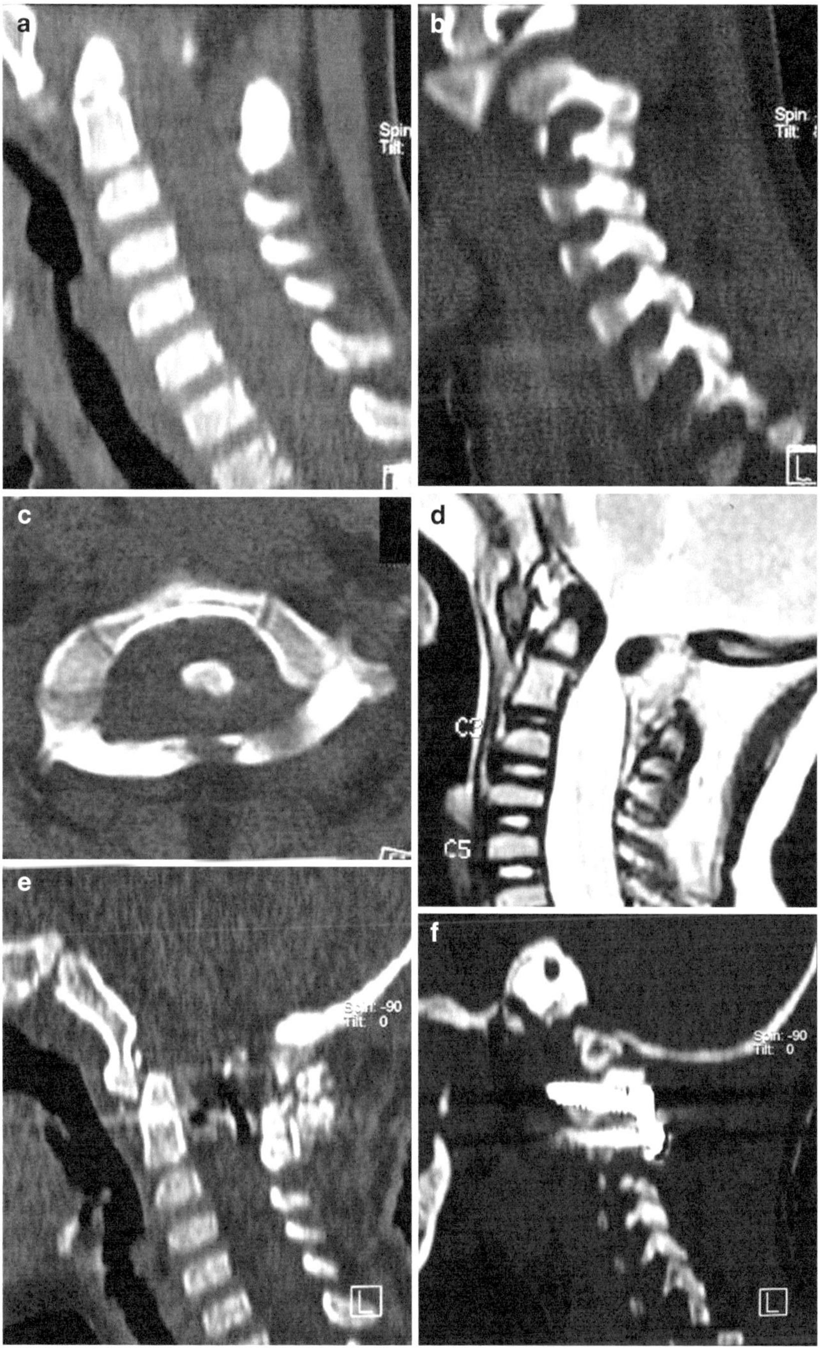

Fig. 7 Images of a 4-year-old boy. (**a**) Sagittal image of CT scan showing basilar invagination. (**b**) CT scan showing listhesis of facet of C1 over the facet of C2. (**c**) Axial view of CT scan showing the atlas bone in multiple segments. (**d**) T2-weighted MRI showing basilar invagination and cord compression. (**e**) Postoperative image showing reduction of the basilar invagination. There is craniovertebral realignment without any bone decompression. (**f**) Lateral sagittal view showing plate and screw fixation of the facets

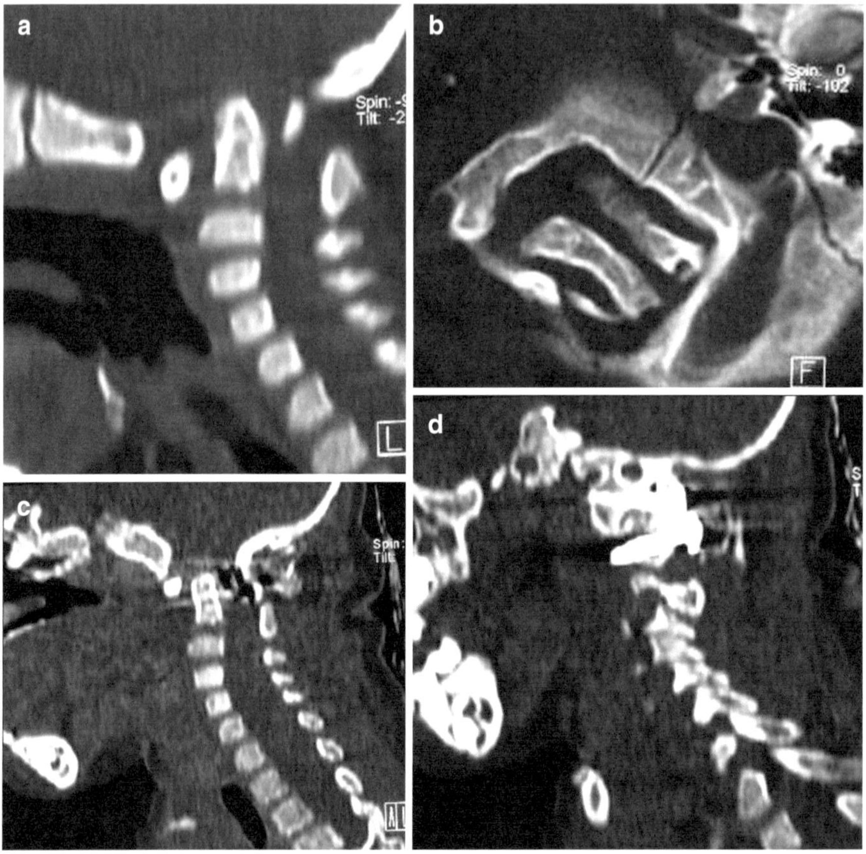

Fig. 8 Images of a 4-year-old girl. (**a**) Sagittal image of CT scan showing a complex craniovertebral anomaly with severe basilar invagination. (**b**) Axial CT scan image showing complex bone alignment at the craniovertebral junction. (**c**) Postoperative image showing craniovertebral realignment. Reduction of basilar invagination can be seen. There is no anterior or posterior bone decompression. (**d**) Lateral cut of sagittal image shows lateral mass plate and screw fixation

Pathogenesis

Several theories have been suggested to elucidate the probable cause and origin of basilar invagination. Most of these theories point towards embryological dysgenesis, genetic abnormalities and viral infections [5, 26, 36, 55, 56]. Several authors, for over a century, have thought that deformation had a mechanical cause and therefore applied the name 'impressio baseos cranii' (Berg and Retzius is cited by Virchow 1857) [55], or basilar impression [5]. Grawitz [36] believed that basilar invagination was often a result of under- or maldevelopment of the craniovertebral transition region. A range of malformations is frequently associated with anomalies of the atlas and axis, some of which may be quite atypical, and with fissures or defects and bone projections from the spinal column in the craniovertebral

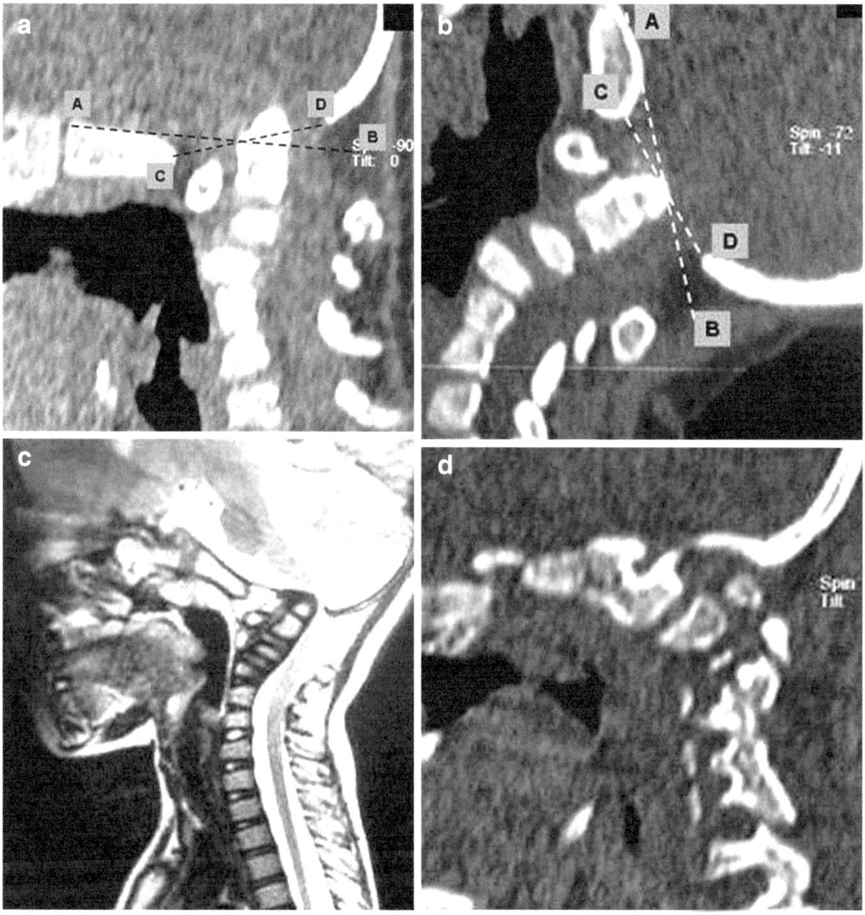

Fig. 9 (**a**) Sagittal image of CT scan with the head in flexed position showing basilar invagination. (**b**) CT scan image with the head in extension showing reduction of basilar invagination. Line *A*, *B* Wackenheim's clival line, Line *C*, *D* McRae's Foramen Magnum line. (**c**) T2-weighted MRI showing basilar invagination. (**d**) Image through the lateral masses showing incompetence of the facets

transition zone. The latter anomalies were grouped together by von Torklus and Gehle as suboccipital dysplasias [56].

Basilar invagination can be secondary to abnormally inclined alignment of the facets of atlas and axis [16, 19, 42]. The progressive slippage of the atlas over the axis secondary to this malalignment, a process similar to spondylolisthesis in the lumbosacral spine, results in invagination of the odontoid process into the craniocervical cord [42]. Short neck, low hairline, web-shaped neck muscles, torticollis, reduction in the range of neck movements and several such physical variations have been described as hallmarks of basilar invagination for over a century. A number of bone fusion deformities and platybasia have also been recorded. Neck pain, muscle spasms and restriction of neck movements are frequently noted and suggest instability of the region

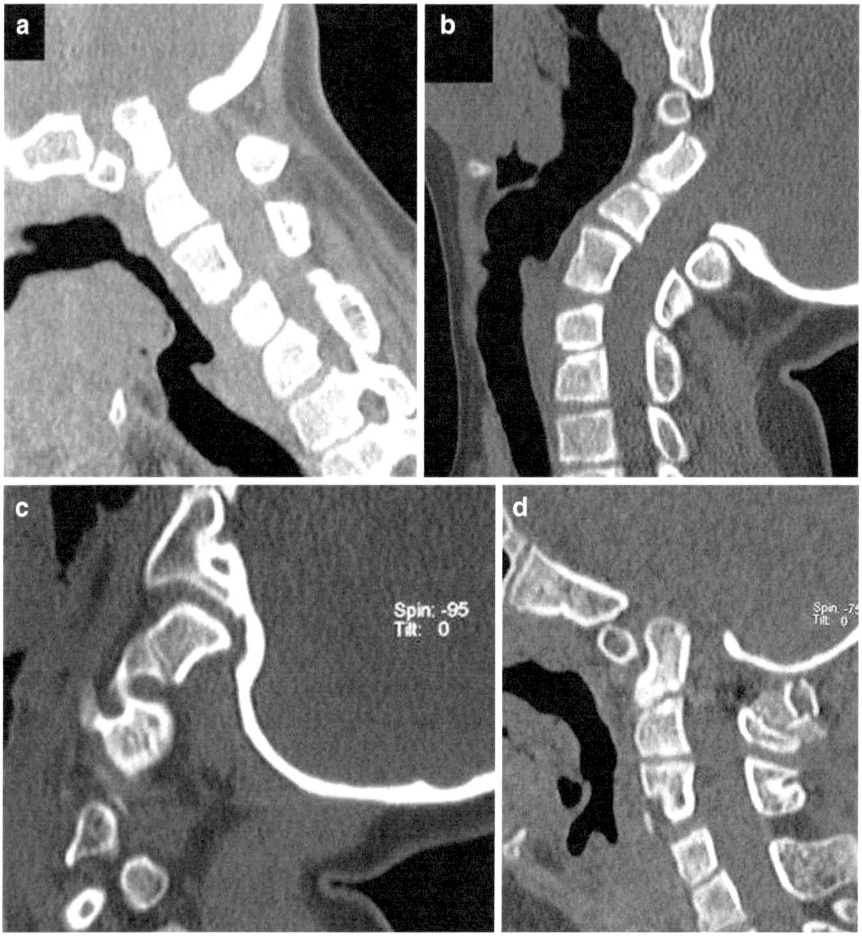

Fig. 10 (**a**) Sagittal view of CT scan with the head in flexed position showing basilar invagination. (**b**) View with head in extension position showing complete reduction of basilar invagination. (**c**) View through the facets showing their abnormal orientation. (**d**) Postoperative view showing reduction of basilar invagination

Classification into Groups I and II

In the year 1997, we presented a classification system for basilar invagination that divided it into two discrete categories. This classification helped in clarifying the understanding of the pathology and pathogenesis of the anomaly, in the selection of the surgical treatment and in prediction of the outcome [16]. Based on a single criterion of the absence or presence of Chiari malformation, the anomaly was classified into Groups I and II, respectively.

Essentially, Group I included cases where there was invagination of the odontoid process into the foramen magnum and it indented into the brainstem. The tip of the odontoid process distanced itself from the anterior arch of the atlas or the inferior aspect of the clivus. The distancing of the odontoid process from the anterior arch suggested the presence of instability of the region and atlantoaxial dislocation. The angle of the clivus and the posterior cranial fossa volume were essentially unaffected in these cases. In Group II, on the other hand, the assembly of odontoid process, anterior arch of the atlas and the clivus migrated superiorly in unison resulting in reduction of the posterior cranial fossa volume, which was the primary pathology in these cases. The Chiari malformation or herniation of the cerebellar tonsil was considered to be a result of reduction in the posterior cranial fossa volume. In the year 1997, Goel first defined the clinical implication of association of small posterior cranial fossa volume and Chiari malformation [16].

Classification into Groups A and B

In our recent study, we identified a subgroup of patients where there was clear radiological evidence of instability of the region that was manifested by distancing of the odontoid process away from the anterior arch of the atlas and the radiological features matching those of Group I cases. Considering this current evaluation we have proposed a *new classification for basilar invagination* into two groups based on parameters that determined an alternative treatment strategy [19]. In Group A basilar invagination, there was a 'fixed' atlantoaxial dislocation, and the tip of the odontoid process 'invaginated' into the foramen magnum and was above the Chamberlain's line [5], McRae's line of foramen magnum [47] and Wackenheim's clival line [54]. The definition of basilar invagination of prolapse of the cervical spine into the base of the skull, as suggested by von Torklus [56], was suitable for this group of patients. Group B basilar invagination was where the odontoid process and clivus remained anatomically aligned despite the presence of basilar invagination and other associated anomalies. In this group, the tip of the odontoid process was above the Chamberlain's line but below the McRae's and the Wackenheim's lines. The radiological findings suggested that the odontoid process in Group A patients resulted in direct compression of the brainstem. Essentially, in Group A basilar invagination, the pathogenesis appeared to be mechanical instability of the region that was manifested by the tip of the odontoid process distancing itself from the anterior arch of the atlas or the lower end of the clivus. In some Group A patients, there was Chiari malformation, and this feature differentiates the present classification from the earlier classification. In this group, the atlantoaxial joints were 'active', and their orientation was oblique as shown in the figure, instead of the normally found horizontal orientation. Similarities of such a position of the C1–2 facets with spondylolisthesis seen in the subaxial spine can be seen. It appears that the atlantoaxial joint in such cases is in an abnormal position, and progressive worsening of the dislocation is probably secondary to increasing 'slippage' of the facets of atlas over the facets of axis. In Group B, the pathogenesis appeared to be congenital dysgenesis, and atlantoaxial joints were normally aligned or were entirely fused. The pathogenesis of basilar invagination appears to be different in the two groups. Understanding of these two types of basilar invagination is crucial in understanding the various involved management issues.

Diagnosis

Radiological Criteria

(a) *Chamberlain's line*: Basilar invagination was diagnosed when the tip of the odontoid process was at least 2 mm above the Chamberlain's line [5]. Measurement of Chamberlain's line on lateral sagittal reconstruction pictures of CT scan and sagittal MRI was seen to be reliable and accurate. The analysis of basilar invagination in the two groups on the basis of Chamberlain's line suggested that the basilar invagination is much more severe in Group B than in Group A.
(b) *Distance between the odontoid tip and the pontomedullary junction*: The distance of the tip of the odontoid from the pontomedullary junction, as observed on MRI, is a useful index to define the reduction of the posterior cranial fossa bone size [16]. The distance was markedly reduced in Group B cases, whilst it was relatively large in Group A cases.
(c) *Atlantodental or clivo-dental interval*: In Group A cases, it was seen that the odontoid process migrated superiorly and posteriorly into the foramen magnum and distanced itself from the anterior arch of the atlas and the inferior end of the clivus. As judged from the atlantodental or clivo-dental interval, there was an element of 'fixed' atlantoaxial dislocation in these cases. Actual mobility of the atlantoaxial joint on flexion and extension of the neck can be infrequently demonstrated with a good quality imaging. In Group B the alignment of the odontoid process with the anterior arch of the atlas and with the inferior aspect of the clivus remains normal and there is no instability.
(d) *Vertical mobile and reducible atlantoaxial dislocation*: There was basilar invagination when the neck was flexed, and the alignment was normal when the head was in extended position [27]. Although such mobility is only rarely identified, it does indicate the need for dynamic flexion–extension studies to preoperatively assess the craniovertebral instability. Vertical dislocation is due to incompetence of the atlantoaxial joint and lateral masses.
(e) *Wackenheim's clival line*: Wackenheim's clival line is a line drawn along the clivus. The tip of the odontoid process was significantly superior to the Wackenheim's clival line in Group A cases. In Group B cases, the relationship of the tip of the odontoid process and the lower end of the clivus and the atlantodental and clivo-dental interval remained relatively normal. In a majority of these cases, the tip of the odontoid process remained below the Wackenheim's clival line [54] and McRae's line of the foramen magnum [47]. The basilar invagination thus resulted from the rostral positioning of the plane of the foramen magnum in relation to the brainstem.

(f) *Platybasia*: A line is drawn along the anterior skull base. The angle of this line to the clivus is referred to as the basal angle. Reduction of the basal angle is referred to as platybasia. *Posterior cranial fossa volume*: The Klaus' height index [56] measured on the MRI was seen to be much more accurate than the conventional measurements based on plain X-rays. The tentorium could be clearly identified on MRI, and the distance of the tip of the odontoid from the line of the tentorium indicated the height of the posterior cranial fossa. On the basis of Klaus' index, the posterior fossa height was found to be markedly reduced in Group B cases, whilst it was only moderately affected in Group A cases.

(g) *Omega angle*: Although not frequently used, the omega angle or the angulation of the odontoid process from the vertical as described by Klaus was found to be a useful guide [56]. We described a modified omega angle as the measurement of the angle from the vertical was affected by the flexion and extension of the neck [16]. A line was drawn traversing through the centre of the base of the axis parallel to the line of the hard palate. The line of the hard palate was unaffected by the relative movement of the head and the cervical spine during the movement of the neck in these 'fixed' craniovertebral anomalies. Facial hypoplasia or hard palate abnormality was not seen in any case in this series and did not affect the measurements. The omega angle depicted the direction of displacement of the odontoid process. The omega angle was severely reduced in Group A cases, whilst it was much larger in Group B cases. The reduction in the omega angle in Group A cases depicted that the odontoid process had tilted towards the horizontal and was posteriorly angulated in Group A cases, whilst it was near vertical and superiorly migrated in Group B cases.

(h) *Brainstem girth*: The effective brainstem girth measured on MRI was a useful additional parameter. Whilst the brainstem girth was markedly reduced in Group A cases, the girth was only marginally affected or unaffected in Group B cases indicating thereby that there was no direct brainstem compression as a result of the odontoid process in the latter group.

(i) *Neck size*: Measurement of craniovertebral height can be done using a modification of Klaus' posterior fossa height index [26]. The cervical height was measured from the tip of the odontoid process to the midpoint of the base of the C7 vertebral body.

(j) *Direct physical measurement* of the neck length: It can be a useful parameter. The parameter of direct physical measurement of the neck length from the inion to the tip of the C7 spinous process can be useful [26].

(k) *Cervical lordosis*: It was evaluated with a modification of the Klaus omega angle [26] and a modified omega angle [16].

Clinical Features

Majority of patients with Group A basilar invagination (58 %) had a history of minor to major head injury prior to the onset of the symptoms [19]. The pyramidal symptoms formed a dominant component. Kinaesthetic sensations were affected in

55 % cases. Spinothalamic dysfunction was less frequent (36 %). Neck pain as a major presenting symptom was in 77 % cases. Torticollis was present in 41 % cases. The analysis of radiological and clinical features suggests that the symptoms and signs were a result of brainstem compression by the odontoid process.

The presentation was relatively acute in Group A cases, whilst it was long-standing and slowly progressive in Group B cases. In Group B cases, the onset of symptoms and their evolution were insidious. Thus, a careful inquiry was needed to pinpoint the timing of appearance of the initial symptoms. In the majority of cases, the time of onset was already forgotten. This made it difficult to establish with certainty the age at which the complaints began. The symptoms and signs in Group B basilar invagination appeared to be directly related to the 'crowding' of neural structures at the foramen magnum. Although the dimensions of the foramen magnum were large and sometimes larger than even in a normal state, the volume of its contents and probably the 'pulsatile' compression of the structures at the foramen magnum resulted in neurological symptoms. The markedly reduced girth of the brainstem in Group A cases clearly showed that direct compression of the brainstem by the odontoid process caused the neurological symptoms. Central cord symptoms and related signs were noted in cases associated with syringomyelia.

Occipitalisation of the atlas: Occipitalisation of the atlas associated with basilar invagination was noted first by Rakitansky [cited by Grawitz [36]] and has since been referred to frequently [36, 47, 54, 55]. Many authors have regarded assimilation as a characteristic feature of basilar invagination. The assimilation of atlas can be partial or incomplete.

Klippel–Feil bone anomaly refers to the triad of observations of extensive cervical vertebral fusions, low hairline, restrictions of neck movements and a short neck.

Trauma of varying severity was a noteworthy precipitating factor in Group A cases [19]. Trauma seldom plays any major role in precipitating the symptoms in Group B cases. The fact that trauma influenced the acute development of symptoms pointed towards an element of instability of the craniovertebral region in Group A patients.

Age factor: Basilar invagination Group A is more often seen in younger patient group, whilst Group B basilar invagination is more frequently encountered in older patient group.

Surgical Management

Craniovertebral Realignment for Group A Basilar Invagination

The conventional form of treatment of Group A basilar invagination is a transoral decompression that is followed by posterior occipitocervical fixation. However, the long-term clinical outcome following the twin operation of transoral decompression followed by posterior stabilisation was seen to be inferior to the clinical outcome following surgery that involves craniovertebral realignment without any bone, dural or neural decompression [15, 16, 19, 27].

The technique of craniovertebral realignment by wide removal of atlantoaxial joint capsule and articular cartilage by drilling and subsequent distraction of the joint by manual manipulation provided a unique opportunity to obtain reduction of the basilar invagination and of atlantoaxial dislocation.

Technique of Facetal Distraction and Craniovertebral Realignment

This operation is suitable for patients with Group A basilar invagination. The exposure of the atlantoaxial joint in cases with basilar invagination is significantly more difficult and technically challenging when compared to a normally aligned atlantoaxial joint encountered during the treatment of posttraumatic instability. The joint is significantly rostral in location and the microscope needs to be appropriately angled. The atlanto-axial facet joints are widely exposed on both sides after sectioning of the large C2 ganglion. The joint capsule is excised and the articular cartilage is widely removed using microdrill. The joints on both sides are distracted using an osteotome. The flat edge of the osteotome is introduced into the joint and it is then turned vertical to effect distraction. The status of the dislocation and of basilar invagination is evaluated by intraoperative radiographic control. Corticocancellous bone graft harvested from the iliac crest is stuffed into the joint in small pieces. Specially designed titanium spacers are used in selected cases as strut graft and impacted into the joints to provide additional distraction and stability. Over the period of our experience, we have realised that bone graft introduction inside the joint cavity and subsequent fixation can suffice, and there is a need for metal spacer only in selected cases. Fixation of the joint with the help of interfacetal screws and a metal plate provided a biomechanically firm fixation and sustained distraction. Holes in the titanium metal spacer provided space for bone fusion. The fixation was seen to be strong enough to sustain the vertical, transverse and rotatory strains of the most mobile region of the spine. Postoperatively the traction is discontinued and the patient is placed in a four-post hard cervical collar for 3 months, and all his physical activities involving the neck are restrained during the period.

Reversibility of Musculoskeletal Changes Following Surgery

A number of bone and soft tissue anomalies are associated with basilar invagination. These include short neck, torticollis, platybasia, cervical vertebral body fusion (Klippel–Feil abnormality) including assimilation of atlas, spondylotic spinal changes and restriction of neck movements. A number of these abnormalities were seen to be reversible following decompression and stabilisation of the region [26]. Considering that several physical features associated with this group of basilar invagination are reversible, it appears that the pathogenesis in such cases may be more due to mechanical factors rather than congenital causes or embryological dysgenesis. The common teaching on the subject is that the short neck and torticollis are a result of embryological dysgenesis and effectively result in indentation of the odontoid process into the cervicomedullary cord. However, it appears that it is the cord compression due to indentation by the odontoid process that is the primary event and all the physical alterations and bony abnormalities, including the short neck and torticollis, are secondary natural protective responses that aim to reduce the stretch of the cord over the indenting odontoid process. Pain, restriction of neck movements and hyperlordosis of the neck indicate the presence of instability of the craniovertebral junction. All of these natural responses probably allow the cord a relatively stretch-free traversal over the indenting odontoid process. Reduction of the disc spaces, osteophyte formation, incomplete and complete cervical fusions and alterations in the craniospinal and cervical angulations appear to be directly related to the reduction in neck length. The reduction in the disc-space height and fusions are more prominently seen in the upper cervical vertebrae. It appears that cervical fusions and assimilation of the atlas may be related to long-standing and progressive reduction in the disc-space height.

Foramen Magnum Decompression for Group B Patients

Foramen magnum bony decompression appears to be ideal for Group B basilar invagination. The procedure resulted in amelioration of symptoms and at least an arrest in the progression of the disability. Driesen reported that during operations for craniovertebral anomalies, he often had to remove noticeably thickened pieces of bone from the posterior edge of the foramen magnum [11]. In our cases, the suboccipital bone and posterior rim of the foramen magnum and the dura overlying the herniated cerebellar tissue were thin in a significant number of cases. This probably was related to the chronic pressure changes secondary to the reduced posterior cranial fossa volume. The bulbous lipping of the posterior rim of the foramen magnum represents the rudiments of the posterior arch of the atlas assimilated into the occipital bone [48]. Various authors have recommended that to achieve maximal decompression, it is necessary to open the dura mater and to cut all constrictive dural and arachnoidal bands. Some authors have recommended leaving the dura open, whilst others have recommended the placement of a graft. Current papers do not recommend resection of the herniating tonsils or even sectioning of adhesions around it. The fact that dural opening was not necessary whilst performing posterior fossa or foramen magnum decompression was first described by Goel in 1997 [16]. This was based on the understanding that the dura is an expansile structure and cannot be a compressive factor [41]. Opening of the dura is not only unnecessary but also subjects the patient to an increased risk of cerebrospinal fluid fistula. It makes an otherwise simple surgery into a relatively complex and dangerous surgical manoeuvre.

Syringomyelia: Pathology and Treatment

Syringomyelia is a frequently encountered clinical and radiological entity. It is associated with a range of pathological conditions that include congenital craniovertebral anomalies, tumours, infections, trauma and spinal deformities. Syringomyelia is rarely or never an acute phenomenon and is generally encountered in long-standing and persistent space-occupying or space-reducing lesions and in situations with subtle but persistent instability. Due to the long-standing and relentlessly progressive nature of the pathology and of clinical symptoms of syringomyelia, it is only rarely encountered in paediatric age group. Obstruction to the normal flow of spinal or cranial CSF by posttraumatic or infective arachnoiditis is also a less frequently encountered cause of syringomyelia. Acute injuries, acute infections, rapidly growing malignant tumours, mobile dislocations and acute posttraumatic deformities are generally not associated with syringomyelia. We recently reported cases of three infants having a mobile and reducible atlantoaxial dislocation having syringomyelia.

Syringomyelia or 'hydrocephalus of the cord' is 'never' a primary phenomenon. It is always 'secondary' to an obvious or an unidentified pathology [17]. The understanding of the pathophysiology of syringomyelia is crucially important to design a suitable treatment strategy and prognosticate the ultimate outcome. All attempts must be made to identify and treat the primary pathological cause. Syrinx drainage as a primary procedure may not be considered as therapeutic option. Syrinx drainage or shunting without dealing with the primary pathology can result in disastrous clinical consequences.

Basilar Invagination and Syringomyelia (Fig. 11): Basilar invagination and the associated basal maldevelopment and the resultant reduction in the posterior cranial

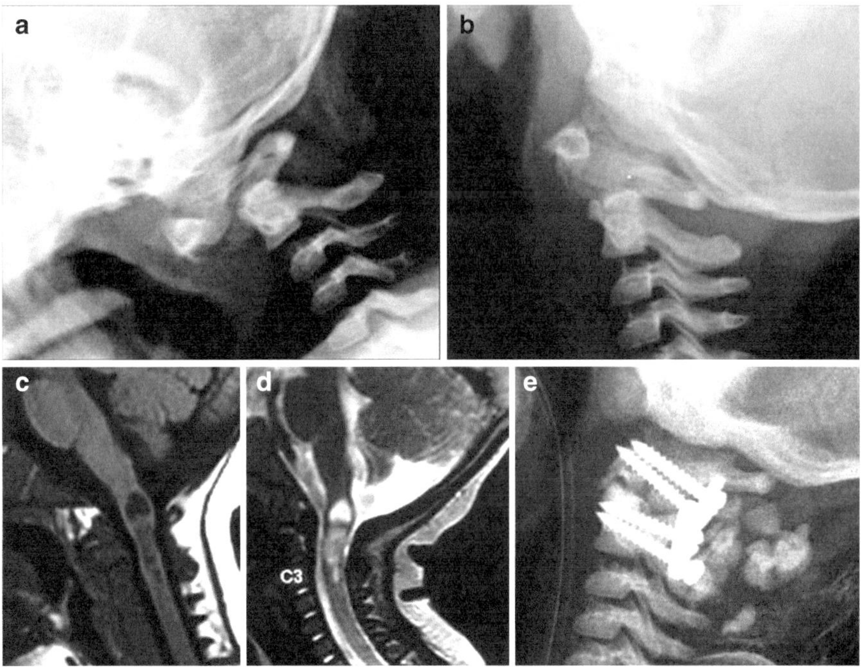

Fig. 11 (**a**) Lateral view of plain X-ray of an infant showing marked atlantoaxial dislocation. (**b**) View with the head in extension showing reduction of dislocation. (**c**) T1-weighted image of MRI with head in flexion showing evidence of cord compression and syringomyelia. (**d**) T2-weighted image with head in extension showing syringomyelia. (**e**) Postoperative X-ray showing plate and screw fixation

fossa volume are the primary events in syringomyelia pathology [22]. There is usually no demonstrable structural abnormality of the brainstem, cerebellar hemisphere or fourth ventricle suggesting that the neural development in these patients remained unaffected in the embryonic dysgenesis. The presence of the normal bulk of the cerebellum in the reduced volume posterior cranial fossa results in the herniation of a part of the cerebellum into the foramen magnum, an entity labelled as Chiari 1 malformation. Essentially it appears that syringomyelia is a tertiary event to the primary basilar invagination and secondary Chiari malformation. Long-standing pulsatile pressure of the herniated tonsil into the foramen magnum can result in compression of the cervicomedullary cord. Apart from physical attempts to increase the volume of the foramen magnum by bone erosion and membranous thinning and expansion, formation of syringomyelia probably provides a cushioning counterbalance of fluid from the spinal end so that the pressure of the tonsils on the cervicomedullary cord is minimised. The signs and symptoms related to the syrinx are more predominant than those related to brainstem compression by the tonsillar herniation. It could be that the primary aim of the entire process of syrinx formation is to reduce the compression of the brainstem at the level of foramen magnum by the herniating cerebellum.

Rationale of Treatment

Treatment strategy in such cases should be directed towards increasing the posterior cranial fossa volume by posterior fossa volume expansion or foramen magnum decompression. Logue reported 75 patients treated with craniovertebral decompressions for Chiari malformations and syringomyelia [45]. The patients were divided into two groups: one treated with bone decompression alone, leaving the arachnoid intact, and one group treated with Gardner's procedure of opening the fourth ventricle and plugging the upper cervical canal. They concluded that muscle plugging did not seem to change the results. Levy et al. also concluded on the same lines [44]. Logue noticed that there was no significant need for performing a syringosubarachnoid shunt following craniovertebral decompression [45]. Various subsequent studies have questioned the need for a syrinx drainage surgery following foramen magnum decompression. Di Lorenzo et al. concluded from their study that 'conservative' craniocervical decompression should be considered the first option in the treatment of syringomyelia–Chiari 1 complex [10]. The routine of opening of the posterior cranial fossa dura, resection of the cerebellar tonsils, arachnoidal sectioning and syringostomy is unnecessary. It appears that if the primary problem of basilar invagination is dealt with early in the course of the disease, the secondary and the tertiary events will spontaneously regress [23]. Craniovertebral realignment by atlantoaxial facetal distraction can be a philosophical approach to treatment in cases having Group A basilar invagination, Chiari malformation and syringomyelia.

Primary syringomyelia, where the cause is not identifiable, is a relatively complex clinical situation. The syringomyelia in such cases simulated 'normal-pressure hydrocephalus'. The intra-syrinx pressure is relatively low in such cases, and the results of any kind of treatment are far from gratifying.

When there is syringomyelia and Chiari malformation but no definite basilar invagination, efforts can be made to identify the cause of Chiari malformation. In such cases, it might be possible that the cerebellar mass is larger than normal. Even in such cases, volume expansion of the posterior cranial fossa is required. The theory that dura or dural bands can act as compressive factor appears unacceptable and does not correlate well with the pathogenic events. The dura is an expansile structure and may never be a compressive factor [17, 41].

Syringomyelia secondary to primary cord pathology like a tumour or kyphosis also appears to be a secondary and a 'protective' phenomenon. Treatment in such cases should be directed towards treatment of the pathology and not towards the treatment of syringomyelia [21]. Our observation is that if the syringomyelia is treated without dealing with the primary pathology, more often than not, the outcome is poor and the patient can be harmed.

Tuberculosis of Craniovertebral Junction (Fig. 12)

Tuberculosis of the craniovertebral junction usually occurs secondary to a primary focus elsewhere in the body. Osteoligamentous destruction and deformities leading to a range of clinical presenting symptoms have been recorded in cases with tuberculosis involving the craniovertebral junction. The understanding of the site of involvement of the tuberculosis in the craniovertebral junction, the pattern of its spread and nature of its pathogenetic effects on the osteoligamentous assembly is crucial for defining the strategy of the management. It has to be understood that tuberculosis involves the bone primarily and ligaments are affected only secondarily. Bones are involved by destruction, whilst the ligaments are involved by displacement and disruption.

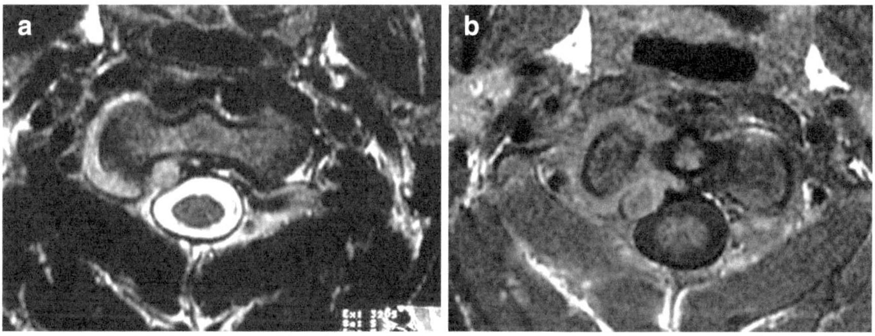

Fig. 12 (**a**) Axial image of a T2-weighted MRI showing tuberculous pus collection around the right side facet of the C2 vertebra. (**b**) Another view showing the unilateral affection of the pus

Natural Course of the Disease

The general pattern of progression of craniovertebral affection secondary to tuberculosis can be divided into three stages [31].

Stage 1: In this stage there is unilateral involvement of the cancellous part of the facet of atlas. There is no destructive deformation in this stage. Less frequently, there may be isolated and unilateral involvement of cancellous part of the facets of axis or of the odontoid process. Inflammatory granulomatous reaction is present, and caseous necrosis may be seen. Granulation tissue is usually located around the involved facet. The other parts of the atlas (or axis) bone and the contralateral facet are not involved.

In this stage, the patient has pain in the neck and restriction of neck movements. Systemic symptoms like loss of weight, loss of appetite and fever are usually present.

Stage 2: In this stage the disease progresses to involve the atlantoaxial joint by destructive necrosis and inflammation. The joint involvement is a result of extension of the inflammatory reaction. The destruction involves the atlantoaxial joint complex, and in addition it extends to other parts of the atlas and/or axis bones. Tuberculous inflammation may extend widely. The contralateral joint is still unaffected in this stage. The incompetence of the joint and osseous destruction and the adjoining ligamentous disruption in such a situation has been known to result in atlantoaxial dislocation. The atlantoaxial dislocation is probably a result of ineffectiveness of the alar and transverse ligaments as their bone attachment site is destroyed. As the contralateral atlantoaxial joint is normal, the atlantoaxial dislocation is of 'fixed' and rotatory variety, and grossly mobile and reducible dislocation is never or seldom encountered. The facet of the atlas may be collapsed. Prevertebral or extradural spinal caseous necrosis or pus formation is usually encountered. On imaging, the joint space on the involved side is seen to be reduced or absent, whilst on the contralateral side it is normal.

In this stage, the patient has pain in the neck, neck muscle spasm and severe restriction of neck movements. Torticollis is characteristic and most prominent symptom. Torticollis appears to be a natural defence process, wherein the neck turns to the contralateral side in an attempt to reduce all weight bearing by the affected lateral mass and the joint and protect the cord from compression by the infective granulation.

In this stage, the patient may or may not have neurological symptoms or deficits.

Stage 3: The disease involves the contralateral atlantoaxial joint and other bones and joints in the region. Evidence of instability of the craniovertebral junction is usually seen.

In this stage, the patient usually has a neurological deficit.

Indications of Surgery

Neurological deficits are notably delayed and less pronounced despite the aggressive destruction and deformation by the disease. The disease is initially unilateral, and the contralateral atlantoaxial joint is spared till late in the disease process. Due to the presence of relatively stable craniovertebral region despite the unilateral facetal destruction and the effectiveness of the modern antituberculous drugs, surgery can be delayed or avoided.

The extent and nature of involvement of the joints are determining factors for need for any kind of surgery for stabilisation of the region. Surgery for evacuation of pus or granulation tissue is seldom required. Despite the extensiveness of the bone destruction and inflammation, the patient is usually neurologically quite stable, and the systemic symptoms are not pronounced, till late in the disease process. In the absence of progressive neurological symptoms and in the presence of intact contralateral atlantoaxial joint, surgery can be avoided. The patient needs to be placed on antituberculous drugs. In addition, the patient will need a firm four-poster cervical collar, and all activities related to neck movements and weight bearing should be avoided for at least 3 months or till there is evidence of bone healing and regression of symptoms.

Surgery is indicated less frequently and may be required in stages 2 and 3 of the disease. The most positive indication of surgery includes presence and progression of neurological deficits. Radiological deformity in the presence of intact neurological condition may only be a marginal indication of surgery. More crucial issue is to identify and relate the problem to tuberculosis and differentiate the lesion from several tumour-like pathological situations.

If the disease is localised to the atlantoaxial region, surgery can involve fixation of the contralateral atlantoaxial joint by the lateral mass plate and screw fixation. Our experience suggests that even if the fixation is done by this method unilaterally, it is strong and provides a stable craniovertebral junction. Incorporation of the occipital bone in the fixation is seldom necessary. However, in the presence of gross and bilateral destructive disease, occipitocervical fixation can be a useful alternative.

Lateral Dislocation of Facet of Atlas Over the Facet of Axis

In the presence of destruction of the facets of atlas and axis on one side, it appears that the alar and transverse ligaments can become unilaterally incompetent [28]. The shift of balance on the contralateral side and the obliquity of the inclination of the facet of atlas in the atlantoaxial joint can result in its lateral dislocation over the facet of axis. Distraction of the facets of the atlas and axis, reduction of lateral dislocation and unilateral fixation of lateral masses can result in effective stabilisation of the region.

Long-Term Outcome After Conservative Treatment

The effectiveness of drugs usually begins in about 3 weeks of treatment. Pain reduces and the systemic symptoms begin to abate. Over the period, the patient recovers in the neurological symptoms and deficits to varying degrees. Fibrous reunion of the region and of the joint usually occurs over the period, and normality of the joint movements is at least partially restored. Patients nonresponsive to drug treatment will usually continue to have progressive destructive necrosis, deformity and instability.

Rotatory Atlantoaxial Dislocation (Figs. 13 and 14)

Rotational types of atlantoaxial dislocations are relatively rare clinical entities encountered more frequently in patients in paediatric age group. Identifying the exact pathological event that causes rotatory atlantoaxial dislocation is crucial to design an appropriate treatment protocol.

Physical neck rotation (or torticollis) is of three types:

Type 1 Positional Torticollis

This is related to positional alteration in the craniovertebral junction over prolonged period of time and is related to the indentation of the odontoid process into the cervicomedullary cord. Such an indentation is seen in cases with Group A basilar invagination. The secondary physical neck alterations simulate the changes in spinal posturing secondary to disc herniation. The torticollis seen in cases with Group A basilar invagination is present in varying degrees in most cases. The long-standing torticollis seen in such cases appears to be a part of protective spinal physical alteration that occurs as an attempt to accommodate the spinal cord from relentlessly and progressively reducing spinal canal. Our recent observations suggest that such a torticollis (and even short neck) is reversible following decompression and stabilisation of the craniovertebral junction [26].

Treatment

Direct manipulation of the atlantoaxial joint, distraction of facets with bone graft, with or without introduction of titanium metal spacers has been shown by us to result in the reduction of basilar invagination and of fixed atlantoaxial dislocation. We have observed remarkable reduction of torticollis by this method of treatment. Differential distraction of the facets can also result in direct reduction of torticollis.

Type 2 Spasmodic Torticollis

The torticollis in this group is related to sternocleidomastoid muscle spasm. The pathology in these cases and the treatment remain controversial. Botulinum injections in the spasmodic muscles have been identified to be a satisfactory treatment modality in resistant cases.

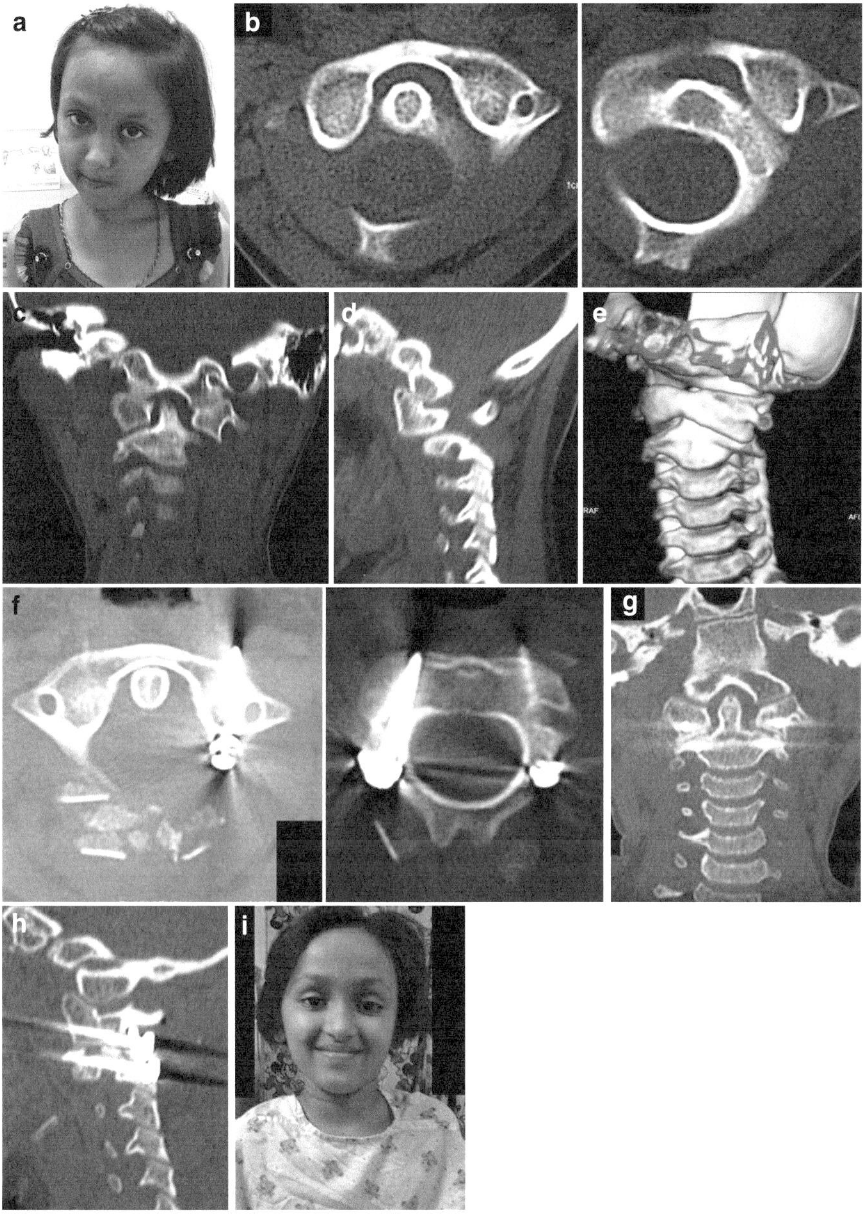

Fig. 13 (**a**) Image of a 5-year-old girl showing torticollis . (**b**) Axial images of C1 and C2 showing rotatory dislocation. (**c**) Coronal view showing the dis-alignment of the facets. (**d**) Sagittal view showing partial alignment of facets on one side. (**e**) 3-D CT scan showing the rotatory atlantoaxial dislocation. (**f**) Postoperative image showing facetal fixation. (**g**) Coronal image showing facetal realignment. (**h**) Sagittal view showing atlantoaxial fixation with facetal realignment. (**i**) Postoperative image showing reversal of torticollis

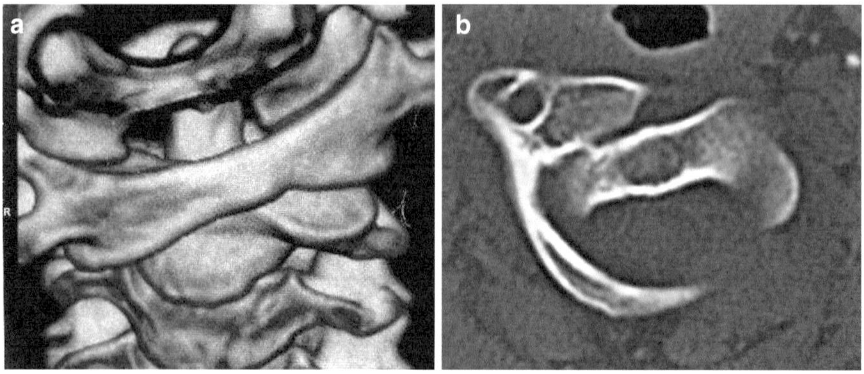

Fig. 14 (**a**) CT scan of a 10-year-old boy showing rotatory atlantoaxial dislocation. (**b**) Axial CT scan showing the rotation

Type 3 Facetal Rotatory Torticollis

Torticollis in this group is related to 'rotatory' atlantoaxial dislocation secondary to rotatory dislocation of facet of atlas over facet of axis. This group forms a discrete entity and is the subject of discussion in this chapter. Locking of the atlantoaxial facets has been identified to result in rotatory atlantoaxial dislocation. Such a dislocation has been identified more commonly in young children. Although several pathogenetic factors have been considered, the exact cause of the phenomenon is unclear. The dislocation is an acute event that usually starts following an episode of relatively minor trauma. Some patients have been identified to be having throat and paranasal sinus infections or tonsillitis at the time of event. However, exact correlation between possible infection, trauma and atlantoaxial dislocation is only speculative.

Historical Background and Nomenclature

Rotatory dislocation of the atlantoaxial joint was first described by Sir Charles Bell in 1830 [2] and Corner in 1907 [6]. Wortzman and Dewar introduced the term atlantoaxial rotatory fixation–subluxation in 1968 [61].

Rotatory atlantoaxial dislocation can be subdivided into *reducible* or *irreducible types*. *Reducible* type rotatory atlantoaxial dislocation is classified as one where the dislocation reduces on dynamic images or after institution of cervical traction. Reducible rotatory atlantoaxial dislocation is usually of incomplete type, when some part of the facet of atlas is in contact with the facet of axis. Complete rotatory dislocation can also reduce on traction, but the possibilities of its reduction are relatively less. Mobile and reducible rotatory dislocation can be treated by conservative observation for about 3 months using halo traction or cervical collar. If during the period the rotatory dislocation reduces and remains reduced on dynamic imaging, there is no need for surgery. Or else, surgical fixation of the rotatory dislocation in reduced position should be performed. In cases with '*irreducible*' rotatory dislocation, an attempt can be made to reduce the dislocation by local distraction and reduction by manual realignment.

The main presenting symptom of rotatory atlantoaxial dislocation is torticollis of the neck and neurological symptoms may only be marginal. The torticollis may be painless. Surgical treatment for rotatory dislocation is to fix the dislocation in the reduced or 'maximally' reduced position. Segmental fixation of the dislocation, even if it is in dislocated position, allows the subaxial spine to move better, and torticollis can be expected to recover.

Biomechanics

The occipitoatlantoaxial joints are the most complex joints of the axial skeleton. This joint complex forms a part of the primary pillar of spine that provides stability and mobility to the head. The primary movement of the atlantooccipital articulation is flexion–extension and of the atlantoaxial joints is rotation. The geometry of the lateral atlantoaxial articular surfaces is such that they are convex with horizontal orientation, thus suitable to permit rotation. The maximum rotation between the atlas and axis is ~45° [58]. When rotation exceeds 45°, the inferior facet of atlas interlocks over the superior facet of axis. If the transverse ligament is deficient, this facet interlock may occur even with rotation of less than 45°. It has also been seen that if the transverse ligament remains intact, anterior arch of atlas will not subluxate over axis unless there is over 65° of rotation.

The alar ligaments limit axial rotation and side bending of the C_0–C_1–C_2 complex. The left alar ligament limits rotation of C_1 and the head to the right, and the right alar ligament limits rotation to the left. The vertebral arteries located in the foramen transversarium are not affected by the extremes of normal rotation, but they can be severely compromised by excessive rotation, especially if combined with anterior displacement [11]. The fact that the vertebral artery has a dynamic relationship with the bones during rotational movements was first discussed by us [4]. The laxity of the vertebral artery in the region assists in facilitating a range of neck movements.

Etiopathogenesis

Predisposing Factors

Several predisposing factors have been identified for rotatory atlantoaxial dislocation including upper respiratory infections, trauma and surgery of the head and neck, genetic diseases and ocular infections [1, 3]. In addition, up to 24 % of cases of rotatory atlantoaxial dislocation can occur without an obvious predisposing cause [9, 50]. Rheumatoid arthritis, Down syndrome, Morquio's disease and an assortment of congenital cervical anomalies have also been associated with it [50, 52, 59, 60]. There is also a definite preponderance of rotatory atlantoaxial dislocation in the paediatric population. The higher incidence of rotatory atlantoaxial dislocation in children may be attributed to the shallower and more horizontally oriented joint surface, the relative elasticity of the ligaments, the not yet fully developed neck muscles and a relatively large head.

The Cause of Fixation

The cause of the fixation remains obscure, since no anatomical or autopsy evidence bearing on this question is available. Wittek [60] suggested that there is an effusion in the synovial joints producing stretching of the ligaments. Coutts [7] proposed the theory that synovial fringes, when inflamed or adherent, may block reduction, whilst Fiorrani-Gallotta and Luzzatti [13] believed that the deformity is due to rupture of one or both alar ligaments and the transverse ligament. Watson Jones [57] postulated hyperaemic decalcification with loosening of the ligaments. Grisel [37] suggested that muscle contracture might follow an upper respiratory tract infection and be a factor. Hess and associates [40] concluded that there is a combination of factors, including muscle spasm, which prevent reduction in the early stages. Wortzman and Dewar [61] postulated damage to the atlantoaxial articular processes of unknown nature. Fielding and Hawking [12] suggested that reduction is probably obstructed in the early stages by swollen capsular and synovial tissues and by associated muscle spasm. If the abnormal position persists because of a failure to achieve reduction, ligament and capsular contractures develop and cause fixation.

Radiographic Features

3-D CT scanning is the gold standard investigation to diagnose and confirm rotational atlantoaxial dislocation. The exact alignment of the facets and their displacement can be evaluated. Dynamic CT scan, with the head and neck in flexed and extended positions, clearly delineates the pathology and assists in determining the appropriate surgical treatment modality.

MRI assists in confirming the findings of CT scan and demonstrates features that would suggest compression and displacement of the neural and vascular structures.

The plain X-ray investigations have now become less relevant with the increasing and popular use of CT scanning and MRI.

The degree of *neck rotation or tilt* in patients having rotatory dislocation is measured as an angle between a line that coursed from the nasion, tip of the nose and symphysis menti to the horizontal. The angle was then expressed as the degree of tilt from the vertical.

Clinical Features

Because of the rarity of the pathology, the infrequency of neurologic involvement and the difficulty in obtaining adequate radiographs, the diagnosis may be difficult to make and is usually delayed. The acuity of the neck deformity in an otherwise healthy and neurologically normal child is the hallmark of the problem. Pain is not a prominent presenting symptom. With more severe degrees of subluxation or dislocation, torticollis may be noted and the patient may present with the typical 'cock robin' posture with the head tilted towards one side and turned (rotated) towards the other and in slight flexion. For example, in a right-sided unilateral anterior rotatory subluxation (right-sided atlas lateral mass subluxated anteriorly), there is *lateral bending* of the head and neck *to the right* and *rotation* of the head *to the left*. When an attempt is made to turn the head opposite to the direction it faces, it is found to be difficult; however, rotating it further in the direction in which it faces is possible. On palpation, the C2 spinous process may be prominent and deviated to the side to which the chin is pointed, as a result of the lateral tilt of the head or from counterrotation of C2; this is done in an attempt to realign the head [12].

In the acute setting it is important to distinguish between true rotatory atlantoaxial dislocation and muscular torticollis. In rotatory atlantoaxial dislocation, the sternomastoid spasm is on the side of the chin, whereas in muscular torticollis the spasm is on the contralateral side. In rotatory dislocation the sternomastoid spasm on the side of the chin is secondary or reflexive, as if the muscle is attempting to correct the deformity [12].

Neurologic involvement is fortunately uncommon; however, occipital neuralgia may occur because the greater occipital nerve runs in close proximity to the C1–C2 facet capsule [12, 49].

Classification

Fielding and Hawkins Classification

Fielding and Hawkins [42] classified rotatory atlantoaxial dislocation into five types:

Type I

Rotatory atlantoaxial dislocation with no anterior displacement of the atlas (ADI of 3 mm or less).

The transverse ligament is intact and the *dens acts like a pivot*. The rotation of the atlas on the axis is greater than 45°. This is the commonest type of rotatory atlantoaxial dislocation.

Type II

Rotatory atlantoaxial dislocation with anterior displacement of the atlas by 3–5 mm.

This type is associated with deficiency of the transverse ligament and unilateral anterior displacement of *one* lateral mass of the atlas, whilst the *opposite joint* is intact and *acts as the pivot*. In these patients there is abnormal anterior displacement of the atlas on the axis, and the amount of fixed rotation is in excess of normal maximum rotation. The rotation usually exceeds 40°.

Type III

Rotatory atlantoaxial dislocation with anterior displacement of atlas by more than 5 mm.

This type is associated with the disruption of both the transverse and alar ligaments. *Both* lateral masses of the atlas are displaced anteriorly, one more than the other thus producing the rotated position. The rotation is more than 40° and the atlas is displaced forward from the odontoid by more than 5 mm.

Type IV

Rotatory atlantoaxial dislocation with posterior displacement of atlas.

This type is rare and occurs when the odontoid process is deficient or fractured. There is a posterior shift of one or both lateral masses of the atlas, one of them shifting more than the other thus causing rotation.

Levine and Edwards [43] added to this classification by describing the extreme injury pattern of rotatory dislocation.

Type V

Frank rotatory atlantoaxial dislocation.

Goel's Classification of Facetal Locking [30]

The facetal locking was divided into two types: rotatory and translatory.

Rotatory Locking

Rotatory locking was when the head was in torticollis or 'rotated' position. Rotatory locking was 'partial' when the facet of atlas of only one side was dislocated anteriorly over the facet of axis. The facet on the contralateral side was not abnormally positioned and acted as a pivot for the dislocation. Rotatory locking was complete when the facets of atlas on both sides were dislocated over the facets of axis in a rotatory fashion. The process resulted in facet of atlas being positioned anterior to facet of axis on one side and posterior to it on the other side.

Translatory Dislocation

Translatory dislocation was described as a condition when facets of atlas on both sides were dislocated anterior to the facets of axis. Such a dislocation resulted in a fixed-flexion neck deformity. Although a posterior translation is also technically possible, but such cases were not encountered.

Treatment

It is important to recognise atlantoaxial rotatory fixation as there may be an underlying compromised atlantoaxial complex with the potential to cause neurological damage or even sudden death.

Traditional treatment guidelines based on the classification of *Fielding and Hawkins* [12] are as follows:

Type I lesion which is the most benign may be treated with cervical spine immobilisation after reduction.

For *type II* lesions if reduction is achieved within 14 days of luxation in children, subsequent immobilisation with halo was recommended. For type II lesions associated with occipitoatlantal dislocation and/or when the diagnosis was delayed for more than 14 days, a posterior atlantoaxial or occipitoatlantoaxial arthrodesis was recommended.

Type III and IV lesions were all treated with posterior arthrodesis after reduction.

Fielding and Hawkins [12] described children in whom the diagnosis of rotatory atlantoaxial subluxation was not made for months and in whom traction was unsuccessful in achieving a satisfactory reduction or relief of the symptoms. They performed an arthrodesis of atlas and axis in these patients and achieved resolution of the torticollis. They made no attempt intraoperatively to realign the atlas on the axis. Manipulative reduction of rotatory atlantoaxial subluxation may be indicated in selected patients with recent onset of torticollis, but there is less risk when reduction is achieved by bed rest or by traction without manipulation.

Phillips and Hensinger [50] recommended a treatment plan that is based on the duration of the torticollis. Patients who have had a rotatory subluxation of less than 1-week duration can be treated with immobilisation in a soft collar and bed rest for a week. Close follow-up is essential. If reduction fails to occur spontaneously, then the patient should be hospitalised and given traction. In patients with rotatory subluxation of more than 1-week duration but less than 1-month duration, hospitalisation and cervical traction are indicated. After reduction, immobilisation for 4–6 weeks is recommended. In patients with subluxation of more than 1-month duration, cervical traction can be attempted for up to 3 weeks. If reduction does not occur, an arthrodesis should be performed.

Pang [49] in a recent review studied the normal biomechanics of atlantoaxial rotation and constructed a physiologic motion curve for relative motions between these joints and introduced new diagnostic criteria for rotatory atlantoaxial dislocation. Fielding and Hawkins [12] described treatment guidelines based on their classification. Depending on the nature of facetal dislocation, we classified the deformity into two groups, rotatory dislocation and translatory dislocation. This classification varies from the ones previously described in that it includes translatory dislocation in the subgroup. Considering that the facetal malalignment was present as an acute phenomenon in a similar clinical setting in both the groups of patients, widening the scope of classification of neck deformity appeared to be reasonable. The rotatory dislocation was further classified into complete rotatory dislocation where facets on both sides were not in their alignment and an incomplete rotatory dislocation where there was only a unilateral facetal malalignment, the facets being in the normal position on the contralateral side. The normally aligned facet acts as a pivot on which the contralateral side rotates. Such a rotatory dislocation has been described earlier [9]. On physical observation, the degree of torticollis was not remarkably different in the two groups. A period of clinical observation ranging from few weeks to 2–3 months and attempts at closed reduction of the dislocation has been uniformly advocated. Some authors advise the use of direct cervical traction or a progressive halo traction for varying periods [53]. Analysis of the result of traction and modifying the surgical strategy is accordingly carried out. However, we observed that most children tolerated traction poorly, and in one of the cases in the presented series, it resulted in a permanent repositioning of the facets to normal alignment. Although long-term outcome of untreated rotatory atlantoaxial dislocation is not elaborately described in the literature, fusion in dislocated position can be expected. Delayed lower and midspinal deformities are possible that will assist the head to look straight ahead.

There are only isolated reports mentioning surgical treatment strategy in cases with locked atlantoaxial facets. Schmidek et al. [51] used a transoral route, and Crockard et al. [8] employed an extreme lateral approach to remove obstructing ligamentous or bone structures within the joint. Goto et al. [35] released the atlantoaxial lateral facet joint by a transoral surgery and followed it up by a posterior fixation using interlaminar clamps. Continuous monitoring of the neurological status of the patient is essential during any manipulative reduction. After reduction some form of cervical immobilisation is used to prevent recurrent subluxation. Immobilisation presumably allows the stretched or edematous ligaments to heal and to return to their normal length. Full, pain-free motion of the neck should be restored before external immobilisation is discontinued.

Some authors have discussed the usefulness of fixation in the abnormal position [35, 50]. They observe that segmental fixation of the dislocation, even if it is in a dislocated position, allows the subaxial spine to move better, and torticollis can be expected to recover. Our technique involves sectioning of the C2 ganglion, wide exposure and opening up of the atlantoaxial joint and unilateral or bilateral manipulation of the atlantoaxial facets [14, 18, 23]. It was observed that external traction may not be successful in relocating the facets, as the effect of traction was dissipated more to the lower neck than to the site of problem in the region of the joint.

Goel's Technique of Craniovertebral Realignment for Cases with Locked Facet

Under anaesthesia, the patient is placed under cervical traction, the weights ranging from 3 to 6 kg. The head end of the table was raised approximately 35° to provide countertraction by the body. The position assisted in reducing the venous congestion in the operative field, particularly in the vein-loaded region of the lateral masses. The exposure of the atlantoaxial joint in cases with facetal malalignment is significantly more difficult and technically challenging when compared to a normally aligned atlantoaxial joint encountered during the treatment of posttraumatic instability. However, it was observed that intraoperative traction had resulted in an improvement in the alignment of the facets in all cases, when compared to their preoperative status. The atlantoaxial facet joints are widely exposed on both sides after sectioning of the large C2 ganglion. Such a wide exposure provided an opportunity to observe the status of the facets and in affecting direct manipulations. The joint capsule is excised and the articular cartilage is widely removed using microdrill. The joints on both sides are distracted using an osteotome. The flat edge of the osteotome is introduced into the joint, and it is then turned vertical to affect distraction and further manipulation. The sizes of the osteotomes could be varied depending on the local situation. The sequence of manipulation of the facets varied, but in general the more affected facet was treated first. Whenever necessary, the distraction was done simultaneously on both sides. Although visualisation of the region with high-definition radiography or intraoperative CT scanning is possible, but such investigations were not performed. Direct observation of the position and alignment of the articular surfaces of the facets of atlas and axis was the key to facetal realignment. Other indicator of successful realignment was the location of the tip of spinous process of the axis in relationship with midline of the arch of atlas. Corticocancellous bone graft harvested from the iliac crest is stuffed into the joint in small pieces. Subsequent fixation of the joint with the help of interarticular screws and a metal plate provided a biomechanically firm fixation and sustained distraction and realignment. In cases where the facet of atlas was dislocated anteriorly and manual realignment was incomplete, the screw (with the plate) was first inserted into the lateral mass of the axis and was tightened. The atlas screw was then tightened over the fixed plate. This variation resulted in posterior movement of the facet of atlas. Similar technique of reduction has been described in the treatment of spondylolisthesis [46]. Larger pieces of corticocancellous bone graft were placed in the midline over the arch of atlas and lamina of axis after appropriately preparing host bone. Postoperatively, the traction is discontinued and the patient is placed in a four-post hard cervical collar for 3 months, and all physical activities involving the neck are restrained during the period. After a 6-month period, all activities, including sports, were permitted in an unrestrictive manner.

Direct distraction of the facets appeared to be the most important component of the operation. Further manipulations of the position of the facets and their realignment were then possible. Opening up of the articular capsule, removal of the articular cartilage and stuffing of the bone graft within the articular cavity resulted in dysfunctioning of the joint and set a stage for its ultimate fusion. The screw fixation in the bones that were otherwise normal was seen to be strong enough to sustain the vertical, transverse and rotatory strains of the most mobile region of the spine. Although reported, we did not locate any broken piece of bone or cartilage or identify the presence of any evidence of infection in the region of the joint in any case. Our long-time experience with the opening of the atlantoaxial joint and of facetal manipulation for the treatment of atlantoaxial dislocation and basilar invagination assisted in the conduct of the operation [14, 18, 23]. Although technically challenging and anatomically precise, the procedure results in excellent restoration of the facetal alignment and neck shape and satisfactory neck movements.

We employed the technique of opening of the joint, distraction and manipulation of the facets and reduction of rotatory atlantoaxial dislocation. The technique is relatively complex and tedious, particularly so in the presence of intact neurological condition of the patient. However, reduction of the rotatory dislocation is possible by this technique. Holding and manipulation of the spinous process of axis, posterior arch of atlas and the facets of atlas and axis can result in reduction of the rotatory dislocation.

Rotatory atlantoaxial dislocation and related neck torticollis can be a physically crippling disorder. The difficulties associated with exposure and manipulation of the atlantoaxial joint for reduction of the rotatory dislocation, particularly in neurologically intact patients, make surgery for this problem a difficult and controversial issue. Locking of the facets and related neck deformity can be a physically crippling disorder. The difficulties associated with exposure and manipulation of the atlantoaxial joint for reduction of the dislocation, particularly in neurologically intact patients, make surgery a formidable technical challenge. The proposed operation necessitates fixation of the joint. A technique that will reduce dislocation and permit movements of the atlantoaxial joint needs to be identified.

Conclusions

Stabilisation of craniovertebral instability poses a therapeutic challenge. Atlantoaxial joint treatment that involves denuding of the articular cartilage, placement of bone graft within the joint cavity and subsequent facetal fixation with metal implants provides a ground for bone fusion. Segmental fixation is crucial in the treatment of atlantoaxial instability in children. Direct facetal manipulation can be used effectively in the management of complex pathology involving the region.

References

1. Beer JV, Hoffman EB, Kieck CF (1990) Traumatic atlantoaxial subluxation in children. J Pediatr Orthop 10:397–400
2. Bell C (1830) The nervous system of the human body. Embracing the papers delivered to the Royal Society on the subject of nerve. Case 143:403
3. Bredenkamp JK, Maceri DR (1990) Inflammatory torticollis in children. Arch Otolaryngol Head Neck Surg 116:310–313
4. Cacciola F, Phalke U, Goel A (2004) Vertebral artery in relationship to C1-C2 vertebrae. An anatomical study. Neurol India 52(2):178–184
5. Chamberlain WE, Basilar impression (platybasia) (1939) A bizarre developmental anomaly of the occipital bone and upper cervical spine with striking and misleading neurologic manifestations. Yale J Biol Med 11:487–496
6. Corner EM (1907) Rotatory dislocation of the atlas. Arch Surg 45:9–26
7. Coutts MB (1934) Atlanto-epistropheal subluxations. Arch Surg 29:297–311
8. Crockard HA, Rogers MA (1996) Open reduction of traumatic atlanto-axial rotatory dislocation with use of the extreme lateral approach. A report of two cases. J Bone Joint Surg Am 78(3):431–443
9. DeRoeck BN (1977) A case of rotatory dislocation of atlas on axis. Radiography 43: 127–130
10. Di Lorenzo N, Fortuna A, Guidetti B (1982) Craniovertebral junction malformations. Clinicoradiological findings, long-term results, and surgical indications in 63 cases. J Neurosurg 56:603–608
11. Driesen W (1960) Findings at operation in the central nervous system in basilar impressions and related abnormalities of the atlanto-occipital region. Acta Neurochir 9:9–68 (Ger)
12. Fielding W, Hawkins RJ (1977) Atlantoaxial rotatory fixation – subluxation. J Bone Joint Surg Am 59:37–44
13. Fiorrani-Gallotta G, Luzzatti G (1957) Sublussazione laterale e sublussazione rotatorie dell'atlante. Arch Ortop 70:467–484
14. Goel A, Laheri VK (1994) Plate and screw fixation for atlanto-axial dislocation, (technical report). Acta Neurochir (Wien) 129:47–53
15. Goel A, Achawal S (1995) Surgical treatment for Arnold Chiari malformation associated with atlantoaxial dislocation. Br J Neurosurg 9:67–72
16. Goel A, Bhatjiwale M, Desai K (1998) Basilar invagination: a study based on 190 surgically treated cases. J Neurosurg 88:962–968
17. Goel A, Desai KI (2000) Surgery for syringomyelia. An analysis based on 163 surgical cases. Acta Neurochir (Wien) 142:293–302
18. Goel A, Desai K, Muzumdar D (2002) Atlantoaxial fixation using plate and screw method : a report of 160 treated patients. Neurosurgery 51:1351–1357
19. Goel A (2004) Treatment of basilar invagination by atlantoaxial joint distraction and direct lateral mass fixation. J Neurosurg Spine 1(3):281–286
20. Goel A, Kulkarni AG (2004) Screw implantation in spinous process for occipitoaxial fixation. J Clin Neurosci 11(7):735–737
21. Goel A, Cacciola F, Muzumdar DP (2005) Trigeminal neurinoma associated with Chiari malformation and syringomyelia. J Clin Neurosci 12(5):608–610
22. Goel A, Sharma P (2005) Craniovertebral junction realignment for the treatment of basilar invagination with syringomyelia: preliminary report of 12 cases. Neurol Med Chir (Tokyo) 45(10):512–518
23. Goel A, Kulkarni AG, Sharma P (2005) Reduction of fixed atlantoaxial dislocation in 24 cases: technical note. J Neurosurg Spine 2(4):505–509
24. Goel A (2007) Double insurance atlantoaxial fixation. Surg Neurol 67(2):135–139
25. Goel A (2007) Atlantoaxial joint jamming as a treatment for atlantoaxial dislocation: a preliminary report. Technical note. J Neurosurg Spine 7(1):90–94

26. Goel A, Shah A (2009) Reversal of longstanding musculoskeletal changes in basilar invagination after surgical decompression and stabilization. J Neurosurg Spine 10(3):220–227
27. Goel A, Shah A, Rajan S (2009) Vertical mobile and reducible atlantoaxial dislocation. Clinical article. Vertical mobile atlantoaxial dislocation. J Neurosurg Spine 11(1):9–14
28. Goel A, Shah A (2010) Lateral atlantoaxial facetal dislocation in craniovertebral region tuberculosis: report of a case and analysis of an alternative treatment. Acta Neurochir (Wein) 152(4):709–712
29. Goel A (2010) Occipitocervical fixation: is it necessary? J Neurosurg Spine 13(1):1–2
30. Goel A, Shah A (2011) Atlantoaxial facet locking: treatment by facet manipulation and fixation. Experience in 14 cases. J Neurosurg Spine 14(1):3–9
31. Goel A, Cacciola F (2011) The craniovertebral junction: diagnosis, pathology, surgical techniques. Georg Thieme Verlag, Stuttgart
32. Goel A, Shah A, Kothari M, Gaikwad S, Dhande PL (2011) Comparative quantitative analysis of osseous anatomy of the craniovertebral junction of tiger, horse, deer, and humans. J Craniovertebr Junction Spine 2(1):32–37
33. Goel A (2011) Cervical ganglion (CG2) neurectomy: a window to the atlantoaxial joint. World Neurosurg(Nov.)
34. Goel A (2012) Is 'Self-to-Self' bone graft ideal for bone fusion after craniovertebral stabilization? World Neurosurg(Jan 28)
35. Goto S, Mochizuki M, Kita T, Murakami M, Nishigaki H, Moriya H (1998) Transoral joint release of the dislocated atlantoaxial joints combined with posterior reduction and fusion for a late infantile atlantoaxial rotatory fixation. A case report. Spine (PhilaPa 1976) 23(13): 1485–1489
36. Grawitz P (1880) Beitrag zur lehre von der basilaren Impression des Schadels. Arch Path Anat Physiol 80:449
37. Grisel P (1930) Enucleation de l'atlas et torticollis naso-pharyngien. Presse Med 38:50–53
38. Grob D, Magerl F (1987) Operative stabilisierung bei Frakturen von C1 und C2. Orthopade 16:46–54
39. Gupta S, Goel A (2000) Quantitative anatomy of lateral masses of the atlas and axis vertebrae. Neurol India 48:120–125
40. Hess JH, Bronstein IP, Abelson SM (1935) Atlanto-axial dislocations. Unassociated with trauma and secondary to inflammatory foci in the neck. Am J Dis Child 49:1137–1147
41. Kothari M, Goel A (2006) Maternalizing the meninges: a pregnant Arabic legacy. Neurol India 54(4):345–346
42. Kothari M, Goel A (2007) Transatlantic odonto-occipital listhesis: the so-called basilar invagination. Neurol India 55(1):6–7
43. Levine AM, Edwards CC (1986) Treatment of injuries in the C1-C2 complex. Orthop Clin North Am 17:31–44
44. Levy WJ, Mason L, Hahn JF (1983) Chiari malformation presenting in adults: a surgical experience in 127 cases. Neurosurgery 12:377–390
45. Logue V, Edwards MR (1981) Syringomyelia and its surgical treatment- an analysis of 75 patients. J Neurol Neurosurg Psychiatry 44:273–284
46. Matthiass HH, Heine J (1986) The surgical reduction of spondylolisthesis. Clin Orthop 203:34–44
47. McRae DL (1953) Bony abnormalities in the region of foramen magnum: correlation of anatomic and neurologic findings. Acta Radiol 40:335–354
48. Menezes AH (1995) Primary craniovertebral anomalies and hindbrain herniation syndrome (Chiari 1): data base analysis. Pediatr Neurosurg 23:260–269
49. Pang D, Li V (2004) Atlantoaxial rotatory fixation: part 1 – biomechanics of normal rotation at the atlantoaxial joint in children. Neurosurgery 55:614–626
50. Phillips WA, Hensinger RN (1989) The management of rotatory atlanto-axial subluxation in children. J Bone Joint Surg Am 71A:664–668
51. Schmidek HH, Smith DA, Sofferman RA, Gomes FB (1986) Transoral unilateral facetectomy in the management of unilateral anterior rotatory atlantoaxial fracture/dislocation: a case report. Neurosurgery 18(5):645–652

52. Sherk HH, Nicholson JT (1969) Rotatory atlanto-axial dislocation associated with ossiculum terminale and mongolism. J Bone Joint Surg Am 51A:957–964
53. Subach BR, McLaughlin MR, Albright AL, Pollack IF (1998) Current management of pediatric atlantoaxial rotatory subluxation. Spine 23:2174–2179
54. Thiebaut F, Wackenheim A, Vrousos C (1961) New median sagittal pneumostratigraphical findings concerning the posterior fossa. J Radiol Electrol Med Nucl 42:1–7
55. Virchow R (1857) Untersuchungen fiber die Entwicklung des Schadelgrundes. Reimer, Berlin
56. Von Torklus D, Gehle W (1972) The upper cervical spine. Regional anatomy, pathology and traumatology. In: Georg Thieme Verlag (ed) A systemic radiological atlas and textbook. Grune & Stratton, New York, pp 1–99
57. Watson Jones R (1932) Spontaneous hyperaemic dislocation of the atlas. Proc R Soc Med 25:586–590
58. White AAA, Panjabi MM (1990) Clinical biomechanics of spine, 2nd edn. Lippincot (Pub), Philadelphia
59. Wilson BC, Jarvis BL, Hayden RC III (1987) Non traumatic subluxation of the atlanto-axial joint: Grisel's syndrome. Ann Otol Rhinol Laryngol 96:705–708
60. Wittek A (1908) Ein Fall von Distensionsluxation im Atlanto-epistropheal-Gelenke. Munch med Wschr 55:1836–1837
61. Wortzman G, Dewar FP (1968) Rotary fixation of the atlantoaxial joint: rotational atlantoaxial subluxation. Radiology 90(3):479–487

Minimally Invasive Posterior Trans-muscular C1–C2 Screw Fixation Through an Anatomical Corridor to Preserve Occipitocervical Tension Band: Surgical Anatomy and Clinical Experience

Roberto Díaz, Miguel E. Berbeo, Luis M. Villalobos, Manuel F. Vergara, and Enrique Osorio

Contents

R. Díaz, MD (✉) • M.E. Berbeo, MD, MSc
Unidad de Neurocirugía, Hospital Universitario San Ignacio,
Pontificia Universidad Javeriana, Carrera 7°, N° 40-62, 6° Piso, Bogotá, Colombia
e-mail: rocadior@yahoo.com

L.M. Villalobos, MD • M.F. Vergara, MD
Neurosurgery Resident Unidad de Neurocirugía,
Hospital Universitario San Ignacio, Pontificia Universidad Javeriana,
Bogotá, Colombia

E. Osorio, MD
Medicine School, Universidad el Bosque, Clínica Reina Sofía, Bogotá, Colombia

C. Di Rocco, N. Akalan (eds.), *Pediatric Craniovertebral Junction Diseases*, Advances and Technical Standards in Neurosurgery 40,
DOI 10.1007/978-3-319-01065-6_8,

Abstract The C1–C2 joint is affected by multiple entities that may produce biomechanical instability. Optimal management for atlantoaxial instability has been searched by ways of different surgical techniques with different results, generating discussion between second effects of a particular treatment. Lateral dissections can place the axial neck musculature and ligaments at risk of neural denervations or vascular compromise. Either of these entities may result in significant postoperative atrophy, pain, and instability. Minimally invasive techniques for the treatment of spinal disorders allow to our patients less morbid procedures with equal or better results compared to conventional surgery. In the following paper, we review the anatomy of the atlantoaxial joint and propose a minimally invasive trans-muscular C1–C2 fusion technique using C1 lateral-mass screws and C2 pedicular screws. We describe cases with surgical, clinical, and radiographic follow-up.

Keywords Atlantoaxial joint • C1–C2 instability • Minimally invasive • Spinal fusion

Introduction

The atlantoaxial complex is formed for the two first cervical vertebrae, their joints, and a few important ligaments. As a product of thin intricate relationship, its architecture allows movement in flexion, extension, lateral bending, and rotation. Atlantoaxial instability is produced when any of the former elements is injured, either by trauma, inflammatory disease, malignancy, or congenital defects [11].

The atlantoaxial complex is responsible for more of the 50 % of the rotatory movement of the head. This is a problem when we speak about fusion rates, compared with subaxial levels [1].

Many techniques have been described trying to solve this problem, from external immobilization to internal anterior-posterior fixation. They all have advantages, risks, and variable success/failure rates [11].

For a long time, the treatment of cervical instability was limited to external immobilization, but the high rates of non-fusion and associated morbidity made imperative the search for other alternatives. In 1910 Mixter and Osgood published the first paper describing surgical treatment for C1–C2 instability. They performed a fixation of the posterior arc of C1 and the spinous process of C2, using thick suture material. Since then other techniques have been developed: in 1939 the Gallie fixation and in 1978 the interlaminar clamp of Brooks and Jenkins, Margerl's trans-articular screw, Harms technique with C1–C2 screw and rod system, and the C2 translaminar technique. Despite simplicity of the Gallie and Brooks-Jenkins fixations, they require considerable bone graft and prolonged postoperative rigid immobilization with HaloVest; this could be uncomfortable specially for polytraumatized and elderly patients with rheumatoid arthritis (RA). When screws are used, only a collar is needed in the postoperative period. Other technique using a trans-articular screw has shown biomechanical superiority above other techniques, with fusion rates near to 100 % [3, 11, 15]. The risk of this procedure consists in potential damage of the vertebral artery that could be as high as 8.2 %, also an apparent higher technical difficulty due to the angulation of the screw [12]. In 1994 Goel described an original technique, used for him from 1988, to C1–C2 fixation, placing individual screws in C1 lateral mass and in C2 pars and fixed them with a plate each side, reducing the risk of vertebral artery injury. In this technique Goel used monocortical screws connected with a large plate [7]. He emphasizes the importance to denuding the articular cartilage and stuffing bone graft to provide a good stability. In addition, also, Goel recommended make section of the C2 ganglion to have a wide exposition of the joint region to perform a good construction and avoid vertebral arterial injury [8]. In 2001 Harms and Cols described a new technique for C1–C2 fixation, placing individual screws in C1 lateral mass and in C2 pedicles and fixed them with a rod on each side, reducing the risk of vertebral artery injury. This construct provides adequate biomechanical stability and is technically less demanding than the trans-articular screw fixation [9, 21].

In the original article the author emphasizes the fact that it is not necessary to place any kind of instrumentation on the posterior arc of C1, and allows intraoperative reduction and stabilization of the atlantoaxial complex. In the Harms series no implant failure or neurological deterioration was reported, no vertebral artery injuries or dural tears occurred, and it was reported solid fusion on radiological evaluation at 6 months [9].

Harms' original technique describes a subperiosteal dissection from the occiput to the subaxial cervical spine, which can lead to postoperative pain and, more important, disruption of the tension band due to the posterior ligaments of the cervical spine [9].

The use of a minimally invasive surgical (MIS) technique [14, 18] to perform posterior C1 C2 fixation, reducing muscle devascularization and denervation, would preserve the medial tension band. This means less intraoperative blood loss, less postoperative pain, and shorter hospital stay.

Surgical Anatomy

With the purpose to evaluate feasibility of a minimally invasive approach to the atlantoaxial joint (C1–C2), we studied the anatomical landmarks of the nuchal musculature at our microsurgical laboratory. After dissection of the posterior cervical muscles, it is necessary to remove the *trapezius* and *semispinalis capitis* muscles to expose the deep musculature. At this plane, 2 cm away from the midline, we found that following a point parallel to C2 spinous process, an anatomical corridor is found, formed by the angle between the posterior major *rectus capitis* and the inferior *obliquus capitis*. This corridor is relatively free of important nervous and vascular structures, but deep during the approach, a venous plexus is reached over the atlantoaxial joint with risk of bleeding (Fig. 1a). The third segment (V3) of the vertebral artery is found 3 cm away from the midline on its lateral trajectory to the

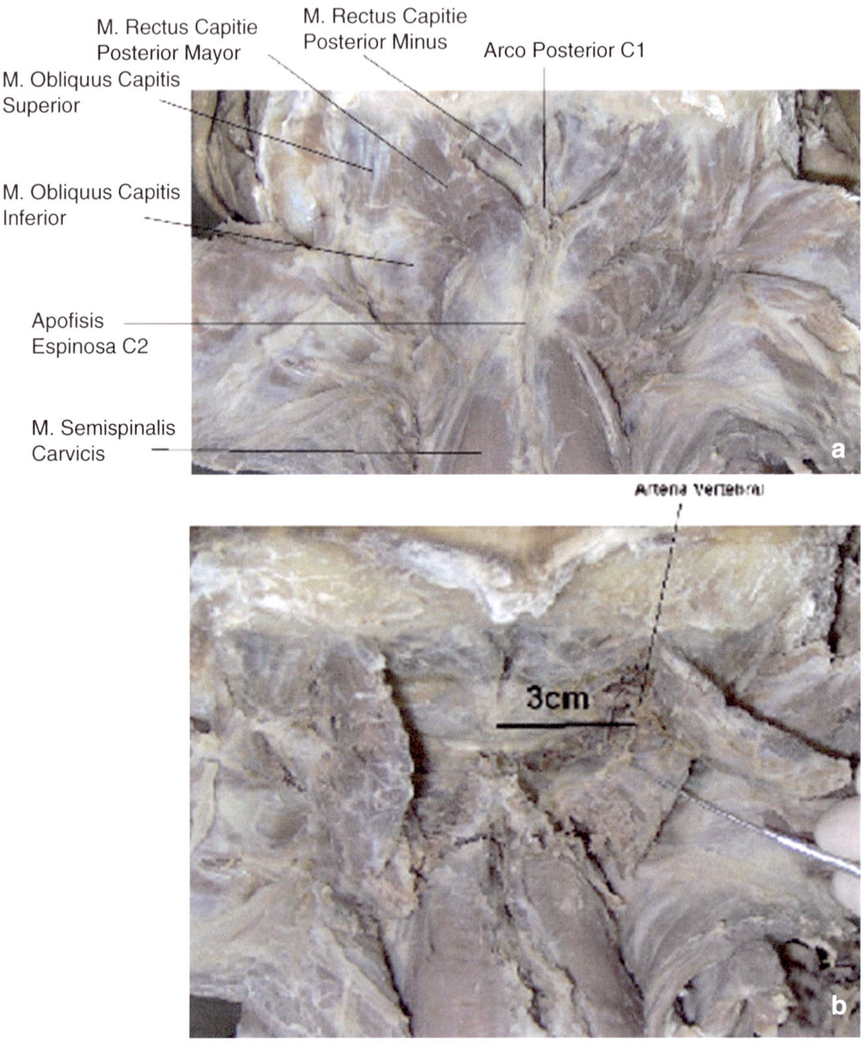

Fig. 1 (**a**) Muscle anatomy of the cranio-cervical junction, we removed trapecius and semiespinalis capitis muscles, you can see an anatomical corridor between rectus capitis posterior maior and obliquus capitis inferior muscles. (**b**) Vertebral artery makes its way approximately 3 cm away midline during vertebral trjectory

C1 posterior arc (Figs. 1b and 2), over which it turns posterior and medial; this is the point where the risk of vascular injury is possible when the C1 lateral-mass screws are inserted.

On the other hand, C1 lateral mass and C2 pedicles were measured, concluding that at least 3.5–4.0 mm diameter screws can be inserted, although this could vary

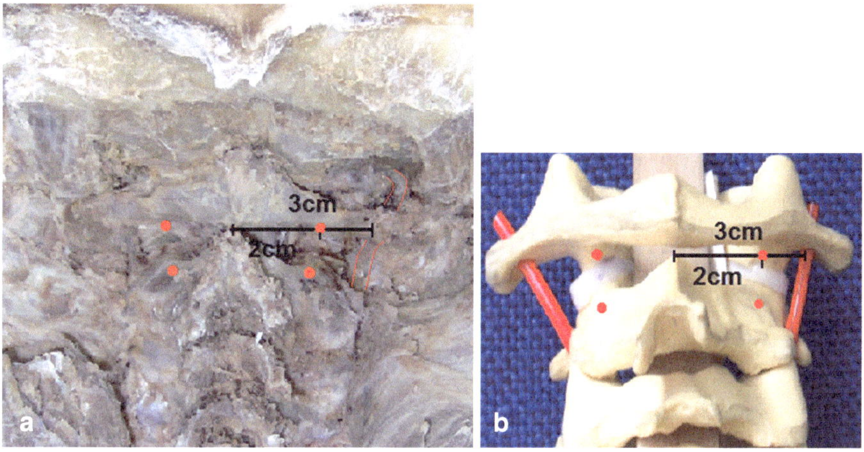

Fig. 2 (**a**) Anatomical entry points of the screws using Harms's technique (*red points*) (**b**) Representation in a cervical spine model of the screws entry points in *red*, you can see the trajectory of the vertebral artery, it is 1 cm approximately away of the screws

from patient to patient making necessary an exhaustive preoperative evaluation and planning, and fluoroscopic confirmation during surgery [9, 10, 20].

Surgical Technique

To preserve the occipitocervical tension band, decreasing morbidity of traditional procedures, and less postoperative pain, we performed a prospective nonrandomized study starting in May 2007 [2] using a minimally invasive trans-muscular approach through a 2.5 cm bilateral paramedian skin incision (Fig. 3a), using the access MIS platform MaXcess® (NuVasive Inc., San Diego, CA, USA) (Fig. 3b), and subsequently placing screws according to the modified Harms technique (Fig. 3c).

This approach uses a progressive tubular dilator system through the superficial nuchal musculature (*trapezius and semispinalis capitis*) and then through the anatomical corridor previously described between the posterior major *rectus capitis* and the inferior *obliquus capitis*. A three-valve spreader MaXcess® with optical fiber light is then placed, allowing good exposure and illumination of the working area (Fig. 3b). Under fluoroscopic guidance, the system is anchored on the access point of the C2 pedicle, trying to avoid obstaculization of the posterior arch of C1 during opening of the retractor. With monopolar cautery the bony surface of C2 is exposed, following it until the lateral border C1–C2 articulation is also visualized. At this point an epidural venous plexus usually bleeds, but it is effectively controlled with a combination of bipolar cautery and Gelfoam®. The C1–C2 bone joint surface is exposed and the C2 root identified and then coagulated and sacrificed to allow adequate insertion of the screw. At this point 3.5 mm diameter polyaxial

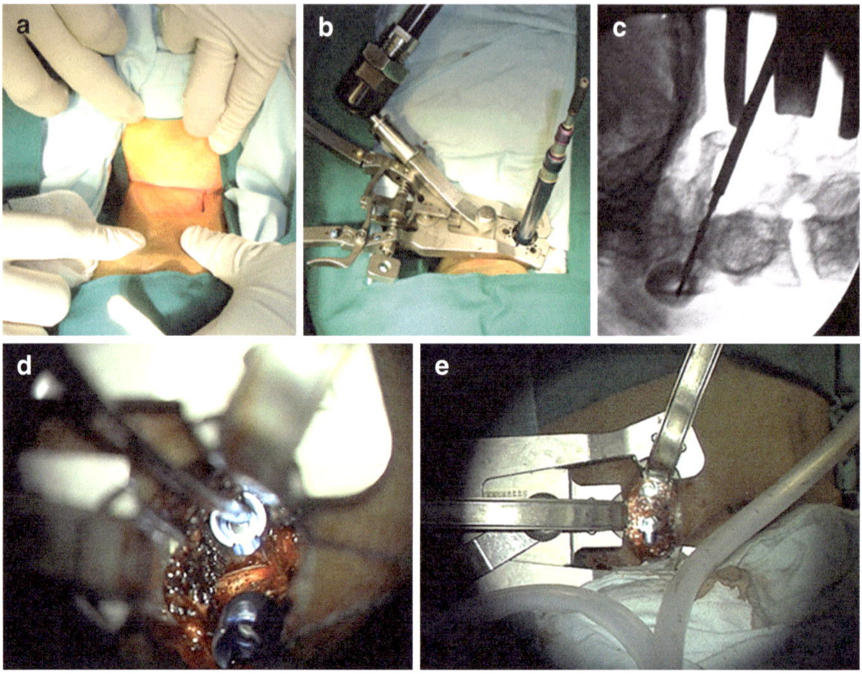

Fig. 3 (**a**) Paramedian posterior cervical incisión (25mm aprox.). (**b**) Intraoperative image of the minimally invasive retractor Maxcess II® (Nuvasive Inc., San Diego, CA, USA. (**c**) Intraoperative x-ray image through the retractor during preparation of C1 screw using the tap. (**d**) Intraoperative close-up image of the screws through the retractor. (**e**) Intraoperative parnoramical view during the procedure

screws are inserted using Harms technique (Fig. 3c, d). The articular surfaces of C1 and C2 are decorticated using micro-curettes and demineralized bone matrix (Grafton® DBM-Putty, Osteotech®, Inc. New Jersey, USA) mixed with bone marrow aspirates (BMA) is placed inside the joint to obtain second fusion (Fig. 3d, e). The same procedure is made in the contralateral side in the same way.

Clinical Experience

Until December 2011 a total of 16 patients were treated using this technique; mean age was 57.5 years old. Eight patients presented unstable C2 fracture and 8 patients atlantoaxial instability secondary to RA. Mean surgical time and blood loss was 193. 7 min and 403. 5 cc, respectively. Patients experienced minimal postoperative pain and were discharged before 46.8 h mean time; also there was no hardware failure.

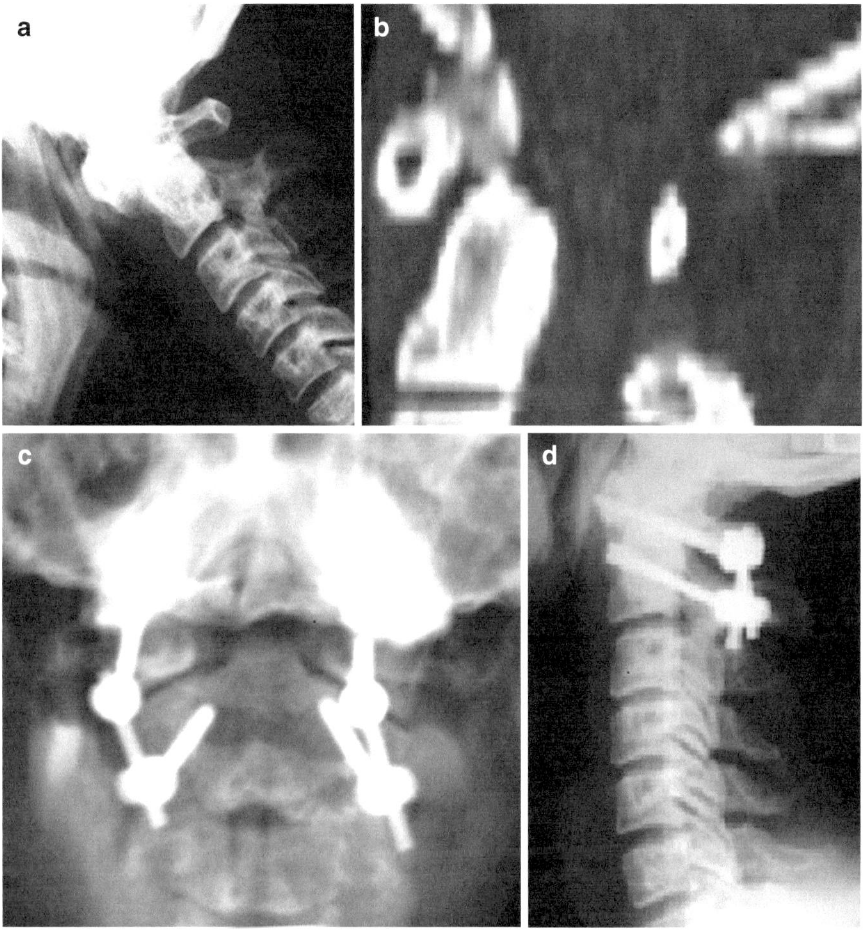

Fig. 4 Case 1. (**a**) Preoperative lateral x-ray film shows type II dens fracture. (**b**) CT scan image confirms dens fracture. (**c**) post-operative AP x-ray view shows C1-C2 construction. (**d**) Post-operative lateral x-ray view of the construction

Clinical Examples

Case 1

A 47-year-old male patient presented with posterior neck pain, occipital headache, and weakness on the left side of the body; 3 days previously the patient had fallen with cervical trauma in flexion.

Neurological exam showed pain on C2 dermatome bilaterally, 4/5 left hemiparesis without Babinski sign, and left patchy distribution hemihypoesthesia for superficial tact.

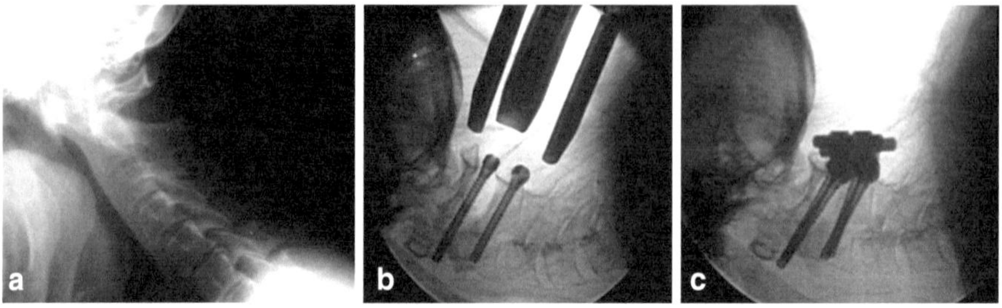

Fig. 5 Case 2. (**a**) Lateral x-ray image of the C1-C2 subluxation secondary to reumathoid arthitis. (**b**) Intraoperative lateral x-ray image shows C1-C2 screws implantation through the retractor. (**c**) Intraoperative lateral x-ray image of the final C1-C2 construction

Cervical x-ray films showed dens fracture type II with instability (Fig. 4a, b).

We performed a minimally invasive C1–C2 fusion procedure using polyaxial 3.5 mm diameter screws in both sides. No intraoperative complications occurred and blood loss was approximately 300 ml. Hospital stay was 43 h and the patient showed motor recovery in the early postoperative period (Fig. 4c, d). After 1 year of follow-up, the patient has neither pain nor weakness and instrumentation looks in good position.

Case 2

A 70-year-old female patient with 30 years history of rheumatoid arthritis, she had noticed a sensation of cervical instability and "cracking" during cervical motion, associated posterior neck pain irradiated to upper dorsal region, numbness, and weakness of the upper limbs.

On exam the patient had bilateral hyperreflexia, as well as Hoffman's sign bilaterally without motor deficit. Magnetic resonance imaging (MRI) scans showed *pannus odontoideum* with posterior lens luxation and compression over the spinal cord without T2 signal of myelopathy. Dynamic x-ray films revealed that the atlanto-odontoid interval reached more than 5 mm in length (Fig. 5a).

A minimally invasive C1–C2 fusion procedure was accomplished using polyaxial 3.5 mm diameter screws in both sides (Fig. 5b). No surgical complications occurred, blood loss was 250 ml, and hospital stay was 48 h. After 1 year of follow-up, the patient has less neck pain and x-ray films showed adequate reduction of C1–C2 instability (Fig. 5c).

Case 3

The patient is an 18-year-old male with history of neck pain. Approximately 3 months before presentation, he had fallen with craniocervical trauma. Neurological

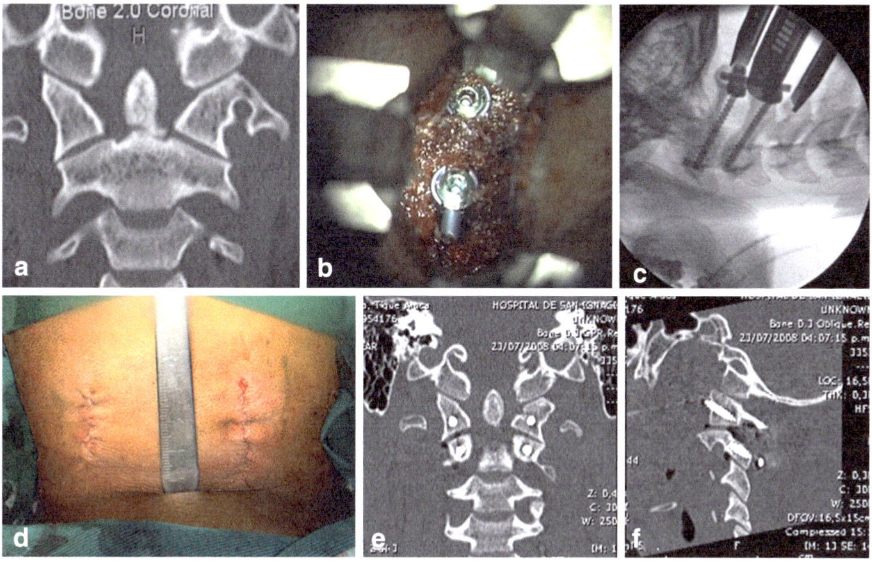

Fig. 6 Case 2. (**a**) Coronal CT scan image showing type II dens fracture. (**b**) Panoramical view through the retractor of the C1-C2 screws combines with bone substitute. (**c**) Lateral intraopertive x-ray image shows C1-C2 construction and retractor. (**d**) Postoperative skin incisions. (**e**, **f**) Coronal and sagital postoperative CT scan shows adequate trajectory of the screws

exam showed no motor or sensory deficit. X-ray films showed dens fracture type II with instability (Fig. 6a).

We performed a minimally invasive C1–C2 fusion procedure using polyaxial 3.5 mm diameter screws in both sides (Fig. 6b, c). He had no intraoperative complications and approximately 280 ml of surgical bleeding. Hospital stay was 36 h (Fig. 6). After last follow-up the patient has pain or weakness and instrumentation looks in good position (Fig. 6d–f).

Discussion

There is no doubt on the multiple potential advantages of a minimally invasive technique for the stabilization of the C1–C2 complex. First of all, the tension band provided by the nuchal musculature and ligaments is preserved, giving additional biomechanical stability to the construct. Second, the patient is not submitted to extensive and painful occipitocervical dissection making the postoperative recovery faster and less morbid [4–6, 10–13, 17, 19].

It is known that there are many surgical options to approach atlantoaxial instability and also that each has pros and cons that must be thoughtfully considered when choosing a specific procedure. On one hand we have the wiring techniques that are simple and less demanding but are associated with poor fusion rates (between 82 and 66 %) and higher risk of pseudoarthrosis (reaching 36.3 % in some series); besides, it requires prolonged postoperative immobilization. Screw fixation provides high fusion rates close to 100 %, lower risk of pseudoarthrosis, and shorter periods of postoperative immobilization, but they are technically more demanding and require the intraoperative utilization of fluoroscopy and the pre-op study of the anatomy, specially concerning the vertebral artery, to lower the risk of vascular injury [1, 3, 15, 16, 21].

Several studies compare different screw fixation techniques: trans-articular C1–C2, C1 lateral mass with C2 trans-pedicular screws, and C1 lateral mass with C2 translaminar screws. Evidence shows no significant differences on fusion rates or complications between one another. On the other hand, biomechanical studies have demonstrated superiority of the C1 lateral mass with C2 trans-pedicular screw technique compared with the C1 lateral mass with C2 translaminar technique when lateral bending and axial rotation were evaluated [1].

In our study, we chose Harms technique, because of the anatomy studies performed at our laboratory that showed a safe surgical access for the minimally invasive approach.

Conclusions

The minimally invasive trans-muscular C1–C2 fusion procedure is a feasible procedure.

Initial experience demonstrates that a MIS trans-muscular C1–C2 approach can be successfully used to fuse C1–C2 complex using C1 lateral-mass screw and C2 pedicular screw bilaterally.

Tension band provided by the nuchal musculature and ligaments is preserved, giving additional biomechanical stability to the construct.

Patient is not submitted to extensive and painful occipitocervical dissection making the postoperative recovery faster and less morbid.

Early clinical results are encouraging. However, only after long-term follow-up it will be confirmed these early favorable results.

Proposals for the Future

As our experience in minimally invasive techniques improves, we can offer our patients less morbid treatment options with similar or better results to those achieved with conventional procedures.

References

1. Claybrooks R, Kayanja M, Milks R, Benzel E (2007) Atlantoaxial fusion: a biomechanical analysis of two C1-C2 fusion techniques. Spine J 7:682–688. Menendez J, Wright N (2007) Techniques of posterior C1-C2 stabilization. Neurosurgery 60 (Suppl 1):103–111

2. Diaz R, Berbeo M, Vergara M, Villalobos L (2009) Minimally invasive posterior C1-C2 screw fixation through an anatomical corridor preserving occipital-cervical tension band. Prospective 21 months clinical and radiological study. Oral presentation, Spine Arthroplasty Society Global symposium on motion Preservation Technology (SAS 9). London
3. Farey I, Nadkarni S, Smith N (1999) Modified Gallie technique versus transarticular screw fixation in C1-C2 fusion. Clin Orthop Relat Res 359:126–135
4. Fessler R, O'Toole J, Eichholz K, Perez-Cruet M (2006) The development of minimally invasive spine surgery. Neurosurg Clin N Am 17:401–409
5. Gala VC, O'Toole JE, Voyadzis JM, Fessler RG (2007) Posterior minimally invasive approaches for the cervical spine. Orthop Clin N Am 38(3):339–349; abstract v
6. Gerszten PC, Welch WC (2006) Spine: minimally invasive techniques. Prog Neurol Surg 19: 135–151
7. Goel A, Laheri V (1994) Plate and screw fixation for atlanto-axial subluxation. Acta Neurochir (Wien) 129:47–53
8. Goel A, Desai KI, Muzumdar DP (2002) Atlanto axial fixation using plate and screw method: a report of 160 cases treated patients. Neurosurgery 51:1351–1357
9. Harms J, Melcher R (2001) Posterior C1-C2 fusion with polyaxial screw and rod fixation. Spine 26(22):2467–2471
10. Joseffer S, Post N, Cooper P, Fremong-Boadu A (2006) Minimally invasive atlantoaxial fixation with polyaxial screw-rod construct: technical case report. Neurosurgery 58(Suppl 2): ONS-375
11. Menendez J, Wright N (2007) Techniques of posterior C1-C2 stabilization. Neurosurgery 60(Suppl 1):103–111
12. Neo M, Sakamoto T, Fujibayashi S, Nakamura T (2005) A safe screw trajectory for atlanto-axial transarticular fixation achieved using an aiming device. Spine 30(9):236–242
13. O'Toole JE, Eichholz KM, Fessler RG (2006) Minimally invasive approaches to vertebral column and spinal cord tumors. Neurosurg Clin N Am 17(4):491–506
14. Powers C, Isaacs R (2006) Minimally invasive fusion and fixation techniques. Neurosurg Clin N Am 17:477–489
15. Reilly T, Sasso R, Hall P (2003) Atlantoaxial stabilization: clinical comparison of posterior cervical wiring technique with transarticular screw fixation. J Spinal Disord Tech 16(3):248–253
16. Shad A, Shariff S, Teddy P (2002) Craniocervical fusion for rheumatoid arthritis: comparison of sublaminar wires and the lateral mass screw craniocervical fusion. Br J Neurosurg 16(5): 483–486
17. Shchedrenok VV, Ivanenko AV, Sebelev KI, Moguchaia OV (2010) Minimally invasive surgery of degenerative diseases of the spine. Vestn Khir Im I I Grek 169(2):102–104
18. Wang M, Levi A (2006) Minimally invasive lateral mass screw fixation in the cervical spine: initial clinical experience with long-term follow-up. Neurosurgery 58:907–912
19. Winder MJ, Thomas KC (2011) Minimally invasive versus open approach for cervical laminoforaminotomy. Le Journal Canadien Des Sciences Neurologiques 38(2):262–267
20. Xiang-Yang M, Qing-Shui Y, Zeng-Hui W, Hong X, Jing-Fa L, Shi-Zhen Z (2005) Anatomic considerations for the pedicle screw placement in the first cervical vertebra. Spine 30(13): 1519–1523
21. Yoshida M, Neo M, Fujibayashi S, Nakamura T (2006) Comparison of the anatomical risk for vertebral artery injury associated with the C2-pedicle screw and atlantoaxial transarticular screw. Spine 31(15):513–517

Os Odontoideum Syndrome: Pathogenesis, Clinical Patterns and Indication for Surgical Strategies in Childhood

Massimiliano Visocchi and Concezio Di Rocco

Contents

M. Visocchi (✉) • C. Di Rocco
Department of Head Neck Diseases,
Institute of Neurosurgery, Catholic University of Rome ,
Largo Gemelli, 8, Rome 0068, Italy
e-mail: mvisocchi@hotmail.com

C. Di Rocco, N. Akalan (eds.), *Pediatric Craniovertebral Junction Diseases*,
Advances and Technical Standards in Neurosurgery 40,
DOI 10.1007/978-3-319-01065-6_9, © Springer International Publishing Switzerland 2014

Abstract Os odontoideum is a rare condition with a controversial pathogenesis and poorly understood natural history. Hypoplasia of the odontoid associated with an independent oval ossicle, with smooth margins widely separated from C2 and well above the superior facets of the axis, is termed "os odontoideum". The neurological manifestations arise from bulbospinal compression both at rest and during motion, due to the craniovertebral junction (CVJ) instability itself. Consequently, the surgical management of os odontoideum should aim at achieving both neural decompression and stabilization of the CVJ. The aims of this paper are to introduce the embryological steps involved in the CVJ development, to underline the updated theories propounded to interpret developmental and congenital disorders of the os odontoideum, to introduce the most updated surgical techniques and to discuss some exemplary cases selected from our personal experience.

Keywords Os odontoideum • Craniovertebral junction • Transoral • Transnasal • Transcervical endoscopic approach • Wiring/screwing instrumentation and fusion

Introduction

Hypoplasia of the odontoid associated with an independent oval ossicle, with smooth margins widely separated from C2 and well above the superior facets of the axis, is termed « os odontoideum ». Two principal theories have been propounded to explain the condition: congenital or acquired [13, 30, 34, 38]. Whichever the aetiology, the affected subjects may develop neurological symptoms and signs in case of a sagittal C2 shift higher than 4.5 mm as evaluated by dynamic x-ray examination. In such an evenience the craniovertebral junction (CVJ) is always unstable [73]. The neurological manifestations arise from bulbospinal compression both at rest and during motion, due to the CVJ instability itself. Consequently, the surgical management of os odontoideum should aim at achieving both neural decompression and stabilization of the CVJ [35–37, 39, 40]. In cases in which accurate preoperative x-ray examinations demonstrate the os odontoideum irreducibility and the associated neural compression, the surgical removal by anterior (i.e. transoral) route of such an ossicle is strongly suggested. On the other hand, when preoperative x-ray examinations demonstrate that the os odontoideum is reducible, neural decompression may be obtained by simply reducing the dislocation ("functional decompression") and by stabilizing the CVJ with a posterior instrumentation, either with wires, claws or screws [67]. The correct surgical treatment should maintain the anatomic alignment while preserving the motion of normal adjacent elements, in order to protect the neural elements [15, 20].

Wiring techniques have been used for instrumentation of the cervical spine widely. They are familiar to most spinal surgeons and the reported results indicate that these procedures are relatively safe in selected patients. A thorough knowledge of the embryological steps leading to the formation of the CVJ and an updated information of the most appropriate techniques required for the correction of its developmental disorders or acquired anomalies are mandatory for the surgical management. Such an expertise is usually acquired only in specialized centres dealing with an adequately high number of patients.

The aims of this chapter are to introduce the embryological steps involved in the CVJ development, to underline the updated theories propounded to interpret developmental and congenital disorders of the os odontoideum, to introduce the most updated surgical techniques and to discuss some exemplary cases selected from our personal experience.

Definition and Pathogenesis

Os odontoideum is defined as an independent ossicle, with smooth margins separated from the base of the odontoid or the axis vertebrae. Usually it does not have the normal shape or size of the dens, often being half the normal size and rounded or oval [13, 30, 31, 34, 38]. Since Giacomini's first description in 1886, the processes leading to the formation of the os odontoideum have remained controversial [18]. Supporters of the congenital aetiology considered the os odontoideum as a segmental anomaly resulting from fusion failure between the odontoid and the axis vertebrae case reports of members of families presenting with os odontoideum support this theory [1, 4, 8, 14, 29, 43, 58]. Indeed, recently, a three-generation family with this type of anomaly has been described [71]. On the other hand, proponents of the acquired aetiology consider the ossicle the result of an unrecognized fracture or cartilage injury of the odontoid. The acquired theory is also supported by numerous observations of previously normal odontoid in subjects developing the os odontoideum after a traumatic injury [72].

The Congenital Theory (see Table 1)

Embryologically, the occipital bone results from the fusion of four occipital sclerotomes, of which the proatlas is the most caudal. The atlas derives from the proatlas and C1 sclerotome. The axis is a complex structure deriving from four primary ossification centres and three sclerotomes: proatlas, C1 and C2. The proatlas, a vestigial bone formation that rarely persists as bony remnant, originates the tip of the dens. C1 gives the body of the dens and C2 the rest of the axis ligaments [9, 30, 34, 38]. The term proatlas stems from the field of comparative anatomy. It is considered to be a rudimentary or vestigial vertebral structure observed in some animals. It is located between the atlas and the occipital bone in animals such as some rodents, reptiles and dinosaurs [43]. The neural arch segment of the proatlas differentiates into two separate regions. The ventral portion creates the anterior margin of the foramen magnum, the occipital condyle and the midline third occipital condyle. The caudal portion gives rise to lateral atlantal masses and the superior portion of the posterior arch of the atlas. Finally, the lateral section of the proatlas condenses to

Sclerotomes	Divisions	Subdivisions	Formations
Occipital 1st			Basiocciput
2nd			
3rd			Exoccipital centers (Jugular tubercles)
4th "Proatlas"	Hypocentrum		Anterior tubercle clivus
	Centrum		Apical ligament Apex of dens
	Neural arch	Ventral Rostral	Occipital condyles,third cond. U-shape of foramen magnum Alar and cruciate ligaments
		Dorsal Caudal	Posterior arch of atlas (C1) Lateral atlantal masses
Spinal 1st	Hypocentrum persists		Atlas anterior arch
	Centrum		Dens
	Neural arch		Posterior inferior atlas arch
Spinal 2nd	Hypocentrum	Disappears	
	Centrum		Body of axis
	Neural arch		Facets, posterior arch of axis

Table 1 The embryological "cascade"

produce the cruciate and alar ligaments [30, 34, 38]. The apex of the odontoid process of the axis is derived from the proatlas.

Usually, proatlas-derived structures can be present in humans upon failure of regression of parts of the proatlas. The most relevant remnants of them are:

1. The Bergman's tubercle (small central ossicle) between the tip of the odontoid process and the foramen magnum. Such a finding in man may be analogous to the centrum of the proatlas in reptiles [43], the prebasilar (hypochordal) arch, third occipital condyle and basilar processes as a consequence of the incorporation of a persistent hypochordal bow in the anterior foramen magnum [26, 43]
2. The median occipital condyle, which is rarely found at the level of the foramen magnum, created by the proatlas
3. The bicoronate dens, due to failure of the two paramedian ossification centres to fuse in the midline. This structural feature appears as a vertical radiolucent line through the dens on AP open-mouth radiographs of the craniovertebral junction.

All these findings represent an interesting phenomena from the embryological point of view but usually have a little clinical significance. However, their knowledge is crucial for the neurosurgeons and radiologists in order to prevent potential misdiagnoses and mistreatments [1, 72].

Persistent Ossiculum Terminale and Os Odontoideum

The possible coexistence of ossiculum terminale and os odontoideum might also further support the congenital theory. The third ossification centre of the odontoid process, known as the ossiculum terminale, arises from the centrum of the proatlas. Usually, it appears by the age of 3 years and fuses by the age of 12 years [55]. A congenital anomaly originates when fusion does not occur, resulting in an *ossiculum terminale persistens*. This can be visualized as a small radiodense ossicle at the tip of the dens [1]. Fusion failure of the ossiculum terminale, also known as Bergman ossicle or « os avis », should not be confused with a type I fracture of the dens [31]. Patients with ossiculum terminale may be unaware of such anomaly since the C1–C2 junction remains stable because the transverse ligament C1–C2 complex is intact. Similar to ossiculum terminale persistens, os odontoideum has been considered as a consequence of a fusion failure between the sclerotomes proatlas and C1.

Sometimes, this anomaly consists in defects of segmentation in the midportion of the dens along with subaxial spine and skeletal anomalies. In ten children, reported in the literature, with os odontoideum, six had skeletal dysplasia, one had C5–C6 fusion and three had no other congenital anomalies [8]. Occasionally os odontoideum may fuse with the clivus. The anterior arch of C1 may be hypertrophic, whereas the posterior arch may be hypoplastic.

Os odontoideum can be isolated or can be also found in other congenital bone and connective anomalies as *spondyloepiphyseal dysplasia congenita, Conradi's disease, and metatropic dwarfism. It* can be associated to chromosomal anomaly as *Down's syndrome* and with metabolic disease as *Morquio's syndrome and other mucopolysaccharidoses* [53].

Spondyloepiphyseal Dysplasia Congenita

Spondyloepiphyseal dysplasia congenita (SED) is a rare form of skeletal systemic disease, characterized by congenital dwarfism with a short trunk and epiphyseal dysplasia in the long bones and vertebral bodies. Patients also frequently suffer from atlantoaxial instability due to os odontoideum. Compression of the spinal cord caused by atlantoaxial instability is a common and serious complication in SED patients, possibly resulting in sudden death [19].

Conradi's Disease

This uncommon condition is also known under a variety of names such as chondrodystrophia foetalis calcificans, stippled epiphyses, or congenital multiple epiphyseal dysplasia. Two main forms are now recognized: the classic, but uncommon, severe rhizomelic type due to an autosomal recessive gene and the more frequent Conradi-Hunermann variety due to an autosomal dominant gene or a mutant gene [53]. Conradi's disease is characterized by the presence of stippled epiphyses at birth in association with other connective tissue disturbances. The spine shows alterations in the form of the vertebral body anomalies often with blunting of its anterior part. The cartilaginous epiphyses show patchy mucoid degeneration and cystic spaces with irregular vascularization. There is scattered calcification with poor alignment of cartilage columns and absence of a zone of provisional calcification. Juxta-articular tissues show ectopic calcification. Atlantoaxial instability due to os odontoideum has been described.

Metatropic Dwarfism

This rare genetic disorder is characterized by an extremely small stature, short limbs and skeletal abnormalities with atlantoaxial instability due to os odontoideum. It is caused by a mutation in the TRPV4 gene, although in most cases the cause has not been elucidated [53].

Down's Syndrome

Down's syndrome (trisomy 21, rarely translocation from 13 to 15 groups to chromosome 21) is the most common chromosomal abnormality occurring in 1 out of 700 live births. Anomalous metabolism of mucopolysaccharides and deficient growth hormone lead to osseous abnormalities [45]. The ligamentous laxity contributes to a high incidence of C0–C1 instability and C1–C2 luxation. The former has been assumed to occur in 10 % and the latter in 15–25 % of patients with Down's syndrome [57]. C1–C2 luxation is « stable » in 44 % of cases whereas 60 % of these patients develop precipitous onset of cervical medullary compression. C1–C2 luxation is «unstable » in 50 % of cases, the average predental space being 8 mm in the neutral position [39]. About one-third of patients with Down's syndrome harbour os odontoideum; 22 % present C1-arch hypoplasia and bifid anterior or posterior arches [62].

A cautious attitude towards the surgical treatment of CVJ instability in patients with Down's syndrome is generally adopted because of a low incidence of associated neurological dysfunctions and a high surgical morbidity. Only subjects with an atlanto-dens interval exceeding 4.5 mm or with other evidence of CVJ instability are considered for operative stabilization [3]. Difficulties encountered in patients with Down's syndrome are widely referred to the immunocompromised state (impaired monocyte and neutrophil chemotaxis, decreased phagocytoses, qualitative deficiency of T lymphocytes) which may facilitate respiratory infections and postoperative complications. Rates of bone fusion may also be lower than in other patients probably for deficient collagen synthesis, which contribute to bone graft resorption [54]. Halo immobilization is instituted early and maintained until objective evidence of bony fusion, which may take as long as 6 months [50].

Morquio's Syndrome

Morquio's syndrome is a genetic mucopolysaccharidosis (type IV) resulting from the absence or the reduced activity of lysosomal hydrolase leading to a pathological collection of mucopolysaccharides in the ligamentous system and consequently hyperlaxity. Children with this syndrome suffer from problems of the lower spine and, more commonly, of the CVJ especially at C1–C2 level. Dysplastic-hypoplastic dens with a detached distal portion (os odontoideum) not always ossified is present in every case. The ring of the atlas tends to be narrowed and thickened [5]. Although C1–C2 instability is mild, severe spinal cord compression can occur because of both anterior extradural soft tissue thickening and invagination of the posterior arch of C1 into the foramen magnum due to condylar hypoplasia. The anterior extradural soft tissue formation is usually reactive ligamentous tissue with or without abnormal deposition of mucopolysaccharides [5]. Decompression remains the main part of the treatment because of the narrow canal and CVJ instability; removal of the posterior arch of C1, widening of the occipital foramen and occipitocervical fusion are required [46]. Interestingly, posterior CVJ fusion results in late disappearance of the soft tissue thickening and normalization of dens development [5].

According to Crockard, every Morquio patient should be investigated for spinal cord compression between 3 and 8 years of age. Treatment aims to prevent neurological damage or, at least, to arrest the progression of the already present neurological disability. Transoral decompression and posterior fusion can be combined in cases with significant anterior compression [5].

The Acquired Theory

The opponents to the congenital theory emphasize that the non-union between the dens and the body of C2 does not appear related to known ossification centres; consequently true os odontoideum due to a failure of development should be quite rare. Furthermore, such non-union may be found in patients having a normal dens before an actual diagnosis of os odontoideum [13]. According to Crockard, os odontoideum should be the product of excessive movement at the time of ossification of the cartilaginous dens [7]. Functionally, this anomaly resembles a C2 fracture at the base of the dens and may leave a weakened C1–C2 complex with a potential or real instability [62]. Thus, os odontoideum probably represents an old non-union fracture or injury to vascular supply of developing odontoid [47, 53].

To support the acquired theory, Verska and Anderson reported two identical twins, one with an os odontoideum after trauma and the other with a normal odontoid and no traumatic history [63]. In the literature, proponents of acquired aetiology also reported 11 patients who had radiographic documentation of a normal odontoid before developing an os odontoideum after a trauma. However, most of those cases of os odontoideum with a pre-traumatic normal radiograph were documented before CT was available. Obviously, only based on plain-film evaluation, the possibility of congenital anomalies cannot be totally excluded [12, 13, 16, 23, 47, 51, 73–75].

Several authors indicated disorders of blood supply as the cause of acquired os odontoideum. In such a direction, Sakaida et al. [49] suggested avascular necrosis after trauma while Hammerstein et al propounded a block of the blood supply to the proximal part of odontoid induced by a trauma as a pathogenetic factor accounting for osseous absorption, in conditions in which the ossiculum terminale continues to receive a normal blood supply, so growing into an os odontoideum [22].

In os odontoideum, hypertrophy of the C1 anterior arch frequently attracted the attention of the investigators. According to Holt et al, hypertrophy of the C1 anterior arch is always associated with os odontoideum and, consequently, it is a useful sign to distinguish os odontoideum from odontoid fracture [26]. In the literature, hypertrophy of the C1 anterior arch was related to an acquired atlantoaxial instability occurring prior to the skeletal maturity and causing the C1 anterior arch hypertrophy [59]. Other authors interpreted the hypertrophy of the C1 anterior arch as the consequence of blood supply preservation at that level after posttraumatic vascular blockage and ischemic necrosis in the watershed area [26, 49].

Clinical Patterns and Indications for Surgical Strategies

The stability of the atlantoaxial articulation depends fundamentally upon the integrity of the odontoid process and the ligaments [9]. Since the reserve space in the atlantoaxial articulation is relatively great in childhood, some patients may not complain of any neurological deficits even when atlantoaxial instability is present. However, if atlantal displacement exceeds the limit of reserve space, clinical symptoms will appear [44]. The neurological manifestations arise from bulbospinal compression both at rest and during motion, due to the CVJ instability itself. The impingement of bulbospinal junction due to os odontoideum may be responsible for myelopathic sensory motor and/or cardiorespiratory disturbances. Lower cranial nerve dysfunctions, bowel and bladder dysfunction, motor weakness up to para- or tetraparesis, hypo-anaesthesia, allodynia, hyperesthesia and hyperalgesia at upper and lower limbs have been described with variable onset (acute or chronic). Recently a sleep apnoea syndrome has been also described as a consequence of CVJ instability associated to os odontoideum [28].

Nevertheless, although there is insufficient evidence to support diagnostic standards/guidelines and treatment standards/guidelines, plain x-rays of the cervical spine (anterior-posterior, open-mouth odontoid and lateral) and plain dynamic lateral x-rays performed in flexion and extension are recommended. TC and/or MRI of the CVJ must be considered mandatory [73, 74].

To date the management of os odontoideum continues to be a subject of debate [4, 56, 75]. The surgical indication is based on the consideration that affected subjects may develop neurological symptoms and signs in case of a C2 shift higher than 4.5 mm, as evaluated by dynamic x-ray examination; indeed, in such a condition the CVJ is always unstable [73].

In the past three decades, increased understanding of spinal biomechanics, proliferation of sophisticated CVJ instrumentation devices, advances in bone fusion techniques, refinement of anterior approaches to the CVJ, and development of microsurgical and minimally invasive methods have made it possible to stabilize every segment of CVJ successfully, regardless of the offending pathology. Accordingly, use of spinal fusion and instrumentation has increased. The question facing the modern spine surgeon is not so much how to stabilize the spine but when to do so. Instability of the CVJ appears to be the key factor for the surgical indication.

Arvin et al recommended the patients with os odontoideum and neurological abnormality or radiological evidence of instability should be offered surgery although cervical arthrodesis in the paediatric age group has the potential for limiting growth potential and causing secondary deformity [4]. In such a condition the surgical management of os odontoideum aims to achieve neural decompression and to stabilize the CVJ [33, 36, 37].

On the other hand Fielding et al reported out of a series of 35 case series with CVJ abnormalities, eight patients without instability who had undergone conservative treatment without any neurological deterioration in a 3-year follow-up period [13].

Other authors underline that patients with os odontoideum, either with or without C1–C2 instability, are at risk for acute spinal cord injury after minor traumatic injury, although without symptoms nor neurological signs prior to the trauma. In order to prevent such an evenience, a preventing treatment fixation and fusion should be undertaken as prophylactic treatment in all cases of os odontoideum [42, 44, 45, 75]. Our personal practice fits with this philosophy.

Surgical Management: Basic Techniques for Posterior Approach

Several surgical options have been described for os odontoideum:

- Anterior resection of the os fragment
- Posterior atlantoaxial onlay fusion
- Posterior atlantoaxial wiring and fusion (Gallie, Brooks, Sonntag techniques)
- Posterior occipitocervical wiring and fusion
- Posterior Magerl screw fixation and fusion
- Harms technique of C1–C2 fusion

Anterior transoral decompression has been suggested in children with preoperative irreducible C1–C2 dislocation harbouring os odontoideum followed by posterior instrumentation and fusion (wiring or screwing); the latter can also be considered a "stand-alone" procedure in case of reducible C1–C2 dislocation. Whereas irreducible C1–C2 dislocation seems to be associated to a significant higher incidence of C1 assimilation and C2–C3 fusion, reducible C1–C2 dislocation appears more frequently associated to os odontoideum; consequently the posterior approach is more indicated in the management of such a pathological condition [50]. The wiring technique is an old-fashioned though effective procedure for paediatric patients [21]. On the other hand, screwing may be technically demanding in this type of population where operative precision and expertise when placing screws in the transarticular C1–C2 space are particularly required [7, 8, 48, 52]. Biomechanical experimental studies have demonstrated that the immediate stability is better achieved after screwing than after wiring [32, 67]. Differences in fusion rates such as 94 % after screwing and 80 % after wiring, which were reported in the past, do not appear to influence the overall final clinical results to determine the choice of the first or the second option. In other terms, as in nearly all the surgical pathologies, the operation should have rather been tailored on the single subject. According to the literature nearly all the procedures tend to reach almost a 100 % rate of fusion [35, 37, 39].

The less invasive C1–C2 wiring instrumentation and bone fusion technique is the Gallie technique which constitutes the oldest variant and incorporates wires or cables under the posterior C1 ring and around the C2 spinous process. An onlay autogenous corticocancellous iliac crest graft is held in place by the wire. In the Brooks technique the wire passes under the C2 lamina, as well as under the C1 ring, and a tricortical bone graft is wedged between the C1 ring and the C2 lamina, blocking extension [24, 25].

While sublaminar wire passage adds surgical risk, the Brooks fusion is more rigid than the Gallie fusion.

The Sonntag technique is somewhat of a blend of the Brooks and Gallie method: one bicortical autologous bone graft is used, the wire is passed sublaminar to C1 only and the bone graft is wedged between C1 and C2 (trapping it between the loops of wire). This technique may have less tendency to pull C1 posteriorly than Gallie and yet avoids the inherent danger of C2 sublaminar wires as in Brooks fusion [17].

The Magerl technique provides posterior C1–C2 screw fixation and is a reliable means of atlantoaxial joint immobilization. While this technique does confer the most rigid fixation, it is technically demanding. The Magerl technique requires a near-anatomic reduction and normal vertebral artery anatomy [61]. Harms technique of fixation to the lateral mass of C1 and the pars or pedicle of C2 has become the most prominent means of stabilization in the adult population [60]. This technique is not as vulnerable to anatomic variability in the course of the vertebral artery as the Magerl technique [71].

Sublaminar wires with different type of autologous bone grafts to treat CVJ instabilities are less incapacitating for children, since the short fixation does not interact with the local and global paediatric spine growing pattern. The inclusion of the occipital bone to perform an occipitocervical fusion in paediatric patients better accomplishes the lever effect by producing a dynamic force pattern with a *pulley-like* mechanism in irreducible C1–C2 dislocations. In other words C1 is attracted by C0 and C2 by including the occiput, and, in our opinion, such a procedure remains the most appropriate treatment when the CVJ instability depends from a progressive genetic-metabolic disease predisposing to possible postoperative cranial settling after C1–C2 fixation [10, 32, 33, 40]. Other studies demonstrate that children older than 4 years, harbouring CVJ instability, can be safely managed with posterior C1–C2 transarticular screw fixation with a high fusion rate [71]. However, whichever the technique utilized, the non-union can occur, also as a consequence of postoperative CSF fistula and wound infection, and it can heal, after the resolution of the infection, with a second bone graft [68].

It is worth to note, however, that the preoperative diagnosis of an irreducible C1–C2 dislocation might be shown to be incorrect intraoperatively during the surgical instrumentation. Indeed, the preoperative apparently "irreducible" C1–C2 dislocation may turn to be reducible under general anaesthesia; curarization, during the instrumentation procedure and anterior decompression, can be avoided [67, 68] (Fig. 1).

Case 1

In this 7-year-old female with Down's syndrome, complaining of neck pain without neurological dysfunction, preoperative dynamic x-ray study showed an irreducible CVJ dislocation more than 8 mm. In O.R., under general anaesthesia, curarization, intraoperative traction and immobilization with a Mayfield head holder, the CVJ dislocation could not be corrected. Nevertheless, it was managed successfully during the instrumentation procedure performed with a light extension of the head on the chest and a soft flexion of the head on the neck. The 5-year follow-up is excellent.

In this and in similar cases, we prefer not to perform the one-stage combined approach, limiting the surgical correction to a unique posterior approach, consequently avoiding the anterior decompression with its possible known complications in the paediatric population [69].

In general most of the authors agree that posterior stabilization in well-selected cases is followed by improvement or at least stabilization of the clinical picture in the great majority of the patients. However, preoperative respiratory deficits, associated to bulbocervical junction myelopathy, tend to have a worse prognosis, especially in children with Down's syndrome in which the recovery, when occurring, is usually very slow (Figs. 2 and 3).

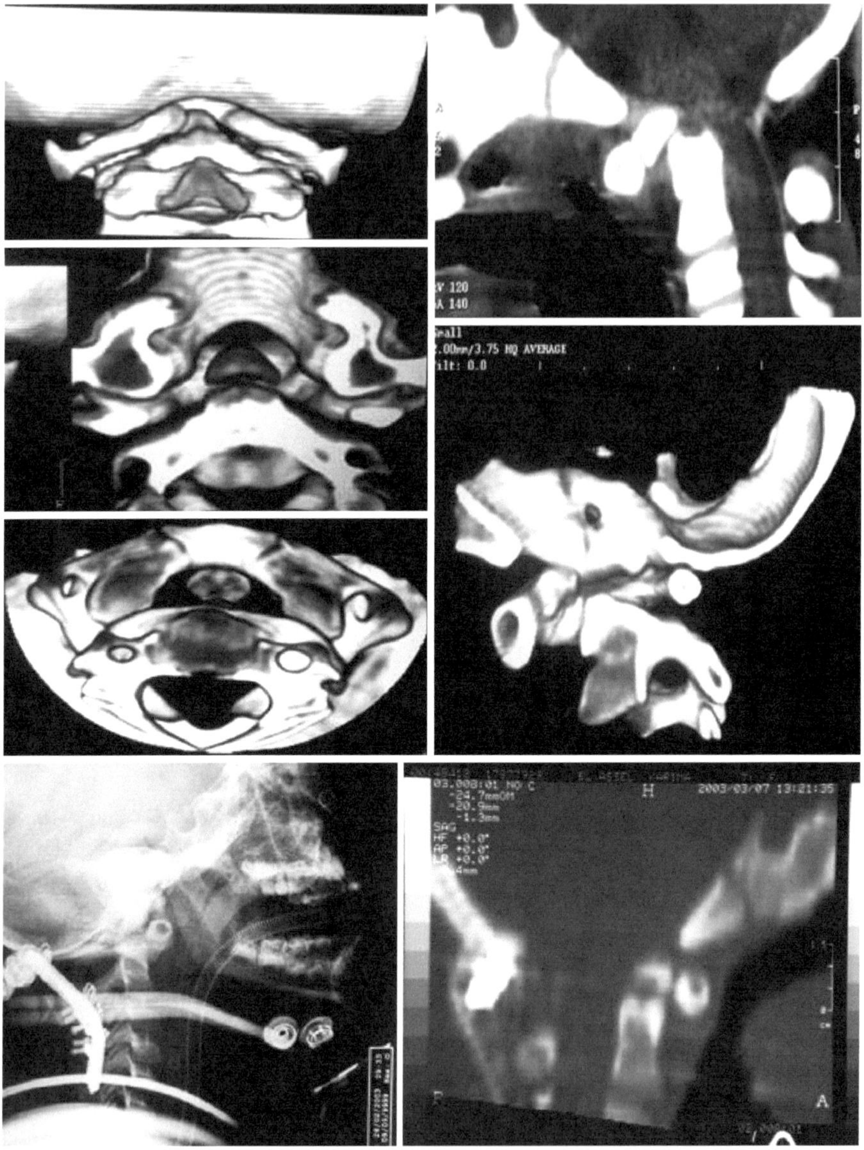

Fig. 1 *Upper* 3D Preoperative CT control showing os odontoideum, C1 bifidum posterior arch and C1–C2 dislocation. *Lower* X-rays and CT postoperative control after intraoperative instrumentation, fusion and reduction

Case 2

In this 8-year-old female complaining of neck pain and presenting with tetraparesis and respiratory dysfunction, preoperative dynamic x- ray study showed a reducible CVJ dislocation more than 6 mm. Soon after surgery the motor

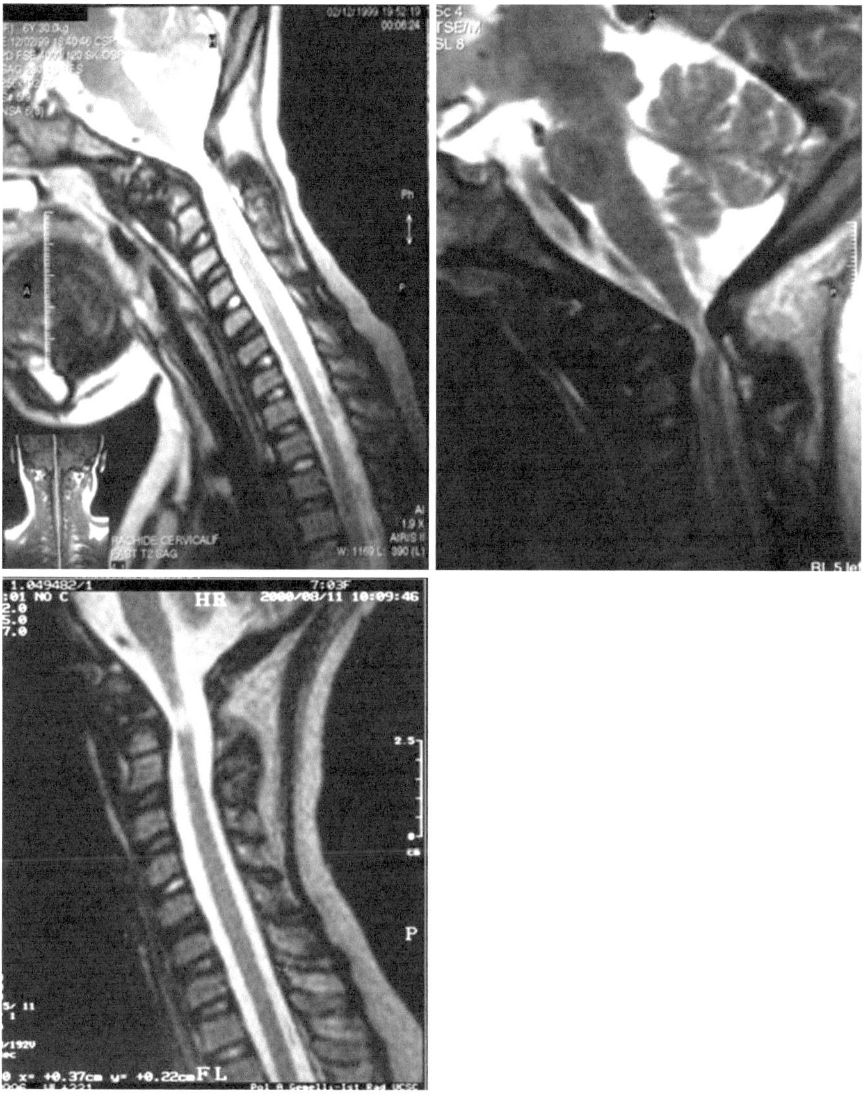

Fig. 2 Down's syndrome. Preoperative dynamic T2-weighted sagittal MR in a case of Down's syndrome with os odontoideum and bulbocervical junction myelopathy associated with respiratory syndrome. *Upper left*: flexion; *upper right*: at rest; *down*: extension

disturbances improved, whereas the respiratory dysfunction recovered completely only 6 months later on.

In most patients who had undergone instrumentation and fusion techniques, late control examinations will not detect postoperative deformity attributable to the surgical treatment.

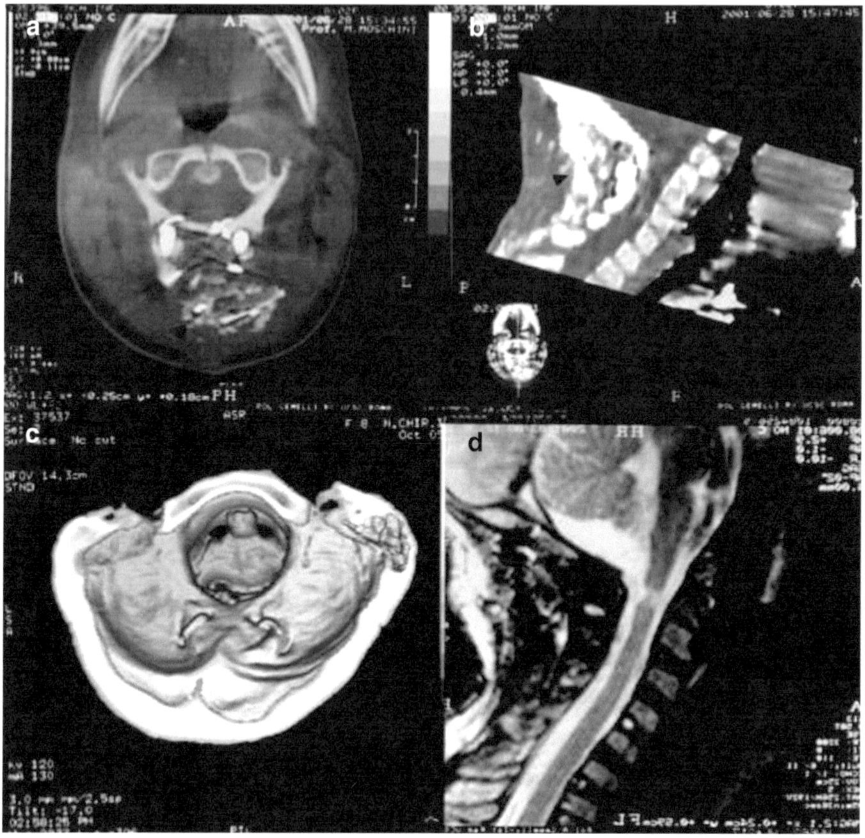

Fig. 3 Down's syndrome. Postoperative axial, sagittal and 3D CT reconstruction of CVJ showing. (**a–d**) The reduction of the os odontoideum. (**a**) The instrumentation with wires and bone fusion. (**d**) Showing the stable decompression of bulbocervical junction myelopathy (MR T2 w sagittal)

Notes on Anterior Surgical Strategies

Transoral-Transpalatopharyngeal Approach

The transoral-transpalatopharyngeal approach can be used for ventral decompression of irreducible os odontoideum [38]. This approach includes a vertical midline incision in the pharyngeal wall over the C1 tubercle followed by a soft palate incision. The soft palate incision is made from the posterior margin of the palatal bone to the superior margin of the uvula. With retraction the longus colli muscles and the longus capitis muscles are exposed and detached from the cervical vertebrae [22]. After the detachment of the muscles, the ventral aspect of the cervical vertebrae is exposed and the bony decompression can be carried out.

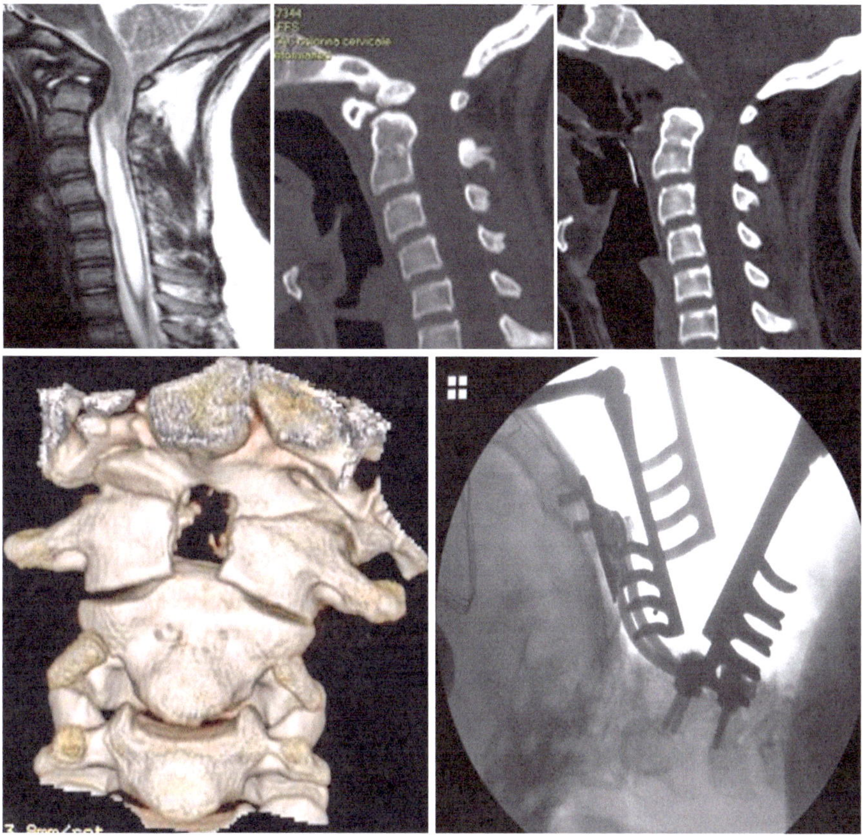

Fig. 4 *Upper right*: preoperative sagittal MR T2-weighted images showing Chiari I malformation and C3–C7 syringomyelia associated with odontoid dysplasia; (*centre*) TC scan (sagittal reconstruction) showing a median occipital condyle, located around and anteriorly to the foramen magnum. *Upper right*: postoperative CT scan (sagittal reconstruction) showing inferior clinoidectomy, median condiloidectomy and anterior C1 archectomy. *Down left*: sagittal postoperative CT showing the odontoid and clival decompression 3D postoperative CT scan. *Down right*: intraoperative lateral x-ray showing the double-staged occipitocervical instrumentation and fusion with median C0, C2 pars and C3 lateral mass screws

In most recent years the surgeon has benefited of endoscopic cameras, light sources and instruments (endoscopic-assisted transoral approach) which allow to perform the traditional approach with a minor traction. Endoscopic-assisted transoral approach is particularly indicated in cases where the traction of incisors cannot be higher than 2.5 cm (Figs. 4 and 5). In general the use of endoscopic tools not only improves the visualization of the oropharyngeal cavity but allows to extend the visualization of the operatory field in the craniocaudal and lateral directions due to the use of angled cameras. The increase in the visual fields allows to better spare the adjacent structures [59, 65, 66, 70].

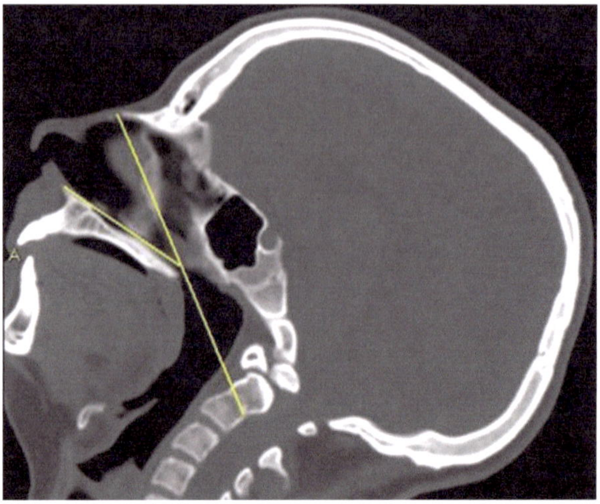

Fig. 5 The *nasopalatine line* is measured by connecting the most inferior point on the nasal bone to the most posterior point on the hard palate in the midsagittal plane

Case 3

This 16-year-old boy showed hypostaturalism and shorter intergluteal cleft. He complained of nystagmus, dysphonia, dysphagia, lower limb hypertonus, hyperreflexia, bilateral Babinski sign, ataxic walking and positive Romberg sign. Occipital condyle, created by the proatlas, is a rare dysmorphism mimicking an os odontoideum. Both microsurgical and endoscopic techniques were used to remove the malformed bone through a transoral approach. At the maximum follow-up (2 years) all symptoms recovered completely.

Endoscopic Transnasal Approach

The endoscopic transnasal approach has been introduced as a further option for the anterior approach mainly to limit the complication related to the transoral approach. The possibility to avoid the incision of the soft palate facilitates the early discharge of the patients because of the shorter period necessary for the surgical wound healing. The technique also avoids velopharyngeal incompetence [2, 6, 27, 41]. The transnasal approach allows accessing the ventral part of C1 and C2 vertebrae in patients who would need additional incisor retraction. The limit of this approach is the "nasopalatine line" (Fig. 5).

The preoperative assessment of this line is crucial when planning to use the endonasal or transoral approaches. The patient's head is placed in the neutral position, in regard to the CVJ, secured with headpins or resting on a horseshoe pad. An intraoperative navigation system is used to increase accuracy of the procedure. The approach is conducted under direct endoscopic visualization only. As the instruments are introduced, the middle turbinates are lateralized and an access hole is

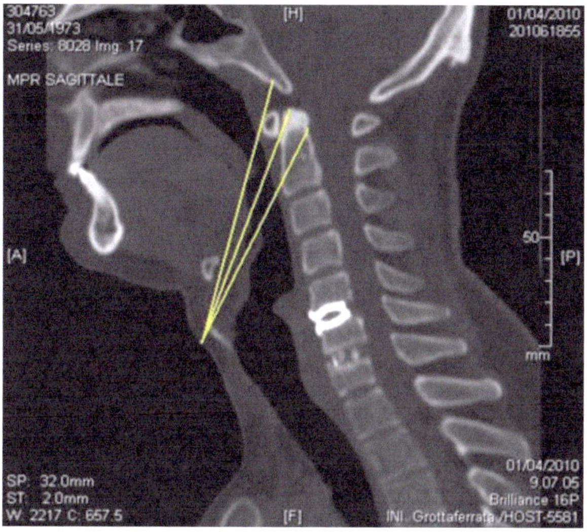

Fig. 6 Oblique laterocervical retropharyngeal surgical route for the transcervical approach (*yellow lines*)

made in the posterior portion of the nasal septum to allow for bilateral access to the nasopharynx. In order to enlarge the working area, the sphenoid sinus is opened. In the nasopharynx an incision of the mucosa is made and the skin is reflected caudally as a flap. With this incision and reflection, the inferior clivus, the ventral arch of the C1 vertebrae and the odontoid are visualized for a bony decompression to be carried out [11, 59, 64, 70].

High Anterior Cervical Retropharyngeal Approach

The high anterior cervical retropharyngeal is an alternative approach to gain access to the ventral aspect of the craniovertebral junction. This approach allows for ventral decompression with anterior cervical fixation/fusion without subsequent posterior fixation. Moreover, this approach avoids the complications that are associated with an oral approach in which the mucosa is disrupted [11, 59] (Fig. 6).

The patient is placed in a supine position with the head extended and rotated to the contralateral side. An incision is made approximately 4 cm inferior and parallel to the mandible in order to avoid injury to the mandibular nerve. This incision exposes the platysma muscle which is divided in order to expose the submandibular gland that is dissected and retracted to gain access to the bellies of the digastric muscles and the facial artery. The digastric muscles are detached and retracted to reveal the hypoglossal nerve which is also retracted exposing the pharyngeal muscles. The pharyngeal muscles are then dissected and retracted medially to expose the anterior portion of the C1 and C2 vertebrae [59].

Conclusions

Os odontoideum is a rare condition with a controversial pathogenesis and poorly understood natural history. As a result, it is difficult for clinicians to decide which patients require surgical fusion to prevent symptomatic progression and potentially devastating neurological injury. The existing literature regarding both asymptomatic and symptomatic os odontoideum and its treatment is very limited, consequently preventing any reliable definitive conclusion. In contrast, the neurosurgeon is offered several techniques and variants to treat the malformation when the surgical indication is established on the basis of the clinical findings and the neuroradiological investigations. All these techniques have indications, advantages/disadvantages, side effects and putative complications:

Transoral-Transpalatopharyngeal Approach

Virtually no surgical limitations do exist for endoscopically assisted transoral approach, compared with the pure endonasal and transcervical approaches.

Endoscopic Transnasal Approach

Pros: *partial isolation of the oral cavity, no need of tracheostomy and reduced need of feeding tube.*

Cons: *oblique approach, only piecemeal removal of CVJ pathology is allowed, not recommended for low-sited os odontoideum.*

High Anterior Cervical Retropharyngeal Approach

Pros: complete isolation of the oral cavity, no need of tracheostomy and feeding tube.

Cons: ob*lique approach, only piecemeal removal of CVJ pathology is allowed, not recommended for obese, barrel-chested and severely kyphotic children.*

CVJ instrumentation and fusion, as a consequence of previous anterior decompression or as "stand-alone" procedure, has the potential for limiting growth and causing secondary deformity in the paediatric age group. Nevertheless, recent advances in image analysis have enabled preoperative planning which is critical to evaluate the size of instrumentation and its relation to the patient's anatomy.

References

1. Al Kaissi A, Chehida FB, Ghachem MB, Grill F, Klaushofer K (2009) Atlanto-axial segmentation defects and os odontoideum in two male siblings with opsismodysplasia. Skeletal Radiol 38:293–296
2. Alfieri A, Jho HD, Tschabitscher M (2002) Endoscopic endonasal approach to the ventral cranio -cervical junction: anatomical study. Acta Neurochir (Wien) 144:219–225
3. American Academy of paediatrics, Committee on Sports Medicine (1984) Atlanto-axial instability in Down syndrome. Paediatrics 74:152–154

4. Arvin B, Fournier-Gosselin MP, Fehlings MG (2010) Os odontoideum: etiology and surgical management. Neurosurgery 66:22–31
5. Ashraf J, Crokard HA, Ransford AO (1991) Transoral decompression and posterior stabilization in Morquio's disease. Arch Dis Child 66:1318–1321
6. Cavallo LM, Messina A, Cappabianca P, Esposito F, de Divitiis E, Gardner P, Tschabitscher M (2005) Endoscopic endonasal surgery of the midline skull base: anatomical study and clinical considerations. Neurosurg Focus 19(1):E2
7. Crockard HA, Stevens JM (1995) Craniovertebral junction anomalies in inherited disorders: part of the syndrome or caused by the disorders? Eur J Pediatr 154(7):504–512
8. Currarino G (2002) Segmentation defect in the midodontoid process and its possible relationship to the congenital type of os odontoideum. Pediatr Radiol 32:34–40
9. Dai L, Yuan W, Ni B, Jia L (2000) Os odontoideum: etiology, diagnosis, and management. Surg Neurol 53:106–108; discussion 108–109
10. Diaz JH, Belani KG (1993) Perioperative management of children with mucopolysaccharidoses. Anesth Analg 77:1261–1270
11. Fielding JW (1978) Acquired os odontoideum. A case report. Clin Orthop Relat Res 135:71–73
12. Fielding JW, Griffin PP (1974) Os odontoideum: an acquired lesion. J Bone Joint Surg Am 56:187–190
13. Fielding JW, Hensinger RN, Hawkins RJ (1980) Os odontoideum. J Bone Joint Surg Am 62:376–383
14. Flemming C, Hodson CJ (1955) Os odontoideum; a congenital abnormality of the axis; case report. J Bone Joint Surg Br 37:622–623
15. Frankel HC, Hancock DO, Hyslop G (1969) The value of postural reduction in the initial management of closed injures of the spine with paraplegia and tetraplegia. Paraplegia 7:179–1932
16. Freiberger RH, Wilson PD Jr, Nicholas JA (1965) Acquired absence of the odontoid process: a case report. J Bone Joint Surg Am 47:1231–1236
17. Garfin SR, Balderston RA et al (eds) (1999) The spine. Lippincott-Raven, pp 242–243. Hensinger RN (1986) Osseous anomalies of the craniovertebral junction. Spine 11(4):323–333
18. Giacomini C (1886) Sull' esistenza dell' 'os odontoideum' nell' uomo. Gior Accad Med Torino 49:24–28
19. Gembun Y, Nakayama Y, Shirai Y, Miyamoto M, Sawaizumi T, Kitamura S (2001) A case report of spondyloepiphyseal dysplasia congenita. J Nippon Med Sch 68(2):186–189
20. Gluf WM, Brockmeyer DL (2005) Atlantoaxial transarticular screw fixation: a review of surgical indications, fusion rate, complications and lessons learned in 67 paediatric patients. J Neurosurg Spine 2:164–169
21. Grob D, Dvorak J, Panjabi MM, Antinnes JA (1994) The role of plate and screw fixation in occipitocervical fusion in rheumatoid arthritis. Spine 15:2545–2551
22. Hammerstein J, Russo S, Easton K (2007) Atlantoaxial dislocation in a child secondary to a displaced chondrum terminale. A case report. J Bone Joint Surg Am 89:413–417
23. Hawkins RJ, Fielding JW, Thompson WJ (1976) Os odontoideum: congenital or acquired. A case report. J Bone Joint Surg Am 58:413–414
24. Hensinger RN (1999) Congenital anomalies of the cervical spine. In: Herkowitz HN, Garfin SR, Balderston RA (eds) The spine. Lippincott-Raven, Philadelphia, pp 242–243
25. Hensinger RN (1986) Osseous anomalies of the craniovertebral junction. Spine 11(4):323–333
26. Holt RG, Helms CA, Munk PL, Gillespy T 3rd (1989) Hypertrophy of C-1 anterior arch: useful sign to distinguish os odontoideum from acute dens fracture. Radiology 173:207–209
27. Kassam AB, Snyderman C, Gardner P, Carrau R, Spiro R (2005) The expanded endonasal approach: a fully endoscopic transnasal approach and resection of the odontoid process: technical case report. Neurosurgery 57(1 Suppl):213; discussion E213
28. Kawaguchi Y, Iida M, Seki S, Nakano M, Yasuda T, Asanuma Y, Kimura T (2011) Os odontoideum with cervical mylopathy due to posterior subluxation of C1 presenting sleep apnea 16(3):329–333

29. Kirlew KA, Hathout GM, Reiter SD, Gold RH (1993) Os odontoideum in identical twins: perspectives on etiology. Skeletal Radiol 22:525–527
30. Klimo P Jr, Kan P, Rao G, Apfelbaum R, Brockmeyer D (2008) Os odontoideum: presentation, diagnosis, and treatment in a series of 78 patients. J Neurosurg Spine 9:332–342
31. Lipson SJ (1977) Fractures of the atlas associated with fractures of the odontoid process and transverse ligamentum ruptures. J Bone Joint Surg Am 59:940–943
32. Magerl F, Seman PS (1987) Stable posterior fusion of the atlas and axis by transarticular screw fixation. In: Kehr P (ed) Cervical spine. Springer, New York, pp 322–327
33. Marcotte P, Dickman CA, Sonntag VHK (1993) Posterior atlantoaxial facet screw fixation. J Neurosurg 79:234–237
34. Matsui H, Imada K, Tsuji H (1997) Radiographic classification of os odontoideum and its clinical significance. Spine 22:1706–1709
35. Menezes AH (1994) Occipito-cervical fusion: indications, technique and avoidance of complications. In: Hitchon PW (ed) Techniques of spinal fusion and stabilisation. Thieme, New York, pp 82–91
36. Menezes AH (1996) Posterior occipital C1 – C2 fusion. In: Principles of spinal surgery. Mc Graw Hill, New York, pp 1051–1065
37. Menezes AH (1996) Rheumatological disorders. In: Principles of spinal surgery. Mc Graw Hill, New York, pp 705–722
38. Menezes AH (1999) Pathogenesis, dynamics, and management of os odontoideum. Neurosurg Focus 6:e2.1065
39. Menezes AH, Van Gilder JC, Cr C (1985) Odontoid upward migration in rheumatoid arthritis: an analysis of 45 patients with cranial settling. J Neurosurg 63:500–509
40. Menezes AH, Ryken TC (1992) Craniovertebral abnormalities in Down's syndrome. Pediatr Neurosurg 18(1):24–33
41. Messina A, Bruno MC, Decq P, Coste A, Cavallo LM, de Divittis E, Cappabianca P, Tschabitscher M (2007) Pure endoscopic endonasal odontoidectomy: anatomical study. Neurosurg Rev 30:189–194
42. Michejda M, Menolascino F (1975) Skull base abnormalities in Down's syndrome. Ment Retard 13(1):24–2
43. Morgan MK, Onofrio BM, Bender CE (1989) Familial os odontoideum. Case report. J Neurosurg 70:636–639
44. No authors listed (2002) Os odontoideum. Neurosurgery 50(3 Suppl):148–155
45. Oda I, Abumi K, Sell LC, Haggerty CJ, Cunningham BW, Mc Afee PC (1999) Biomechanical evaluation of five different occipito-atlanto-axial fixation technique. Spine 24:2377–2382
46. Pouliquen JC, Pennecot GF, Beneux J, Chadoutaud F, Lacert P, Duval – Beaupere G, Durand J (1982) Craniovertebral junction and Morquio disease. A propos of 6 cases. Chir Pediatr 23(4):247–255
47. Ricciardi LE, Kaufer H, Louis DS (1976) Acquired os odontoideum following acute ligament injury. J Bone Joint Surg Am 58:410–412
48. Ryken TC, Menezes AH (1995) Abnormalities of the craniovertebral junction in Down's syndrome. In: Principles of spinal surgery. Mc Graw Hill, New York, pp 395–409
49. Sakaida H, Waga S, Kojima T, Kubo Y, Niwa S, Matsubara T (2001) Os odontoideum associated with hypertrophic ossiculum terminale. Case report. J Neurosurg 94:140–144
50. Salunke P, Behari S, Kirankmar MV, Sharma MS, Jaiswal AK, Jain VK (2006) Paediatric congenital atlantoaxial dislocation: differences between the irreducible and reducible varieties. J Neurosurg 104(2 Suppl):115–122
51. Schuler TC, Kurz L, Thompson DE, Zemenick G, Hensinger RN, Herkowitz HN (1991) Natural history of os odontoideum. J Pediatr Orthop 11:222–225
52. Segal LE, Drummond DS, Zanotti RM (1991) Complications of posterior arthrodesis of the cervical spine in patients who have Down syndrome. J Bone Joint Surg Am 73:1547–1554
53. Sherk H, Nicholson J, Chung S (1978) Fractures of the odontoid process in young children. J Bone Joint Surg Am 60:921–924

54. Sherman L (1994) The craniovertebral junction in Rao KCVG. In: MRI and CT of the spine. Williams & Wilkins, Baltimore, pp 71–97
55. Smoker WR (1994) Craniovertebral junction : normal anatomy, craniometry and congenital anomalies. Radiographics 14(2):255–277
56. Spierings EL, Braakman R (1982) The management of os odontoideum. Analysis of 37 cases. J Bone Joint Surg Br 64:422–428
57. Stevens JM, Kendall BE, Crokard HA, Ransford A (1991) The odontoid process in Morquio – Brailsford's disease. The effects of occipitocervical fusion. J Bone Joint Surg (Br) 73:851–858
58. Stevens CA, Pearce RG, Burton EM (2009) Familial odontoid hypoplasia. Am J Med Genet A 149:1290–1292
59. Stevens JM, Chong WK, Barber C, Kendall BE, Crockard HA (1994) A new appraisal of abnormalities of the odontoid process associated with atlanto-axial subluxation and neurological. Fielding JW (1978) Acquired os odontoideum. A case report. Clin Orthop Relat
60. Stulík J, Vyskocil T, Sebesta P, Kryl J (2005) Harms technique of C1-C2 fixation with polyaxial screws and rods. Acta Chir Orthop Traumatol Cech 72(1):22–27
61. Takakuwa T, Hiroi S, Hasegawa H (1994) Os odontoideum with vertebral artery occlusion. Spine 19(4):460–462
62. Tippets RH, Alvis MA (1996) Treatment of axis fractures. In: Menezes AH, Sonntag VHK (eds) Principles of spinal surgery. Mc Graw Hill, New York, pp 871–883
63. Verska JM, Anderson PA (1997) Os odontoideum. A case report of one identical twin. Spine (Phila Pa 1976) 22:706–709
64. Visocchi M (2011) Advances in videoassisted anterior surgical approach to the craniovertebral junction. Adv Tech Stand Neurosurg 37:97–110
65. Visocchi M, Della Pepa GM, Doglietto F, Esposito G, La Rocca G, Massimi L (2011) Video-assisted microsurgical transoral approach to the craniovertebral junction: personal experience in childhood. Childs Nerv Syst 27(5):825–831
66. Visocchi M, Doglietto F, Della Pepa GM, Esposito G, La Rocca G, Di Rocco C, Maira G, Fernandez E (2011) Endoscope-assisted microsurgical transoral approach to the anterior craniovertebral junction compressive pathologies. Eur Spine J 1518–152
67. Visocchi M, Di Rocco F, Meglio M (2003) Craniocervical junction instability: instrumentation and fusion with titanium rods and sublaminar wires. Effectiveness and failures in personal experience. Acta Neurochir (Wien) 145:265–272
68. Visocchi M, Fernandez EM, Ciampini A, Di Rocco C (2009) Reducible and irreducible os odontoideum treated with posterior wiring, instrumentation and fusion. Past or present? Acta Neurochir (Wien) 151(10):1265–1274
69. Visocchi M, Pietrini D, Tufo T, Fernandez E, Di Rocco C (2009) Preoperative irreducible C1–C2 dislocations: intraoperative reduction and posterior fixation. The always posterior strategy. Acta Neurochir 151(5):551–559
70. Visocchi M (2010) The craniovertebral junction: posterior and anterior approaches. State of art. Crit Rev Neurosurg WFNS 1:1–11
71. Wang J, Vokshoor A, Kim S, Elton S, Kosnik E, Bartkowski H (1999) Pediatric atlantoaxial instability: management with screw fixation. Pediatr Neurosurg 30(2):70–78
72. Wang S, Wang C (2011) Familial dystopic os odontoideum: case report. J Bone Joint Surg Am 93(9):e44
73. Wang S, Wang G (2012) Acquired os odontoideum. A case report and review of the literature. Childs Nerv Syst 28(2):315–319
74. White AA, Panjabi M (1990) Kinematics of the spine. In: White AA (ed) Clinical biomechanics of the spine. JB Lippincott, Philadelphia, pp 85–126
75. Zhang Z, Zhou Y, Wang J, Chu T, Li C, Ren X, Wang W (2010) Acute traumatic cervical cord injury in patients with os odontoideum. J Clin Neurosci 17(10):1289–1293

Craniovertebral Junction Anomalies in Achondroplastic Children

Vincent Reina, Genevieve Baujat, Brigitte Fauroux, Vincent Couloigner, Elise Boulanger, Christian Sainte-Rose, Philippe Maroteaux, Martine Le Merrer, Valérie Cormier-Daire, Laurence Legai-Mallet, Michel Zerah, and Federico Di Rocco

Contents

V. Reina, MD • E. Boulanger, MD • C. Sainte-Rose, MD • M. Zerah, MD, PhD
F. Di Rocco, MD, PhD (✉)
Pediatric Neurosurgical Departement, Hôpital Necker-Enfants Malades, APHP, 149, Rue de Sèvres, Paris 75743, France

G. Baujat, MD, PhD • P. Maroteaux, MD • M. Le Merrer, MD, PhD
V. Cormier-Daire, MD, PhD • L. Legai-Mallet, PhD
Genetic Department, National Reference Centre for Congenital Bone Diseases, Hôpital Necker-Enfants Malades, INSERM U781, Paris, France

B. Fauroux, MD
Otorhinolaryngology Department, Hôpital Necker-Enfants Malades, Paris, France

Unité de ventilation non-invasive et du sommeil de l'enfant, INSERM U 955, Hôpital Necker-Enfants Malades, Paris, France

V. Couloigner, MD, PhD
Otorhinolaryngology Department, Hôpital Necker-Enfants Malades, Paris, France

C. Di Rocco, N. Akalan (eds.), *Pediatric Craniovertebral Junction Diseases*, Advances and Technical Standards in Neurosurgery 40,
DOI 10.1007/978-3-319-01065-6_10,

Abstract The natural history of CVJ stenosis in achondroplastic children is only partially known. Achondroplastic children have a foramen magnum that is significatively smaller at birth, and it does not follow the normal growth during the first 18 months of life, leading to CVJ stenosis and, for the most severe of them, to neurological and developmental impairment and delay and even sudden death due to cervicomedullary narrowing. We reviewed our experience based on 37 patients operated for cervicomedullary decompression between 1970 and 2010 and performed a literature review. The indication for surgery should be taken on very strict clinical and radiological parameters as well as sleep studies. Under those criteria, surgical decompression of CVJ leads to neurological and developmental improvement, despite non-negligible mortality and morbidity.

Keywords Achondroplasia • Cranio-cervical junction • Sudden death • Foramen magnum decompression

Introduction

Achondroplasia is the most common form of short-limb dwarfism. Its prevalence is estimated at 1/15,000 newborns per year. This condition is caused by a mutation in FGFR3 gene. In more than 99 % of the cases, the same amino acid substitution (G380R) is found, resulting in a constitutive activation of the receptor independent from its ligands [33, 38, 40]. FGFR3 plays a key role in the ossification processes, and its alteration has multiple effects in craniofacial and vertebral development especially at the level of the craniovertebral junction (CVJ) [7, 12].

Normal Bone Growth and Embryology of CVJ [22]

The normal growth of CVJ begins around the end of the fourth week of development, when 42 somites originate from the mesenchyma under notochord's mediation and regulation. Among those somites that will give rise to the spine, the 4 occipital somites and the first 2 cervical somites will take part in the formation of the CVJ [20, 21].

At the spinal level, each somite will divide in three parts: a dorsal dermatome, a cranial myotome and a sclerotome. The sclerotome surrounds the notochord, which is central and remains the element that regulates the whole process, then appears a central cleft in each sclerotome (called "Ebner's cleft") dividing each sclerotome into 2 halves, 1 superior and 1 inferior. The gap between the 2 halves will be invaded by cells that will give the intervertebral disc. Progressively, the superior half of one sclerotome will merge with the inferior half of the sclerotome that is just above, leading to the formation of the spine.

At the level of the CVJ, the process is quite different. The first three occipital sclerotomes will not divide. The first two occipital sclerotomes will give the basi-occiput. The third one will form the jugular tubercles.

Table 1 Summary of the four occipital and first two cervical sclerotomes segmentation and evolution

Sclerotome	Division	Subdivision	Formation
1st occipital	No	No	Basi-occiput
2nd occipital	No	No	Basi-occiput
3rd occipital	No	No	Jugular tubercles
4th occipital	Hypocentrum	No	Anterior tubercles of clivus
"proatlas"	Centrum	No	Apical ligament, apex of odontoid
	Neural arch	Rostral	Occipital condyles, alar and cruciform ligaments
		Caudal	Posterior arch and lateral masses of C1
1st cervical	Hypocentrum	No	Anterior arch of C1
	Centrum	No	Odontoid process
	Neural arch	No	Postero-inferior arch of C1
2nd cervical	Hypocentrum	–	–
	Centrum	No	Vertebral body of C2
	Neural arch	No	Posterior arch and articular facets of C2

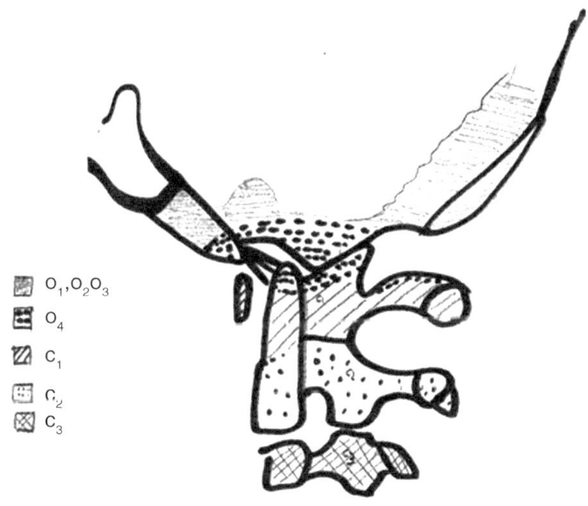

Fig. 1 Embryology of the craniovertebral junction. *O* occipital sclerotome, *C* cervical sclerotome (Adapted from Menezes et al. [44] and Thompson and Pang [45])

The fourth occipital sclerotome and the first two cervical sclerotomes will divide into three parts called hypocentrum, centrum and neural arch.

The fourth occipital sclerotome is of particular importance and called "proatlas" because of its crucial role in the formation of C1.

Concerning the proatlas, the hypocentrum will give the anterior tubercles of the clivus; the centrum will generate the apical ligament and the apex of the odontoid process. The neural arch will itself divide into one rostral contingent from which the occipital condyles, the alar and cruciform ligaments will rise and into one caudal contingent giving the posterior arch and the lateral masses of C1.

The first cervical sclerotome will give the anterior arch of C1 (hypocentrum), the odontoid process (centrum) and the inferior aspect of the posterior arch of C1 (neural arch).

At last, from the second cervical sclerotome will rise the vertebral body (centrum) and posterior arch and articular facets (neural arch) of C2.

All those elements are summarised in Table 1 and Fig. 1.

Craniovertebral Junction Development in Achondroplasia

Bone Growth and Embryology of the CVJ

Intra-membranous and Endochondral Ossification

There are two mechanisms of ossification at the level of the skull: intra-membranous and endochondral (Fig. 1). During the intra-membranous ossification, the bony tissue will develop by direct differentiation of mesenchymal cells that lie in the mesenchymatous matrix. Those cells will differentiate into osteoblasts and build a new, rich, osseous tissue which will grow.

In the endochondral ossification, mesenchymal cells build a cartilaginous matrix that will secondary become osseous through different stages.

Ossification of the Skull

Ossification of the skull vault and the face is principally intra-membranous (Fig. 1). There are numerous sites (called the ossification points) situated in the mesenchymal matrix that lie between the dura mater and the skin, where the ossification process begins. Bone growth is due to addition of numerous plates of ossification that grow in a centrifugal way from the ossification points and tend to merge together. The frontier between two plates represents a suture where remains a very thin band of mesenchymal tissue.

Ossification of the skull base is principally endochondral (Fig. 2). Several regions called synchondrosis can be described in the skull base (spheno-occipital synchondrosis, for example). In those regions, some mesenchymal cells differentiate into chondrocytes and constitute a cartilaginous plate that is central, whereas cells that are located at the periphery differentiate into primitive osteoprogenitors and begin the ossification process. Bone growth is due to the very active production of the cartilaginous plate. The principal receptor that is implicated in achondroplasia, FGFR3, is expressed quasi exclusively in the proliferative and prehypertrophic zone of the cartilaginous plate [4].

CVJ Bone Growth in Achondroplastic Children

Molecular and Histologic Characteristics of Achondroplasia

Achondroplasia is the most frequent of the diseases caused by different mutations of the gene that codes for the fibroblast growth factor receptor 3 (FGFR3) [33, 38]. Mutations in FGFR3 can lead to many other forms of chondrodysplasia such as the hypochondroplasia or thanatophoric dysplasia [13] or SADDAN and even some

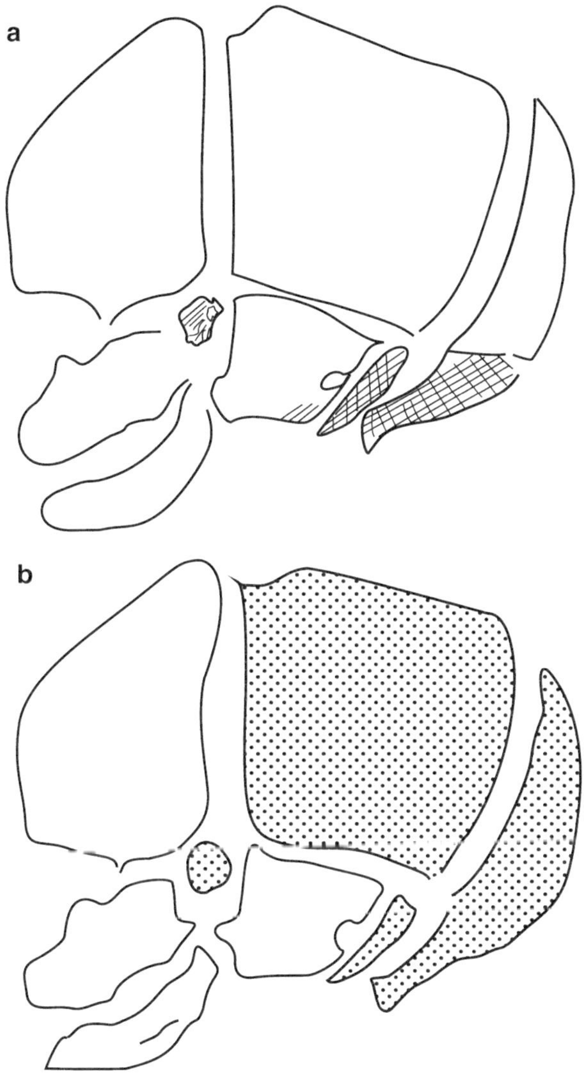

Fig. 2 Bone growth and embryology of the skull. (**a**) Membranous ossification (*white*) and endochondral ossification (*shaded*). (**b**) Neural crest origin (*white*) and mesoderm (*dotted*) (Adapted from Helms et al. [11])

craniostenosis such as the Muenke-Lajeunie syndrome [18, 25, 30, 35] or the Crouzon syndrome with acanthosis nigricans [24, 32]. Even if many progresses have been made since the discovery of those mutations in early 1990s, the exact molecular consequences of the mutation and the exact mechanism for each disease remain a matter of debate. Mutations of FGFR3 in those diseases have been shown to cause a gain of function of FGFR3, the receptor becoming constitutively activated. At the end, FGFR3 is thought to be one of the most important of bone growth regulators. Its activation results in an inhibition of bone growth, by altering the proliferation and the differentiation of the chondrocytes that are active in the cartilaginous growth plate of endochondral sites of ossification. With the receptor being

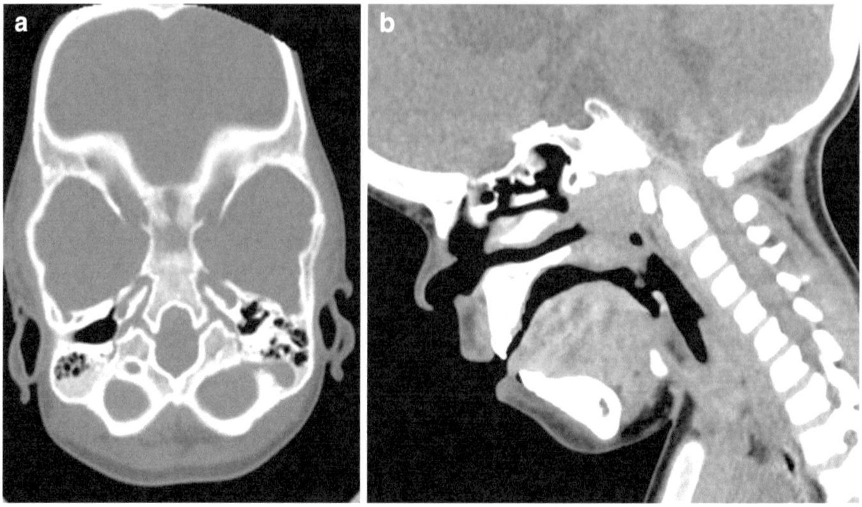

Fig. 3 Craniovertebral junction in an achondroplastic child. Axial (**a**) and sagittal (**b**) reconstruction showing the abnormal shape of the clival bone

constitutively activated in achondroplasia, this leads to a major dysfunction of the cartilaginous growth plate and bone growth [14].

Those elements are confirmed by the histologic characteristics of the cartilaginous growth plate of achondroplastic children. The chondrocytes that normally constitute the growth plate show a very poor organisation in those patients. The normal organisation in cells columns separated by collagenous septa is hardly outlined in achondroplastic subjects. Furthermore, the collagenous septa are hypertrophic, leading sometimes to the constitution of true zones of fibrosis in the cartilaginous plate [39].

Endochondral ossification is the principal mechanism of ossification occurring in long bones, in the spine and in the skull base. This explains why achondroplastic children suffer from dwarfism and lumbar stenosis and may have signs of cervicomedullary compression due to a too narrow CVJ.

At the level of the skull base, the spheno-occipital synchondrosis is particularly affected. In fact it is typically absent in achondroplastic children and replaced by ossified tissue. Such alteration is associated to an abnormal clivus that can be observed at CT or MR imaging (Fig. 3). The clival bone is, in fact, reduced in size, especially in the anterior-posterior dimension, thus participating to the midface retrusion found in these children.

Foramen Magnum (FM) Stenosis in Achondroplasia

The FM of achondroplastic children is known to be small [5, 19], but a quantification of the extent of this stenosis has been lacking until the 1980s. In two major studies published in 1985 and 1989 [8, 10], Hecht et al. performed computerised tomography studies of the foramen magnum in achondroplastic and non-achondroplastic children. They compared the sagittal and transversal measures of the FM in achondroplasia with those in the general population and then the same measures in symptomatic (i.e. achondroplastic children that presented signs of cervicomedullary compression) and asymptomatic achondroplastic children. The authors could demonstrate (1) that all achondroplastic children have a foramen magnum that is significantly smaller at birth, both in the transversal and sagittal diameters; (2) that the FM in achondroplastic children does not follow the outstanding growth during the first 18 months of life as the FM of normal children does; and (3) that in adulthood the FM is on average equivalent to the one of a normal newborn on the transversal diameter and to the one of a normal 2-year-old child on the sagittal diameter, meaning that the stenosis is greater along the transverse dimension. They could also show that (4) symptomatic achondroplastic children have a significantly smaller FM than asymptomatic achondroplastic children.

Actually, when the measures of achondroplastic and normal children are reported together, the curves obtained by Hecht et al. showed that whatever the clinical status is, the FM size of achondroplastic children is at least within -5SD of the mean for the transverse measure and within – 4SD for the sagittal dimension. Moreover, the authors proved that symptomatic patients had significantly smaller FM than asymptomatic ones, both transversally and sagittally ($p<0.0005$ for each dimension). This last element confirms that the higher the stenosis is, the worse the clinical consequences are.

The results of the studies by Hecht et al. are confirmed by the work of Keiper et al. [16], who followed 11 initially asymptomatic achondroplastic children prospectively between 1988 and 1995. At the time of first MRI evaluation (mean age 23 weeks), the mean values of the FM were 7.9 mm (6–10 mm) for the sagittal dimension and 9.09 mm for the transverse dimension (6–12 mm). Out of these 11 patients, 4 needed to be operated for CVJ stenosis. They had a smaller mean value of 6.7 mm for the sagittal dimension and of 7.5 mm for the transverse dimension.

In our experience based on the retrospective analysis of 37 achondroplastic children that needed surgical cervicomedullary decompression between 1981 and 2010 (mean age at surgery 29.3 months), we reached the same conclusions. The mean values of FM measured on CT scan and/or on MRI were 6,01 mm for the sagittal dimension and 9.3 mm for the transversal one (Table 2). Those values are consistent with those presented by Keiper et al. [16] and slightly inferior to those described by Hecht et al. [8]. One explanation for this observation might be that in our evaluation as well as in Keiper's one, the measures were performed using MRI, whereas in Hecht's study the measures were obtained by CT scan. Nevertheless, all measures in achondroplastic children were far below those observed in unaffected children.

However, the specific impact of the sagittal and of the transverse alterations was questioned by King et al. who performed 20 surgical decompressions in 18 achondroplastic children between 1958 and 2008 (mean age of 23 months at the time of the surgery) [17]. They evaluated the FM on CT scan examinations sagittally and transversally in seven symptomatic patients and compared them to eight

Table 2 Characteristics of the 37 patients operated between 1981 and 2010 at Necker-Enfants Malades, Paris

Child	Age at surgery (months)	Sagittal measurement before surgery (mm)	Transverse measurement before surgery (mm)	Sagittal measurement after surgery (mm)	Transverse measurement after surgery (mm)
C.Z.	18	7	5	9	10
E.F.S.	7	4	9	7	9
M.M.	180	10	12	12	12
R.A.	20	8	10	8	10
K.S.	7	4	7	7	9
G.K.	13	–	–	9	11
W.L.	132	–	–	7	–
R.S.	18	5	8	9	7
L.I.	16	3	8	9	9
M.E.	5	6	9	9	8
M.S.	20	5	10	7	9
A.O.	19	5	–	8	10
Z.S.	17	6	9	8	9
V.J.	17	6	9	8	10
W.J.	20	3	10	7	8
R.T.	6	–	–	–	–
D.M.	8	7	8	–	–
A.A.	19	–	–	7	9
H.P.H.	13	7	9	10	10
B.O.	16	–	–	–	–
N.C.	17	5	9	9	–
S.P.L.	23	6	9	9	10
L.J.	12	5	9	9	11
P.L.	14	5	6	8	9
D.T.O.	15	5.5	8	9	9
P.L.	18	5	14	8	–
G.L.	81	12	13	11	20
B.P.	58	–	–	8	10
T.N.	13	–	–	7.5	10
O.H.E.	13	4	10	–	–
F.J.	7	–	–	–	–
N.S.	7	–	–	7.5	8.5
D.J.	14	4	10	9	12
H.C.	42	7.1	10.3	8.6	9.1
A.L.	20	5.7	9	8	9.2
K.M.	162	7.2	12.1	8.8	11.9
Mean	29.3	6.01	9.32	8.98	9.98

asymptomatic patients that did not required surgery. Symptomatic children had significantly smaller transverse dimension of the FM than the asymptomatic ones (13.5 vs. 18.8, $p=0.03$), but there was no significant difference between the two groups concerning the sagittal diameter.

Yamada et al. proposed a different evaluation of the extent of FM stenosis [42]: they measured the sagittal dimension of the brainstem at three levels – (a) at the level of the pontomedullary junction, (b) at the level of the FM and (c) at the level of C3. Seven patients were assessed this way, using MRI T1 sagittal imaging. Importantly, five of these patients needed surgical opening of the FM on clinical follow-up. The authors then defined three ratios. FM stenosis was regarded as severe by the authors if the ratio b/a was <0.6 and/or if the ratio b/c was <1. In the remaining two cases, with higher ratios the stenosis was defined as mild. All the five children with a severe FM stenosis based on these criteria needed surgical FM opening and decompression. The work of Yamada et al. is an interesting and probably more complete way to evaluate the sagittal stenosis of FM as it adds two further measurements to the traditionally utilised transversal and sagittal measurements introduced by Hecht et al. In the clinical practice, however, the compression of the spinal cord in achondroplastic children is essentially localised at the level of the FM, and the absolute value of the sagittal diameter has a greater clinical relevance than other measurements such as the ratio b/a or b/c. Thus, most if not all clinical teams dealing with achondroplastic children continue to use the simple sagittal and transversal measures presented by Hecht et al.

CVJ Stenosis in Achondroplasia and Related CSF Dynamics Alteration

The occurrence of an enlarged head size and the presence of large ventricles on CT scanner or MRI are frequent features in achondroplastic children. Dandy first observed this phenomenon and related it to the small volume of the posterior fossa, leading to a communicating hydrocephalus. In 1980, Friedman et al. presented two achondroplastic children who both had enlarged head circumference, tense fontanels and thin scalp skin with dilated veins [6]. The first one had severe quadriparesis and had suffered a respiratory arrest. Both had mild ventriculomegaly on CT scan. Both children underwent cerebrospinal fluid (CSF) shunt placement and measurements of the ventricular pressure and the venous pressure in the superior sagittal sinus, which were high. Both of them recovered after shunt placement. In one of them a cerebral angiography showed narrowing of the sigmoid sinuses. The authors suggested that an impairment in venous outflow due to such an obstruction could be the cause of the hydrocephalus associated to achondroplasia. However, whether the presence of macrocrania is a sign of active hydrocephalus is still matter of debate. Indeed, some authors [5] prefer to use the term ventriculomegaly instead of active hydrocephalus. Sainte-Rose et al. recorded simultaneously the cerebrospinal fluid pressure (CSFP), sagittal venous pressure (SSVP) and jugular venous pressure (JVP) at baseline and during removal and reinjection of CSF in infants with achondroplasia and fixed partial obstruction of the lateral sinuses [36]. The authors showed that CSF removal induced a fall in CSF pressure, but no change in SSVP, and that the SSVP remained always higher than the JVP. They concluded that the

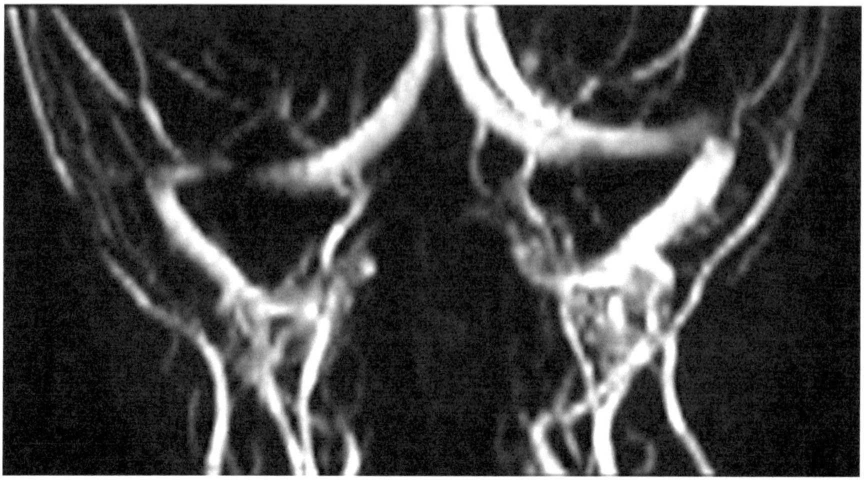

Fig. 4 MRI in an achondroplastic child. Venous study at MRI showing the stenosis of the jugular veins and collateral vascularisation

elevated SSVP was due to a fixed obstruction of the lateral sinuses as showed in venography and angiography (Fig. 4).

Furthermore, the relation between increased venous pressure and hydrocephalus is not linear [36, 37]. Some authors state that in adults the narrowed transverse sinuses lead to an increase in CSF pressure and not to hydrocephalus, in other words to the occurrence of the so-called benign intracranial hypertension. The same alteration in children with non-rigid skull, would, in the other hand, result in macrocrania but not necessarily in an active hydrocephalus.

In a previous study from our institution [28], Pierre Kahn et al., studying 25 achondroplastic children, found that 92 % of them (23/25) had enlarged ventricles, whereas only 60 % (15/25) presented with a macrocrania. Concerning the degree of ventricular dilatation, using the Evan's ratio, in our recent series of 37 patients, we found that the mean Evan's ratio was normal (mean = 0.37) in 24 (64 %) children who showed a ventriculomegaly. Four out of the 37 children of the series (10 %) had a borderline ratio (between 0.4 and 0.5), and only one child presented a ratio superior to 0.5, suggesting an active hydrocephalus.

However, even though any increase in ventricular volume, especially when associated to an increased intracranial pressure, may add an abnormal pressure gradient component to the anatomical anomalies of the posterior fossa and craniovertebral junction, the treatment of the putative hydrocephalus is seldom performed. Of the 56 achondroplastic children that were operated in our Pediatric Neurosurgical Department from 1971 to present, only three underwent a CSF diversion procedure (2 %). Out of 156 achondroplastic children described by King et al. between 1988 and 2008, only 7 had a CSF shunt insertion (4.3 %) [17].

Conversely, the degree of stenosis of the FM seems to play a little role on the ventricular size. In fact, when measuring the Evan's ratio before and after FM decompression, we found no significative difference in our recent series.

Clinical Implications of CVJ Anomalies in Achondroplasia

The principal clinical manifestations of FM stenosis are neurocognitive developmental delay, neurological impairment, cardiorespiratory and sleep dysfunction and the most dreadful evolution: sudden death [3, 26, 41, 43].

Though all achondroplastic children have a small FM, the spectrum of clinical symptoms and signs is very broad. Some patients present with no signs neither radiological nor clinical of cervicomedullary compression. Some have radiological signs of CVJ compression without clinical manifestations, whereas some present with a dramatic clinical status and need surgical decompression. In 1987, Reid et al. [29] estimated that 60 % of achondroplastic children had radiological signs of significant FM stenosis and cervicomedullary compression, but only 35 % of them had relevant clinical signs (neurological and/or cardiorespiratory). However, the actual consequence of the CVJ stenosis might be difficult to evaluate because as stated by Pauli et al., every achondroplastic child has a neurological history and/or a neurodevelopmental examination that is "virtually always abnormal" [27]. Nevertheless, other authors have suggested that symptoms and signs referred to CVJ stenosis may amend spontaneously during growth [31]. Thus, the indication for surgical decompression still remains a matter of debate.

Neurological and Developmental Impairment

Neurological signs of severe CVJ stenosis are those of cervical myelopathy. Those signs include lower limb hyper-reflexia and/or clonus, upper limb hyper reflexia (less common), limb weakness and cranial nerve palsy. Developmental delay can also occur, with decreased truncal tone and delayed or absent ability to walk [27].

In our 37 patients, 28 presented hypotonia (75.6 %), 12 had signs of myelopathy (32.4 %) and 5 presented other signs of developmental delay.

Respiratory Complications

In achondroplasia several abnormalities may predispose to respiratory difficulties especially during sleep. These include not only the CVJ stenosis and compression of the brain stem but also the short cranial base and the relative hypoplastic middle third of the face, as well as chest hypoplasia and deformity.

Snoring and apnoea are the usual respiratory signs in achondroplasia, together with signs of hypoxia. In a recent study from Julliard et al. [15] that included 29 children, the prevalence of snoring and witnessed apnoeas was 83 and 34 %, respectively. The prevalence of polysomnographic abnormalities was also very high (93 %). In achondroplastic patients, those signs can be related to CVJ stenosis (“central sleep apnoea”) but also to adenoid and tonsil hypertrophy (“peripheric apnoea”) [15]. In the work by Pauli et al. [27], among the 53 patients prospectively assessed, 14 (27 %) presented with observed apnoea, but in 35 children that were evaluated by polysomnography, as much as 14 (40 %) had mild, moderate or severe central apnoeas (11 mild, 2 moderate and 1 severe). Menezes [23, 34] and King et al. [17] have reported a higher rate of respiratory signs in the patients that needed surgery (4 out of 6 for Menezes, 12 out of 18 (66.5 %) patients for King).

Sudden Death

The actual risk of sudden death for an achondroplastic child remains a matter of debate. Pauli et al. suggested that sudden death might be in relation with the damages of respiratory centres that are located in the inferior medulla, “either directly or from ischemic damage secondary to compression of the vascular supply of the medulla” [26]. It is supposed to occur mostly in the first year of life. In their study of 1983, the authors reviewed 13 cases of achondroplastic children that had died in the first year of life and for whom the cause for death had been labelled as newborn sudden death. In those 13 cases, the authors assumed that they all suffered from subacute or chronic cervicomedullary compression and that the initial diagnostic of “usual” newborn sudden death was highly questionable.

In 1987, Hecht et al. [9] evaluated the risk of sudden death in achondroplasia at 7.5 % in the first year of life and at 2.5 % between 1 and 4 years old, which is three times more than in the general population. Hecht et al. related this overrated sudden death to the degree of FM stenosis.

However, those assumptions are challenged by Rimoin [31]. Out of 200 patients followed in their institution, only 9 needed a surgical decompression of the FM, and there was only one spontaneous death. Based on their data, the authors evaluated the risk of sudden death related to FM stenosis was between 0.5 and 5 %, depending on whether one assumes that the children who needed surgery would have died from sudden death without surgery or not.

Management of CVJ Anomalies in Achondroplasia

Clinical, Radiological and Polysomnographic Assessment of Achondroplastic Children

As the controversy between Rimoin et al. [31] and Pauli et al. [27]shows, the natural history of achondroplastic children remains unknown, with regard to the risk of sudden death or permanent neurological impairment.

This limitation has a relevant impact on both the family and the caretaker. Both Pauli et al. [27] and Rimoin et al. [31] recommend to focus on specific clinical and radiological signs which indicate a high degree of CVJ stenosis, in order to avoid sudden death, permanent neurological dysfunction or developmental delay. However, the identification of these signs is again a point on which they disagree.

Furthermore, CVJ stenosis can have clinical consequences not only in the first 2 years of life but all life long. Even though cervicomedullary compression that leads to severe clinical signs and may require surgery is well known to occur mainly in the first 24 months of life, a second "peak" of clinical manifestations has been observed to occur after 5 years of age. It was noted by King et al. [17] (3 patients of 9 years old out of the 18 that needed surgical decompression), Ryken and Menezes [34] (2 patients of 7 and 10 years and even 1 patient of 30 years out of their 6 operated patients) and Bagley et al. [2] (43 patients had cervicomedullary decompression with a mean age at surgery of 5.8 years, the oldest being 16 years old). In our series of 37 operated patients, we had five subjects older than 5 years.

Ultimately, in many cases, the most challenging difficulty for the neurosurgeon might be the indication for posterior fossa decompression rather than performing the surgical procedure. Having said that, the rate of "operated patients" versus "non-operated patients" could offer an interesting point for discussion. Reid et al. [29] and Francomano et al. [1] performed a surgical decompression in more than a fourth of their cases (34.6 % for Reid et al., 42.2 and 25.8 % in the two series of the John Hopkins Hospital), while Pauli et al. [27], King et al. [17] and Menezes et al. [23] operated in less than 15 % of their cases (13.3, 7.4 and 7.6 %, respectively). Rimoin et al. [31] performed surgery on 9 patients out of "more than 200" achondroplastic patients that followed (4.5 %).

In our opinion, surgical decompression of CVJ should be performed when there is evidence of:

- Clinical severe neurological impairment or developmental delay
- Evidence of significative central apnoea or hypopnea at polysomnography *and* lack of peri medullary subarachnoid spaces or intra-medullary T2 hypersignal in achondroplastic subjects with a small FM

Surgical Treatment

In our institution as well as in many others, the surgical procedure is standardised. It consists of a limited suboccipital craniectomy with a C1 laminectomy (Fig. 5).

Out of the 37 patients operated since 1981, 32 procedures were performed in the prone position and 5 in the semi-sitting position. Only in 2 cases we performed also a C2 laminectomy because of an ectopic position of the cerebellar tonsils with dural opening. For these 2 patients, a posterior arthrodesis by grafting and immobilisation was performed as well, and for one of them, an anterior decompression by a trans-oral approach was necessary.

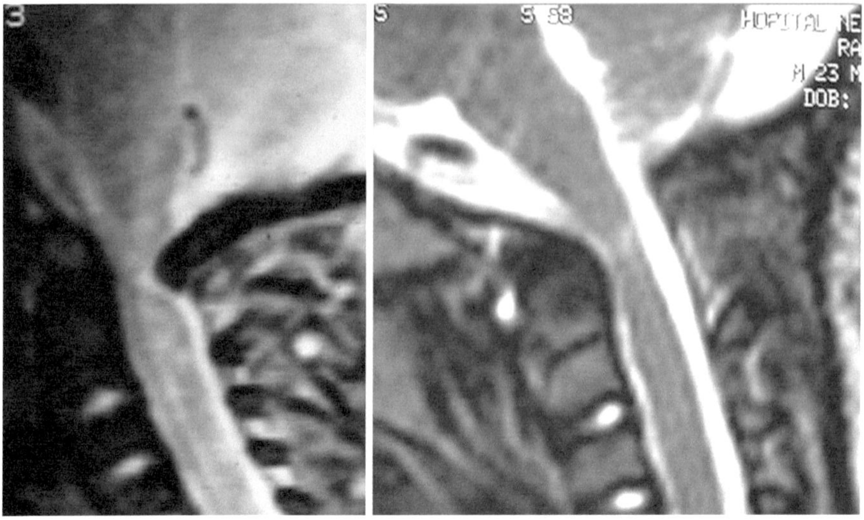

Fig. 5 Sagittal MR before and after a surgical decompression. Note the hypersignal of the spinal cord best visible after the decompression

The dura mater was opened once and a duroplasty was performed (a cervicodorsal syringomyelia was associated to the FM compression). In 5 cases, the dura mater was thinned by taking out the external dural sheet.

No prophylactic external ventricular drainage (EVD) was performed. Only one patient had a previous ventriculoperitoneal shunt (VPS) inserted but 14 years prior to the cervicomedullary decompression.

During our procedure, we did not assess the upper extremity somatosensory evoked potentials, as Aryanpur et al. and Bagley et al. did in the two series of the John Hopkins Hospital [1, 2].

This surgical procedure is similar to the one described by King et al. On the 20 CVJ decompression performed, there was no need for prophylactic EVD. The dura was opened only twice in patients who presented with impairment of conscious state. Menezes et al. opened the dura in 3 of the 6 patients of his series in 1993 and five shunts for CSF drainage were performed [23, 34]. Interestingly, in the 13 patients that needed CVJ decompression between 1993 and 2009, only one had a shunt. Keiper et al. performed no duroplasty in their 4 patients [16].

In the two series presented by Aryanpur [1] and King [17], the authors used to open the dura routinely. The procedure was modified after the first 6 cases because of several cases of CSF leakage. On the next 37 patients remaining, an EVD was performed just before CVJ decompression for those that showed radiological signs of hydrocephalus (8 patients), and a VPS was made if the patient showed clinical as well as radiological evidence of hydrocephalus (9 patients).

We believe that opening the dura is rarely necessary for a good CVJ decompression, and we also consider that such procedure can lead to CSF leaks and wound infection, which can be dreadful complications of the surgical operation. Furthermore, many achondroplastic children present with enlarged ventricles and FM stenosis. As we said previously the presence of enlarged ventricles does not necessarily mean active hydrocephalus, and many achondroplastic patients clinically improved after CVJ decompression despite keeping enlarged ventricles.

Overall, we had four surgical complications during the procedure: accidental dural lacerations (3 cases) and venous bleeding from an ectopic sinus (1 case). All those events were easily controlled at the time of the surgical procedure.

Recently, we added the use of ultrasonic echography to the surgical procedure. We found it helpful to confirm the extent of the decompression objectively. To our opinion, the demonstration of the reappearance of the subarachnoidian spaces around the spinal cord at the end of the procedure testifies the good quality of the decompression.

As for the majority of surgeons, CVJ surgical decompression was rewarding also in our experience. We observed a complete or partial clinical improvement at the last follow-up examination in 29 out of the 37 operated patients, with a mean follow-up of 67, 4 months.

Those results are similar to those presented by many authors. The 5 patients who were prospectively assessed by Pauli et al. [27] and who needed surgery "demonstrated (usually dramatic) improvement of neurological function". On the contrary, the five that were directly sent to surgery after the symptoms appearance "often were left with significant residual disability".

Bagley et al. [2] state in their abstract that all patients had total or partial improvement of symptoms. King et al. [17] assert that all patient "did very well, only one failing to improve clinically". Unfortunately, none of those authors described their patients with precise clinical and radiological features.

Nevertheless, though the procedure can be rewarding, it is weighted by a significant surgical morbidity and even mortality. We had seven complications (20 %), including two post-operative deaths (5.4 %), one related to an epidural hematoma and a second which remained unexplainable.

The other complications were 1 subdural hematoma that had no clinical consequence, 1 empyema that needed surgical evacuation, 2 extubation delays and 1 one transient laryngeal palsy.

Our death rate is similar to that of King et al. (5 %) and minor of that Reid et al. (11.1 %) [17, 29]. Rimoin, Bagley, Francomano, Menezes, Keiper and Yamada [1, 2, 16, 23, 31, 42] had no death, but their surgical series were smaller.

In summary, the high complication rate associated to cranio-spinal decompression in achondroplastic children suggests a cautious attitude, especially considering the controversial experiences reported in the literature. As Rimoin et al. [31] stated, the postsurgical death rate is not negligible and must be taken into account when a surgical CVJ decompression is decided. Indeed, it should be pointed out that the exact "neurological natural" death rate remains unknown and is evaluated between 0.5 and 7.5 % of achondroplastic children.

Breathing Therapies

Concerning the respiratory complications of achondroplastic children, many therapeutic interventions are possible. For central sleep apnoeas due to CVJ stenosis, the treatment is the standard surgical decompression of the CVJ as previously described. For peripheric apnoeas due to an anatomic obstruction (such as hypertrophy of the adenoids, tonsils and/or turbinates), upper airway surgery can be indicated. Adenoidectomy, turbinectomy and tonsillectomy can be performed. In the study of Julliand et al. [15], such procedures were performed in 4 patients, with clinical and polysomnographic improvement in all. In cases of nocturnal alveolar hypoventilation, non-invasive positive pressure ventilation (NPPV) can be proposed. In the same study by Julliard et al., 5 patients were treated this way and all of them improved with a median nocturnal use of NPPV of 8 h.

However, as Julliand et al. showed, achondroplastic children can have apnoeas related to CVJ compression as well as peripheric obstruction or alveolar hypoventilation. This means that every child must have a pluridisciplinary evaluation concerning the breathing complications, with at least one neurosurgeon, one ENT surgeon and one pneumologist. Furthermore, it is not rare that one patient may have benefit from CVJ decompression as well as upper airway surgery, in case of mixed apnoea.

Conclusion

The treatment of CVJ stenosis in achondroplastic children remains a challenging problem.

The natural history of CVJ stenosis is only partially known. A risk of sudden death exists. However, the surgical decompression is weighted by non-negligible morbidity and mortality rates.

The indication for surgery should be taken on clinical and radiological parameters and sleep studies. Every patient should be sent to a skeletal dysplasias' reference centre, in order to perform a precise and multidisciplinary evaluation by geneticists, orthopaedic surgeons, neurosurgeons, ENT surgeons and pneumologists.

References

1. Aryanpur J, Hurko O, Francomano C, Wang H, Carson B (1990) Craniocervical decompression for cervicomedullary compression in pediatric patients with achondroplasia. J Neurosurg 73:375–382
2. Bagley CA, Pindrik JA, Bookland MJ, Camara-Quintana JQ, Carson BS (2006) Cervicomedullary decompression for foramen magnum stenosis in achondroplasia. J Neurosurg 104:166–172

3. Colamaria V, Mazza C, Beltramello A, Polo A, Boner A, Antoniazzi F, Polo M, Luchini P, Sgrò V, Dalla Bernardina B (1991) Irreversible respiratory failure in an achondroplastic child: the importance of an early cervicomedullary decompression, and a review of the literature. Brain Dev 13:270–279
4. Delezoide AL, Benoist-Lasselin C, Legeai-Mallet L, Le Merrer M, Munnich A, Vekemans M, Bonaventure J (1998) Spatio-temporal expression of FGFR 1, 2 and 3 genes during human embryo-fetal ossification. Mech Dev 77:19–30
5. Dennis JP, Rosenberg HS, Alvord EC Jr (1961) Megalencephaly, internal hydrocephalus and other neurological aspects of achondroplasia. Brain 84:427–445
6. Friedman WA, Mickle JP (1980) Hydrocephalus in achondroplasia: a possible mechanism. Neurosurgery 7:150–153
7. Harada D, Yamanaka Y, Ueda K, Tanaka H, Seino Y (2009) FGFR3-related dwarfism and cell signaling. J Bone Miner Metab 27:9–15
8. Hecht JT, Nelson FW, Butler IJ, Horton WA, Scott CI Jr, Wassman ER, Mehringer CM, Rimoin DL, Pauli RM (1985) Computerized tomography of the foramen magnum: achondroplastic values compared to normal standards. Am J Med Genet 20:355–360
9. Hecht JT, Francomano CA, Horton WA, Annegers JF (1987) Mortality in achondroplasia. Am J Hum Genet 41:454–464
10. Hecht JT, Horton WA, Reid CS, Pyeritz RE, Chakraborty R (1989) Growth of the foramen magnum in achondroplasia. Am J Med Genet 32:528–535
11. Helms JA, Amasha RR, Leucht P (2007) Bone voyage: an expedition into the molecular and cellular parameters affecting bone graft fate. Bone 41:479–485
12. Horton WA, Hall JG, Hecht JT (2007) Achondroplasia. Lancet 370:162–172
13. Horton WA, Degnin CR (2009) FGFs in endochondral skeletal development. Trends Endocrinol Metab 20:341–348
14. Iwata T, Hevner RF (2009) Fibroblast growth factor signaling in development of the cerebral cortex. Dev Growth Differ 51:299–323
15. Julliand S, Boulé M, Baujat G, Ramirez A, Couloigner V, Beydon N, Zerah M, Di Rocco F, Lemerrer M, Cormier-Daire V et al (2012) Lung function, diagnosis, and treatment of sleep-disordered breathing in children with achondroplasia. Am J Med Genet A 158A:1987–1993
16. Keiper GL Jr, Koch B, Crone KR (1999) Achondroplasia and cervicomedullary compression: prospective evaluation and surgical treatment. Pediatr Neurosurg 31:78–83
17. King JAJ, Vachhrajani S, Drake JM, Rutka JT (2009) Neurosurgical implications of achondroplasia. J Neurosurg Pediatr 4:297–306
18. Lajeunie E, El Ghouzzi V, Le Merrer M, Munnich A, Bonaventure J, Renier D (1999) Sex related expressivity of the phenotype in coronal craniosynostosis caused by the recurrent P250R FGFR3 mutation. J Med Genet 36:9–13
19. Marin-Padilla M, Marin-Padilla TM (1977) Developmental abnormalities of the occipital bone in human chondrodystrophies (achondroplasia and thanatophoric dwarfism). Birth Defects Orig Artic Ser 13:7–23
20. Menezes AH (2004) Evaluation and treatment of congenital and developmental anomalies of the cervical spine. Invited submission from the Joint Section Meeting on Disorders of the Spine and Peripheral Nerves, March 2004. J Neurosurg Spine 1:188–197
21. Menezes AH (2005) Honored guest presentation: craniocervical developmental anatomy and its implications. Clin Neurosurg 52:53–64
22. Menezes AH (2008) Craniocervical developmental anatomy and its implications. Childs Nerv Syst 24:1109–1122
23. Menezes AH (2009) Editorial. Achondroplasia. J Neurosurg Pediatr 4:295–296; discussion 296
24. Meyers GA, Orlow SJ, Munro IR, Przylepa KA, Jabs EW (1995) Fibroblast growth factor receptor 3 (FGFR3) transmembrane mutation in Crouzon syndrome with acanthosis nigricans. Nat Genet 11:462–464
25. Muenke M, Gripp KW, McDonald-McGinn DM, Gaudenz K, Whitaker LA, Bartlett SP, Markowitz RI, Robin NH, Nwokoro N, Mulvihill JJ et al (1997) A unique point mutation in

the fibroblast growth factor receptor 3 gene (FGFR3) defines a new craniosynostosis syndrome. Am J Hum Genet 60:555–564
26. Pauli RM, Scott CI, Wassman ER Jr, Gilbert EF, Leavitt LA, Ver Hoeve J, Hall JG, Partington MW, Jones KL, Sommer A (1984) Apnea and sudden unexpected death in infants with achondroplasia. J Pediatr 104:342–348
27. Pauli RM, Horton VK, Glinski LP, Reiser CA (1995) Prospective assessment of risks for cervicomedullary-junction compression in infants with achondroplasia. Am J Hum Genet 56:732–744
28. Pierre-Kahn A, Hirsch JF, Renier D, Metzger J, Maroteaux P (1980) Hydrocephalus and achondroplasia. A study of 25 observations. Childs Brain 7:205–219
29. Reid CS, Pyeritz RE, Kopits SE, Maria BL, Wang H, McPherson RW, Hurko O, Phillips JA 3rd, Rosenbaum AE (1987) Cervicomedullary compression in young patients with achondroplasia: value of comprehensive neurologic and respiratory evaluation. J Pediatr 110:522–530
30. Renier D, El-Ghouzzi V, Bonaventure J, Le Merrer M, Lajeunie E (2000) Fibroblast growth factor receptor 3 mutation in nonsyndromic coronal synostosis: clinical spectrum, prevalence, and surgical outcome. J Neurosurg 92:631–636
31. Rimoin DL (1995) Cervicomedullary junction compression in infants with achondroplasia: when to perform neurosurgical decompression. Am J Hum Genet 56:824–827
32. Di Rocco F, Collet C, Legeai-Mallet L, Arnaud E, Le Merrer M, Hadj-Rabia S, Renier D (2011) Crouzon syndrome with acanthosis nigricans: a case-based update. Childs Nerv Syst 27:349–354
33. Rousseau F, Bonaventure J, Legeai-Mallet L, Pelet A, Rozet JM, Maroteaux P, Le Merrer M, Munnich A (1994) Mutations in the gene encoding fibroblast growth factor receptor-3 in achondroplasia. Nature 371:252–254
34. Ryken TC, Menezes AH (1994) Cervicomedullary compression in achondroplasia. J Neurosurg 81:43–48
35. Sabatino G, Di Rocco F, Zampino G, Tamburrini G, Caldarelli M, Di Rocco C (2004) Muenke syndrome. Childs Nerv Syst 20:297–301
36. Sainte-Rose C, LaCombe J, Pierre-Kahn A, Renier D, Hirsch JF (1984) Intracranial venous sinus hypertension: cause or consequence of hydrocephalus in infants. J Neurosurg 60: 727–736
37. Sainte-Rose C, Servant JM, Mayer M, Hirsch JF (1989) Hydrocephalus of venous origin. Neurochirurgie 35:383–389, 410
38. Shiang R, Thompson LM, Zhu YZ, Church DM, Fielder TJ, Bocian M, Winokur ST, Wasmuth JJ (1994) Mutations in the transmembrane domain of FGFR3 cause the most common genetic form of dwarfism, achondroplasia. Cell 78:335–342
39. Stanescu R, Stanescu V, Maroteaux P (1990) Homozygous achondroplasia: morphologic and biochemical study of cartilage. Am J Med Genet 37:412–421
40. Velinov M, Slaugenhaupt SA, Stoilov I, Scott CI Jr, Gusella JF, Tsipouras P (1994) The gene for achondroplasia maps to the telomeric region of chromosome 4p. Nat Genet 6:314–317
41. Yamada H, Nakamura S, Tajima M, Kageyama N (1981) Neurological manifestations of pediatric achondroplasia. J Neurosurg 54:49–57
42. Yamada Y, Ito H, Otsubo Y, Sekido K (1996) Surgical management of cervicomedullary compression in achondroplasia. Childs Nerv Syst 12:737–741
43. Yang SS, Corbett DP, Brough AJ, Heidelberger KP, Bernstein J (1977) Upper cervical myelopathy in achondroplasia. Am J Clin Pathol 68:68–72
44. Pang D, Thompson DN. Embryology and bony malformations of the craniovertebral junction. Childs Nerv Syst 2011;27(4):523–64
45. Menezes AH. Craniocervical developmental anatomy and its implications. Childs Nerv Syst 2008;24(10):1109–22

Craniovertebral Junction Pathological Features and Their Management in the Mucopolysaccharidoses

Erik Pietro Sganzerla, Carlo Giussani, Marco Grimaldi, Rossella Parini, Pablo Ingelmo, Andrea Trezza, and Massimiliano Visocchi

Contents

E.P. Sganzerla, MD (✉) • C. Giussani • A. Trezza
Clinica Neurochirurgica, Università degli Studi Milano-Bicocca,
Ospedale San Gerardo, via Pergolesi 33, Monza (MB) 20900, Italy
e-mail: erikpietros@tiscali.it

M. Grimaldi
Dipartimento di Neuroradiologia, Servizio di Radiodiagnostica,
Ospedale San Gerardo, via Pergolesi 33, Monza, Italy

R. Parini
Clinica Pediatrica, "Fondazioni Mariani" per le Malattie Metaboliche,
Università degli Studi Milano-Bicocca, Fondazione Monza Brianza per il Bambino e la Mamma,
Ospedale San Gerardo, via Pergolesi 33, Monza, Italy

P. Ingelmo
Anestesia e Rianimazione, Servizio di Anestesia Pediatrica,
Università degli Studi Milano-Bicocca, Ospedale San Gerardo, via Pergolesi 33, Monza, Italy

M. Visocchi
Dipartimento di Neurochirurgia, Università Cattolica del Sacro Cuore,
Policlinico Universitario "Agostino Gemelli", largo A, Gemelli 8, Rome, Italy

C. Di Rocco, N. Akalan (eds.), *Pediatric Craniovertebral Junction Diseases*,
Advances and Technical Standards in Neurosurgery 40,
DOI 10.1007/978-3-319-01065-6_11, © Springer International Publishing Switzerland 2014

Abstract The mucopolysaccharidoses (MPS) are multisystemic inherited metabolic diseases caused by the deficiency of the enzymes involved in the degradation of glycosaminoglycans (GAGs), which variably involve the central nervous system, heart, lungs, and bones.

Undegraded or only partly degraded GAGs accumulate in the extracellular matrix, joint fluid, and connective tissue leading to widespread tissue and organ dysfunction.

The introduction of hematopoietic stem cell transplantation (HSCT) and enzyme replacement therapy (ERT) has positively affected the natural history of MPS patients and their life expectancy. However, the presence of spinal abnormalities and deposition of GAGs in soft tissues remains nearly unaltered.

Abnormalities of the craniovertebral junction (CVJ) and GAG deposits can result in spinal cord compression with slowly progressive myelopathy or acute posttraumatic tetraplegia.

The current paper discusses neuroimaging findings in a consecutive series of 42 MPS patients followed at our Center for Metabolic Diseases and their neurosurgical issues.

Current recommendations for decompression and fusion will be discussed according to our experience and review of the literature.

Keywords Mucopolysaccharidoses • Craniovertebral junction • Occipitocervical stabilization • Pediatric neurosurgery • Rigid internal fixation • Spinal cord compression • Diagnostic imaging

Introduction

The mucopolysaccharidoses (MPS) are a group of inherited autosomal recessive lysosomal storage diseases (with the exception of MPS II inherited as sex-linked recessive) caused by the deficiency of the enzymes involved in the degradation of glycosaminoglycans (GAGs), a major component of the ground substance of connective tissue [4, 21].

Involvement of the craniovertebral junction (CVJ) is common in children with MPS, especially in Morquio's disease (MPS IV) [33, 44], and is potentially life-threatening or progressively invalidating [14, 22, 25, 46, 50].

Abnormalities of the CVJ with stenosis of the spinal canal should be recognized early in the course of disease as they may result in slow and progressive myelopathy or sudden posttraumatic tetraplegia and respiratory failure [23, 29, 46].

Preventive surgical treatment with decompression and fusion in asymptomatic children is still a matter of debate but has been especially recommended in all individuals affected by MPS IV (Morquio's disease) with MRI evidence of stenosis and instability at the CVJ, with canal narrowing >50 % [42, 53].

Mucopolysaccharidoses: Mechanisms of the Disease and Principles of Therapy

Undegraded or only partly degraded GAGs like heparan sulfate, dermatan sulfate, keratan sulfate, chondroitin sulfate, or hyaluronan accumulate in the extracellular matrix, joint fluid, and connective tissue leading to widespread tissue and organ dysfunction. Exceeding GAGs are excreted in the urine where they can be collected for diagnostic purposes [6, 34, 49]. Biochemical confirmation can be obtained by testing blood and cultured fibroblasts [27]. The recent introduction of enzyme replacement therapy (ERT) in MPS I, II, and VI [9, 17, 35] and hematopoietic stem cell transplantation (HSCT) [32, 40] in MPS I has altered the natural history of some of these metabolic diseases and the life expectancy of affected individuals, otherwise destined to premature death [34].

Although HSCT and ERT improve many of the systemic effects of MPS, the deposition of metabolites in bone is less influenced than that in soft tissues, and spinal abnormalities remain more or less unaltered [20, 22, 25].

MPS are rare conditions, with an incidence of all types of MPS estimated of 1 in 25,000–45,000 live births [37]. They are classified as types I (three subtypes), II, III, IV, VI, VII, and IX and are variably characterized by ENT and airway obstructions [43], skeletal abnormalities and joint disease [28, 30, 38, 45, 52], central nervous system involvement, hydrocephalus, and soft tissue disorders [4, 15, 19, 23, 28, 30, 48, 49, 54].

The longer life expectancy of these patients has increased medical and surgical efforts to correct invalidating organ dysfunctions, which participate by themselves in increasing the disabilities of these difficult-to-treat patients.

Involvement of the craniovertebral junction (CVJ) is common in children with MPS, especially in Morquio's disease (MPS IV), and is progressively invalidating or even potentially life-threatening [12, 14, 44–46].

Unrecognized upper cervical cord compression, aggravated by physiological movements of the occipitocervical and atlantoaxial joints, may indeed result in slow and progressive myelopathy or sudden, unexpected posttraumatic tetraplegia [23, 29, 46] and respiratory failure.

Therefore, in the diagnostic work-up of MPS patients, it is mandatory to assess the cervical spine early in the course of the disease and at regular scheduled intervals, paying particular attention to the occipitocervical junction, which is electively affected in MPS [28].

Radiological Features and Their Incidence in the Various MPS Subtypes

Magnetic resonance imaging (MRI) of the cervical spine including active dynamic flexion and extension scans is the most powerful imaging technique for detecting spinal cord compression at the CVJ in MPS. It may clearly evidence the presence

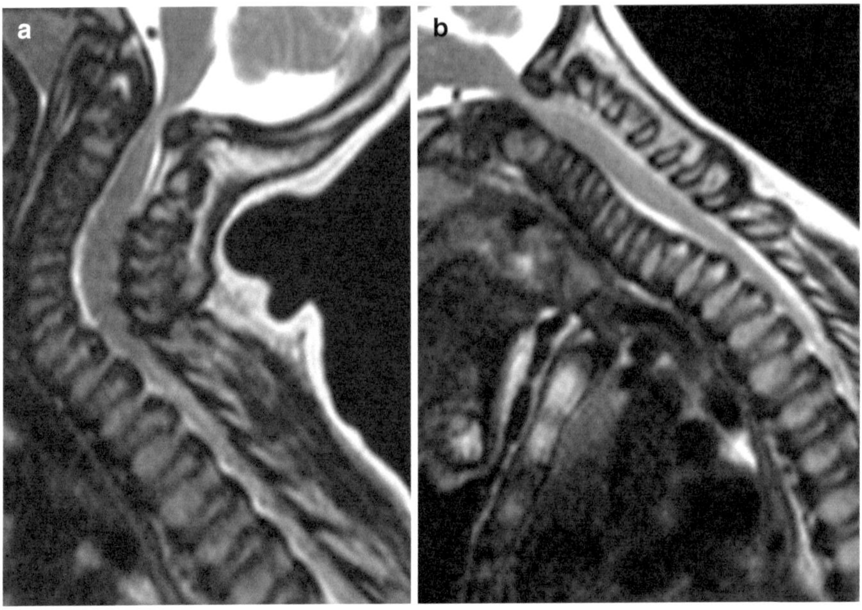

Fig. 1 (**a**, **b**) Flexion/extension MRI study in a MPS IVA case, showing increased cord compression during flexion

of spinal canal narrowing, signs of spinal cord compression, and spinal cord signal alteration [25, 28, 30]. Dynamic flexion and extension scans can evidence abnormal movements of the involved bony segments with the resultant dynamic spinal cord compression.

T1-weighted axial and sagittal and T2-weighted axial and sagittal MRI scans are usually performed. Steady-state free procession (SSFP)-producing images with increased signal from fluid can be used for studying the presence of subarachnoid cerebrospinal fluid in the narrowed upper cervical canal [13] and to define the severity of the stenosis with the Space Available for the Cord (SAC) scale [30, 47].

Although obvious atlantoaxial (C1/C2 subluxation) or occipito-atlantoaxial instability, as defined by classical criteria (atlantoaxial subluxation with atlanto-dental interval >5 mm) [41], is seldom observed in MPS [14, 23, 38, 42], dynamic studies may nonetheless evidence increasing canal stenosis and cord compression during head flexion or extension (Fig. 1).

Main features to consider in MPS are: the presence of odontoid hypoplasia, periodontoid soft tissue masses due to GAG accumulation behind the odontoid process and cartilage/fibrocartilage reactive hypertrophy compounded by hypertrophy of dura and ligamentum flavum [3], spinal canal narrowing, and spinal cord compression with/without MRI signs of cervical myelopathy (Fig. 2).

In addition to high cervical stenosis, multilevel subaxial stenosis has been reported in MPS VI (Maroteaux-Lamy) [22]. Posteriorly protruding intervertebral discs, thickened dura, and hypertrophy of the ligamentum flavum are the most relevant features of subaxial canal narrowing [36].

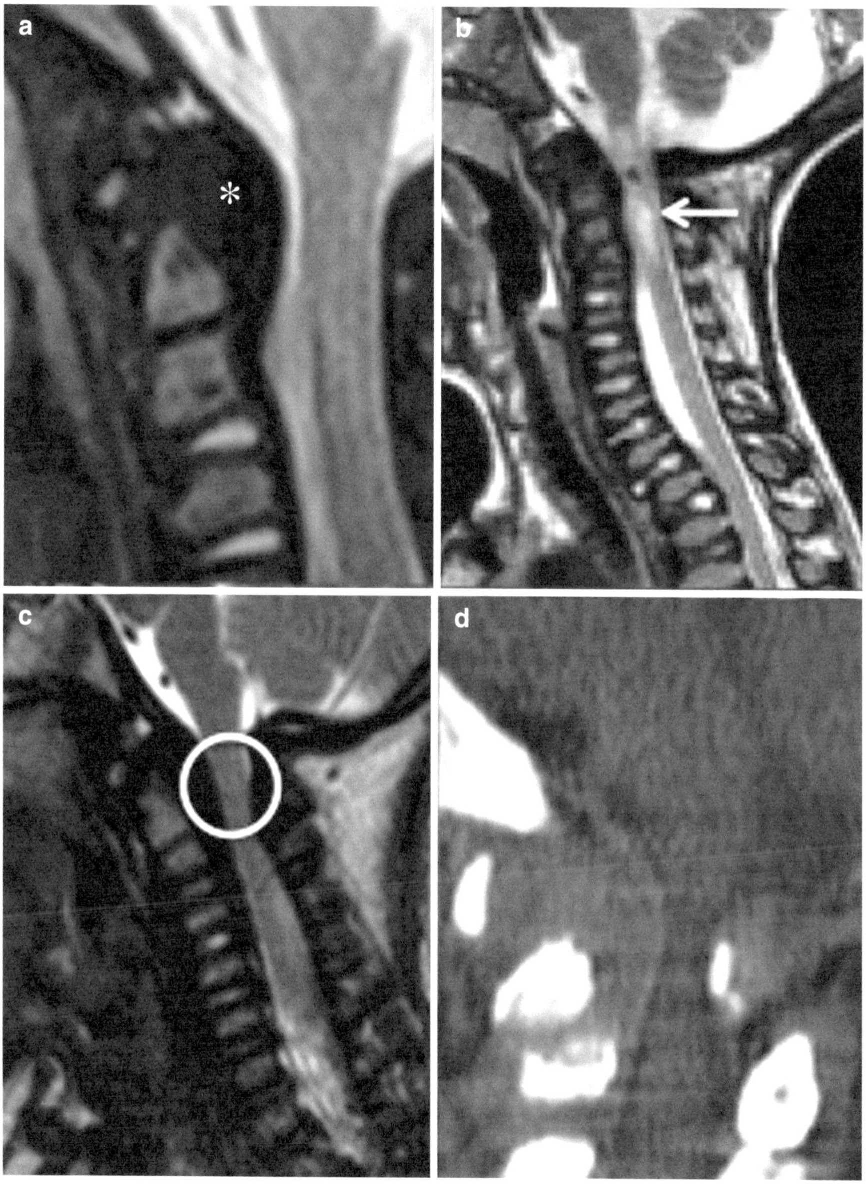

Fig. 2 MRI showing severe dens dysplasia and periodontoid tissue thickening (*asterisk*) in MPS II (**a**), acute posttraumatic myelopathy (*arrow*) in MPS IV (**b**), and severe spinal stenosis (*circle*) in MPS VI (**c**). Preoperative CT scan showing severe cord compression, dens dysplasia, and periodontoid tissue thickening in MPS IV (**d**)

We have recently reviewed radiological features of the CVJ in a consecutive series of 42 MPS patients followed at our Center for Metabolic Diseases: 12 MPS I, 15 MPS II, 2 MPS III, 9 MPS IV, and 4 MPS VI.

MRI studies have been scored according to following MRI features: dens dysplasia, periodontoid tissue thickening, spinal stenosis, myelopathy, and instability on dynamic MRIs [30].

Spinal stenosis in neutral position was classified according to the SAC scale, and the difference between the mean diameter of the subaxial cervical canal and the diameter of the cervical canal at the CVJ expressed in %. Presence or absence of signs of instability was determined by the presence or not of modifications of the SAC score and/or canal diameter during flexion/extension MRI studies at the occipitocervical junction.

CVJ abnormalities were frequent in the whole series of MPS patients, with a reduced diameter of the spinal canal at the CVJ in 17/42 children. The most severe spinal canal stenosis and cord compression were observed in MPS IV (3/9) and MPS VI (2/4). Reduction >50 % of the cervical canal diameter was observed in 5/42 patients. MRI signs of myelopathy were present in 3/42 cases, all affected by MPS IV. Dens hypoplasia was overall present in 33/42 cases and was a constant feature in MPS IV and VI. Due to the very young age of some of the children, hypoplastic dens nevertheless could still be in some case an expression of incomplete development of the C2 dens. Slight modifications of canal diameter during dynamic MRI studies were observed in 9/32 cases, confirming how clear-cut radiological signs of instability are seldom documented in MPS patients. Increased canal stenosis during dynamic MRI studies in flexion and extension was evidenced in 6/9 MPS IV patients.

These observations confirm how in Morquio's disease severe CVJ abnormalities are more frequent and should be screened and controlled at scheduled intervals in all patients [33].

To avoid potentially harmful radiations, computed tomography (CT) scan studies of the CVJ should be reserved for children in whom MRI has evidenced significant pathological features and some surgical procedure is considered.

Fine-cut CT with coronal and sagittal 3-D reconstructions is a powerful tool for imaging the bone and clearly delineates anatomical features of C0–C1–C2 and possible associated bony abnormalities at the CVJ (Fig. 3).

Moreover, the dimensions of a single vertebra (height, width, length) can be easily calculated.

The recognition of heterogeneous anatomical features of the CVJ in MPS patients and the exact determination of bone geometry and diameters is of paramount importance for the selection of the most appropriate hardware placement in tailored surgical procedures with screwing techniques. In selected cases angio-CT delineating the course of vertebral arteries may be indicated, especially if suitability of C1/C2 transarticular screws is evaluated.

Indications to Surgery

The clinical evidence of acute or progressive myelopathy associated with radiological evidence of spinal cord compression at the CVJ is a strong indication to surgery as the natural history of untreated patients is invariably characterized by

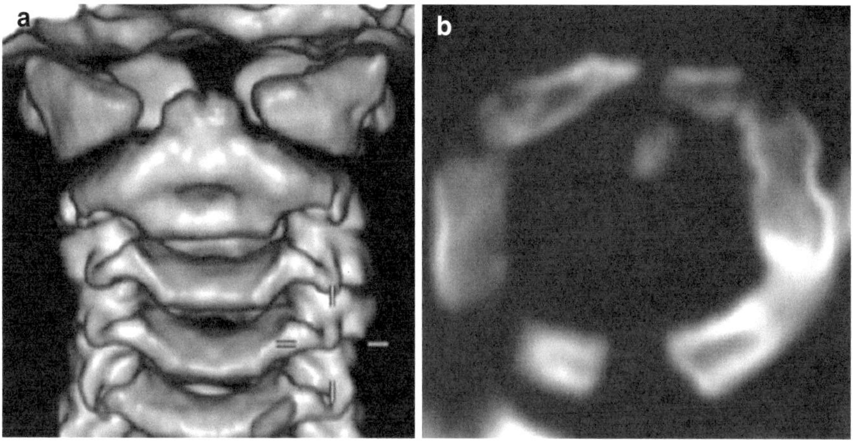

Fig. 3 3-D CT reconstruction (**a**) of the CVJ of a child affected by MPS VI, displaying anterior and posterior midline failure of ossification of the C1 ring; axial CT (**b**) showing similar features in another MPS VI case

increasing neurological deficits and functional impairment [1, 12, 14, 22, 25, 38, 42, 46].

Preventive surgical treatment with decompression and fusion in asymptomatic children is still a matter of debate but has been especially recommended in all individuals affected by MPS IV (Morquio) with MRI evidence of stenosis and instability at the CVJ, with canal narrowing >50 % [38, 42, 44].

In our department we recommend prophylactic surgery in asymptomatic children with severe spinal canal narrowing and complete obliteration of perimedullary subarachnoid spaces (SAC< 1 mm), 50 % or more reduction of the cervical canal at CVJ, and MRI signs of instability (spinal canal stenosis and cord compression). Whenever possible, in very small children, we suggest to await for sufficient bone maturation, operating at the age of at least 3 years, although surgery can be feasible, if clinically necessary, even at a younger age as demonstrated in a 17-month-old symptomatic boy by Dickerman and coworkers [12].

Surgical Techniques

Even if the past surgery of the CVJ in small children was considered challenging and characterized by a high incidence of postoperative neurological complications, the improvement of preoperative radiological work-ups, the accurate preoperative CT identification of individual anatomical bone features, the availability of various techniques for instrumented bone fusion, and the improvement of multidisciplinary evaluations and anesthesiological techniques in these difficult patients, often affected by multiorgan disorders, have made this surgery safe and rewarding if the associated medical problems and anesthesiological challenges are recognized and managed appropriately.

Although some authors considered simple posterior decompression of the CVJ in MPS other than Morquio when dynamic radiological studies did not clearly evidence atlantoaxial or occipito-atlantoaxial instability [26, 39], we recommend decompression and fusion in all cases. Indeed, posterior decompression alone, without fusion, can actually expose these patients to acute posttraumatic myelopathy, even following a minor trauma in flexion, as evidenced in one of our children (case 1).

Ransford et al. [42] already evidenced how odontoid dysplasia with a partially cartilaginous and softer dens, the frequent finding of incomplete anterior or posterior or both ossification of the C1 ring (Fig. 3), and ligamentous laxity can result in complex CVJ instability allowing harmful translatory movements, which may be increased by posterior decompressive surgeries without stabilization.

In fact, decompression is a partly destabilizing technique in patients with pathological ligamentous laxity, as it needs removal of the posterior ring of C1, of the thickened ligamentum flavum, and of the occipito-atlantal membrane.

Recent advances in rigid fixation technologies have enhanced the ability to achieve stable posterior cervical fusions with a variety of screwing techniques, adaptable to the individual anatomical features of these usually very small children, and they should be preferred for their superior biomechanical stability [2, 7, 8, 16, 18, 55].

C1/C2 transarticular screws, C1 lateral mass screws, C1 Olerud clamps, C2 pars screws, C2 translaminar screws, or a combination of them as anchor for occipitocervical U-loop constructs can be taken in consideration on the basis of fine-cut preoperative CT studies [2]. Iliac crest graft, or rib graft, or calvarial bone graft [5] will be used to augment posterior fixation and achieve biological bone fusions. Rigid screwing techniques have also reduced or eliminated the need for external halo orthoses and their complications [2, 10].

Although we consider segmental screw fixation in the pediatric spine superior to posterior wiring techniques and external halo orthosis, the latter techniques do not need to be completely abandoned in selected cases as they still can afford good clinical results with long-term stabilization and fusion of the CVJ, as evidenced by Visocchi [51].

Clinical Results

Recent reports of surgery of the occipitocervical junction in children, comprising small series of MPS, evidence the feasibility, safety, and stability of screwing techniques with good clinical long-term outcomes after instrumented rigid implants [14, 31, 42, 44, 46].

Also in our cases, no asymptomatic patient had new postoperative neurological deficits, and all symptomatic patients improved their Ranawat score during follow-up and maintained stable constructs and solid bone fusion on neuroimaging studies at last follow-up examination.

Case Studies

Case 1: Acute Posttraumatic Myelopathy

H.M., a 6-year-old girl with MPS IVA. She had previously undergone CVJ decompression at another institution for severe canal stenosis and mild myelopathy, with removal of the posterior arch of C1 and of the thickened atlantooccipital membrane and ligamentum flavum. After a backward fall from a child's chair, she developed an acute quadriplegia with respiratory failure (Ranawat IIIB) and was admitted to our neurological intensive care unit. MRI showed an impressive alteration of the spinal cord signal at C0–C1 (Fig. 4a). This patient was initially stabilized with an external halo orthosis and submitted to inpatient rehabilitation for some weeks afterward. After an initial neurological improvement and cardiorespiratory stability, she underwent internal stabilization with C2 pars screws (Fig. 4b) anchored to an occipitocervical U-loop and occipito-C2 calvarial bone graft. At 4-year follow-up examination, she was able to walk with crutches (Ranawat IIIA). Radiological follow-up examinations revealed wide canal decompression and a stable construct (Fig. 4c, d).

Case 2: Progressive Myelopathy

R-B.G., a 6-year-old male with MPS VI. After a minor fall he experienced a transient tetraparesis with quick recovery of deambulation. In the following months he experienced repeated urinary tract infections. Cervical MRI was characterized by severe stenosis and cord compression at the CVJ with spinal cord signal alterations (Fig. 5a). Physical exam evidenced brisk tendon reflexes at all four limbs, and a urodynamic study was diagnostic for a neurological bladder. He was therefore submitted to posterior cervical decompression and internal stabilization with C2 pars screws anchored to an occipitocervical U-loop and calvarial bone graft. Postoperative course was uneventful with slow recovery of bladder function and normal daily activities. Radiological follow-up examination revealed good canal decompression, stable construct (Fig. 5b, c), and steady neurological conditions.

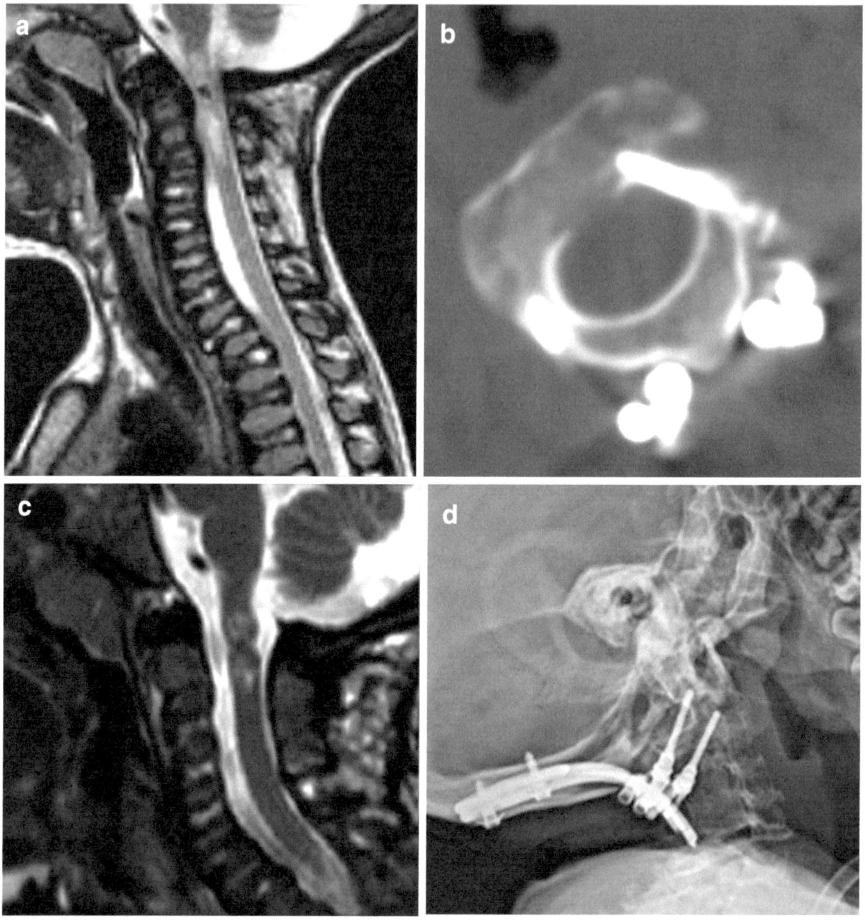

Fig. 4 (**a**) MRI showing severe posttraumatic myelopathy after a minor backward fall in a previously simply decompressed MPS IV child. (**b**) C2 pars screws, (**c**) postoperative MRI, and (**d**) plain X-rays at 4-year follow-up

Case 3: Preventive Surgery

P.M., a 2-year-old boy with MPS IVA. During routine neuroradiological work-up, severe canal stenosis at the CVJ was observed. As there were no signs of major instability and the child was completely asymptomatic with no radiological signs of myelopathy, the case was discussed with the parents and the pediatrician in charge with particular regard to the possible risk of sudden onset of neurological symptoms after trauma. Due to the small dimensions and incomplete development of bony structures at the CVJ and the increased risks of general anesthesia at that age,

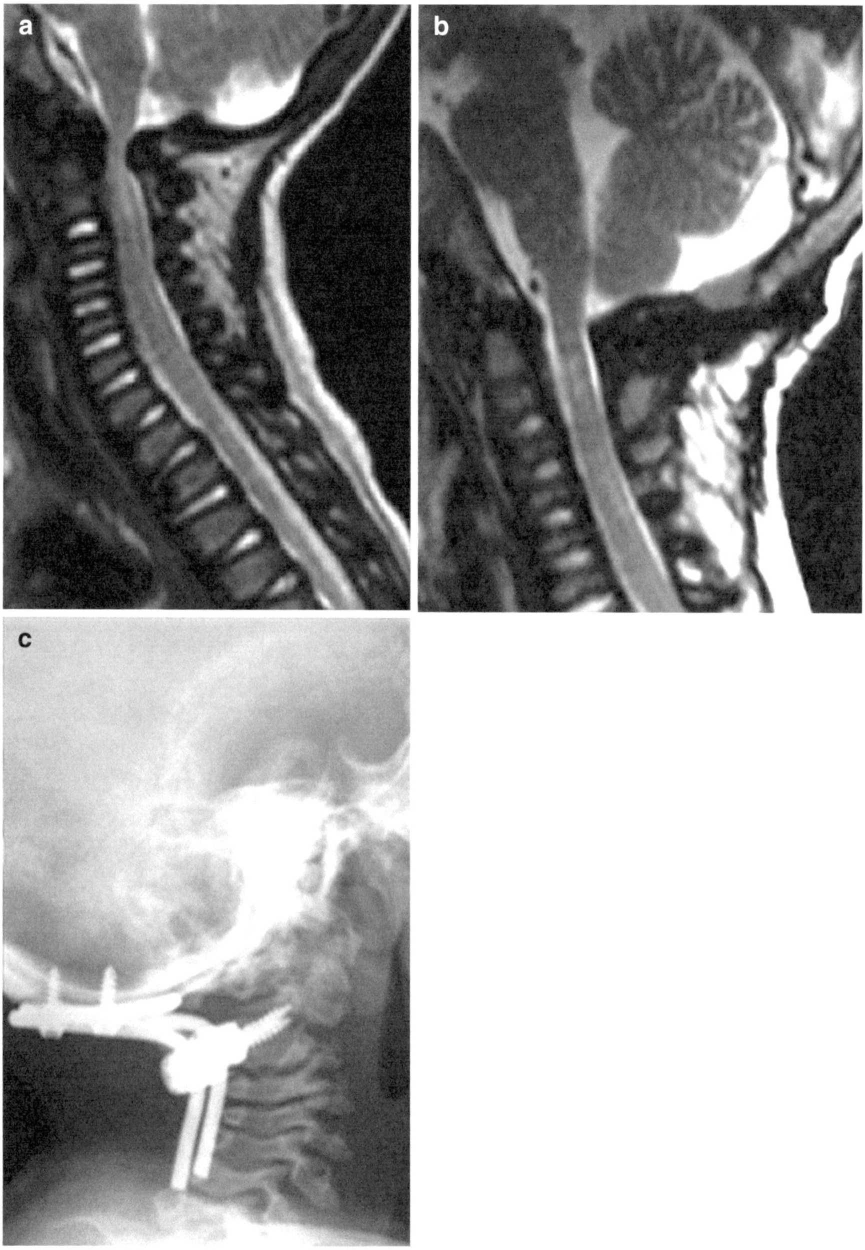

Fig. 5 (**a**) Preoperative MRI in a MPS VI child showing severe canal stenosis and cord compression. (**b**) Postoperative MRI and (**c**) plain X-rays showing good canal decompression and a stable construct at 2-year follow-up

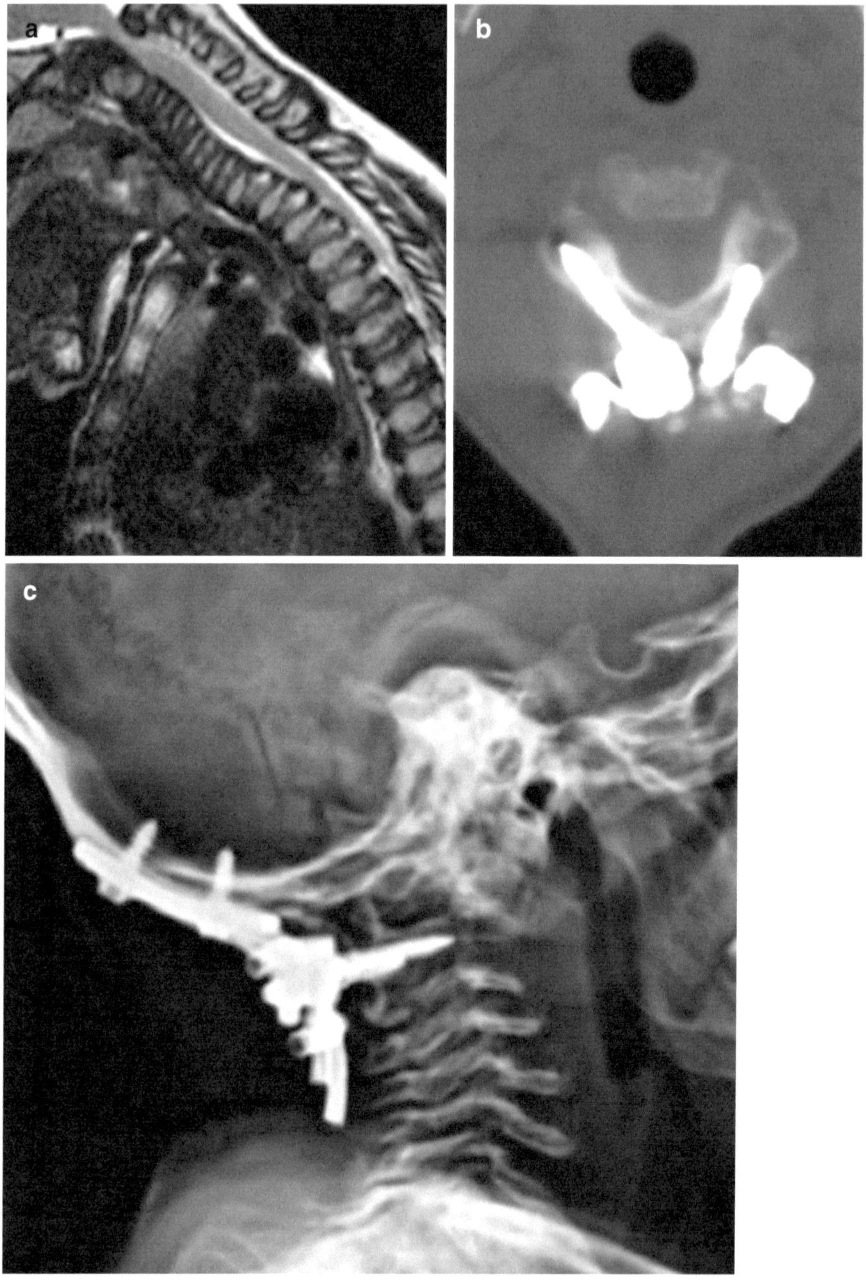

Fig. 6 MRI showing severe cord compression during head flexion in MPS IVA (**a**), laminar screws (**b**), and postoperative plain X-rays at 2-year follow-up (**c**)

it was decided to schedule surgery at 3 years of age. After a follow-up MRI now evidencing increasing cord compression during flexion (Fig. 6a) and a thorough preoperative CT study, we performed preventive CVJ decompression and internal fixation with C2 laminar screws (Fig. 6b) anchored to an occipitocervical loop augmented with calvarial bone. Also in this case postoperative course was uneventful and radiological follow-up controls showed a stable construct (Fig. 6c).

Case 4: Stabilization with Sublaminar Wires

C.V., an 8-year-old child with MPS IV. Mild canal stenosis and dens dysplasia at the CVJ (Fig. 7a, b), partial C0–C1 assimilation, and C2–C3 fusion with signs of C1/C2 instability on plain X-rays in flexion (Fig. 7c) were documented during

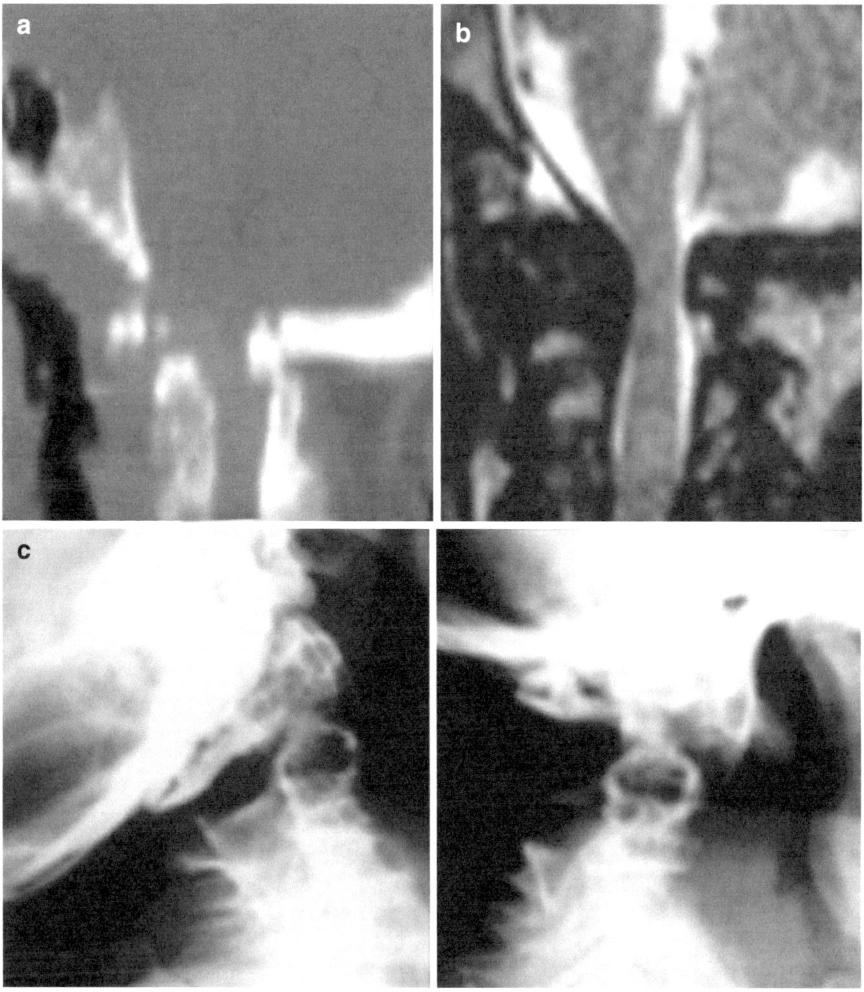

Fig. 7 (**a**) CT and (**b**) MRI showing mild canal stenosis, dens dysplasia, C0–C1 assimilation, and C2–C3 fusion. (**c**) Plain dynamic X-rays showing C1–C2 instability. (**d**) Postoperative plain X-rays

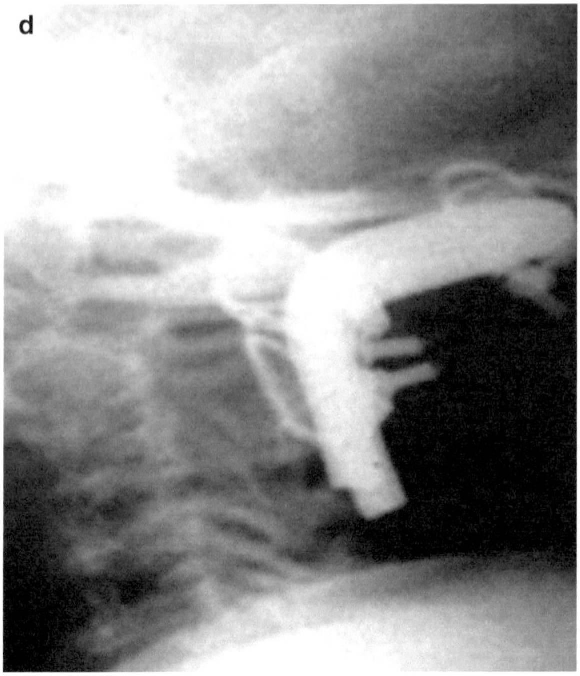

Fig. 7 (continued)

standard neuroradiological work-up. Although the child was asymptomatic with no radiological and clinical signs of myelopathy, the radiological evidence of CVJ stenosis and instability urged us to operate the patient in order to prevent a possible neurological deterioration. CVJ decompression was associated to occipitocervical fusion with U-shaped titanium rods and sublaminar wires at C0–C3 and autologous bone harvested from the iliac crest (Fig. 7d). The patient harbored a SOMI brace system for 6 months. After a 17-year follow-up, the patient does not complain any neurological signs or symptoms or major functional impairments.

Discussion

In a database analysis of 5,300 patients with symptomatic craniovertebral abnormalities among which 2,000 were children, MPS formed only a smaller group [31].

Nonetheless, it is of paramount clinical importance to recognize early in the course of the MPS the presence or not of upper cervical stenosis, cord compression, and instability as, if unrecognized, it can severely affect the natural course of these patients already invalidated by multiorgan disorders.

ERT and HSCT may improve many of the systemic effects of some of the metabolic disorders but have unclear effects on the prevention of cervical myelopathy [22, 25]. According to Horovitz et al. [22] ERT may even increase joint mobility and cervical instability in MPS VI.

A recent report by Miebach et al. [32] however suggests that successful HSCT may have an early positive influence on the CVJ for MPS I H (Hurler syndrome) with improvement of the underdeveloped axis after successful engraftment. Adequate enzyme levels in transplanted patients seem to play a relevant role in dens development.

The increased life expectancy obtained by ERT and HSCT compels the early recognition and treatment of CVJ abnormalities, and preventive treatments should be considered if a reduction of 50 % or more in the sagittal spinal cord diameter can be demonstrated [11, 39, 42, 44].

The incidence of CVJ abnormalities is particularly high in Morquio-Brailsford syndrome (MPS IV). The International Morquio A Registry [33], with a total of 326 patients enrolled in the registry program, showed that 51 % of the patients were eventually submitted to cervical surgery due to progressive cord compression at the CVJ.

Reports describe symptomatic cervical stenosis in MPS VI (Maroteaux-Lamy syndrome) [46], MPS I (Hurler syndrome) [25], MPS II (Hunter syndrome) [26, 50], and MPS VII (Sly syndrome) [12].

MPS patients often present formidable anesthetic challenges for the presence of severe associated upper and lower airway obstruction and cardiac disorders. Hypertrophic and inflamed mucosae, short neck, tonsil and adenoid hyperplasia, macroglossia, high epiglottis, narrowing of larynx and trachea, and valvular cardiac disease all combine to increase technical challenges [24, 38]. Preoperative accurate cardiac assessment, fine-cut CT studies of the respiratory tract [15], and fiber-optic study of airways are thus of vital importance for a successful cervical surgery in these patients [24]. General anesthesia is even more hazardous in MPS patients who also have unstable CVJ abnormalities and should be conducted by expert pediatric anesthesiologists aware of the multiple peculiarities of patients with metabolic diseases.

Surgical techniques have dramatically progressed in recent years, and experiences acquired in adult patients have been successfully transferred to children [2, 7, 8, 16, 18, 55]. Traditionally, occipitocervical fusion in children has been achieved with posterior wiring techniques and an external halo orthosis, and many surgeons have been reluctant to recur to rigid internal fixations with screwing techniques because of the smaller physical size and variable bone anatomy in this population.

Wiring techniques, due to their intrinsic microinstability, should however be considered semirigid constructs and usually need large bone autografts and external orthoses for adequate bone fusion [2].

In particularly difficult cases or in case of unfamiliarity of the surgeon with the use of instrumentation for the pediatric cervical spine, wiring techniques can nonetheless still afford good clinical results [51].

Rigid internal fixations performed using screwing techniques have demonstrated to provide superior biomechanical stability and obviate the need for halo orthoses [2, 10]. The safety of rigid internal fixations even in very young patients has furthermore been well demonstrated [2], and abnormal cervical spine growth was not seen in children who underwent CVJ stabilization below the age of 5 [1].

Anatomical heterogeneity of the CVJ is no more an obstacle as different screw fixation techniques are available and can be variably adapted to individual patients and bone anatomies and personal expertise of the surgeon. According to fine-cut CT studies, surgical strategy can be preoperatively determined and even virtually performed on CT images or on three-dimensional full-scale bone models of the CVJ [56].

Surgery should be performed as soon as possible in all symptomatic patients as neurological functions inevitably decline in untreated children. In asymptomatic patients preventive surgery should be always considered when neuroradiological examinations evidence severe stenosis and cord compression at the CVJ. In children less than 3 years old, we await for sufficient bone maturation after an exhaustive illustrative talk with the parents.

According to published reports and our personal experience [14, 31, 42, 44, 46], clinical and radiological results have been rewarding with no neurological complications in asymptomatic patients and a constant improvement of neurological symptoms in symptomatic patients and radiological stability of the construct with bone fusion at follow-up in absence of noticeable complications.

In summary, CVJ abnormalities have to be recognized early in the course of the disease in patients affected by MPS as unrecognized cord compression at the CVJ can result in progressive myelopathy or sudden, unexpected traumatic cord damage.

Preventive surgery should be considered in asymptomatic patients, especially if affected by Morquio's disease, whenever MRI studies evidence severe canal stenosis and cord compression.

Rigid constructs realized with screwing techniques are to be preferred for their superior biomechanical stability, although wiring techniques have not to be completely disregarded in selected cases.

In all patients a thorough investigation of associated medical problems is of paramount importance for the conduction of a safe general anesthesia.

Conclusions

MPS are inherited metabolic disorders characterized by multiorgan involvement. Modern treatment protocols and the introduction of HSCT and ERT have changed the once limited life expectancy of these children who nowadays need a multidisciplinary approach, a comprehensive diagnosis, and the timely correction of all disabling associated conditions. Skeletal involvement is a well-known feature of MPS, and unrecognized CVJ abnormalities, especially in MPS IV and VI, can progress to chronic or acute myelopathy. Screening of the CVJ with scheduled MRIs and the early treatment of cervical canal stenosis and cord compression is of paramount importance in these patients. Surgery should be conducted in these difficult-to-treat patients by expert multidisciplinary teams well aware of the associated cardiac and respiratory problems.

References

1. Ahmed R, Traynelis VC, Menezes AH (2008) Fusions at the craniovertebral junction. Childs Nerv Syst 24(10):1209–1224
2. Anderson RC, Ragel BT, Mocco J, Bohman LE, Brockmeyer DL (2007) Selection of a rigid internal fixation construct for stabilization at the craniovertebral junction in pediatric patients. J Neurosurg 107(1 Suppl):36–42
3. Ashraf J, Crockard HA, Ransford AO, Stevens JM (1991) Transoral decompression and posterior stabilisation in Morquio's disease. Arch Dis Child 66(11):1318–1321
4. Astarita L, Sibilio M, Andria G (2010) Lysosomal storage disorders: commonalities and differences. In: Parini R, Andria G (eds) Lysosomal storage diseases, early diagnosis and new trcbrseatment, Mariani Foundation Paediatric Neurology Series. John Libbey Eurotext, Montrouge, p 23
5. Bauman JA, Hardesty DA, Heuer GG, Storm PB (2011) Use of occipital bone graft in pediatric posterior cervical fusion: an alternative paramedian technique and review of the literature. J Neurosurg Pediatr 7(5):475–481
6. Bellettato CM, Tomanin R, Scarpa M (2010) Pathophysiology aspects of lysosomal storage disorders. In: Parini R, Andria G (eds) Lysosomal storage diseases, early diagnosis and new treatment, Mariani Foundation Paediatric Neurology Series. John Libbey Eurotext, Montrouge, p 23
7. Brockmeyer D, Apfelbaum R, Tippets R, Walker M, Carey L (1995) Pediatric cervical spine instrumentation using screw fixation. Pediatr Neurosurg 22(3):147–157
8. Brockmeyer DL, Apfelbaum RI (1999) A new occipitocervical fusion construct in pediatric patients with occipitocervical instability. Technical note. J Neurosurg 90(2 Suppl):271–275
9. Clarke LA, Wraith JE, Beck M, Kolodny EH, Pastores GM, Muenzer J, Rapoport DM, Berger KI, Sidman M, Kakkis ED, Cox GF (2009) Long-term efficacy and safety of laronidase in the treatment of mucopolysaccharidosis I. Pediatrics 123(1):229–240
10. Couture D, Avery N, Brockmeyer DL (2010) Occipitocervical instrumentation in the pediatric population using a custom loop construct: initial results and long-term follow-up experience. J Neurosurg Pediatr 5(3):285–291
11. Crockard HA, Stevens JM (1995) Craniovertebral junction anomalies in inherited disorders: part of the syndrome or caused by the disorder? Eur J Pediatr 154(7):504–512
12. Dickerman RD, Colle KO, Bruno CA Jr, Schneider SJ (2004) Craniovertebral instability with spinal cord compression in a 17-month-old boy with Sly syndrome (mucopolysaccharidosis type VII): a surgical dilemma. Spine (Phila Pa 1976) 29(5):E92–E94
13. Facon D, Ozanne A, Fillard P, Lepeintre JF, Tournoux-Facon C, Ducreux D (2005) MR diffusion tensor imaging and fiber tracking in spinal cord compression. AJNR Am J Neuroradiol 26(6):1587–1594
14. Giussani C, Roux FE, Guerra P, Pirillo D, Grimaldi M, Citerio G, Sganzerla EP (2009) Severely symptomatic craniovertebral junction abnormalities in children: long-term reliability of aggressive management. Pediatr Neurosurg 45(1):29–36
15. Grimaldi M, Di Marco D, Remida P (2010) Mucopolysaccharidosis: radiologic findings. In: Parini R, Andria G (eds) Lysosomal storage diseases, early diagnosis and new treatment, Mariani Foundation Paediatric Neurology Series. John Libbey Eurotext, Montrouge, p 23
16. Haque A, Price AV, Sklar FH, Swift DM, Weprin BE, Sacco DJ (2009) Screw fixation of the upper cervical spine in the pediatric population. Clinical article. J Neurosurg Pediatr 3(6): 529–533
17. Harmatz P, Whitley CB, Waber L, Pais R, Steiner R, Plecko B, Kaplan P, Simon J, Butensky E, Hopwood JJ (2004) Enzyme replacement therapy in mucopolysaccharidosis VI (Maroteaux-Lamy syndrome). J Pediatr 144(5):574–580
18. Hedequist D, Proctor M (2009) Screw fixation to C2 in children: a case series and technical report. J Pediatr Orthop 29(1):21–25

19. Hinek A, Wilson SE (2000) Impaired elastogenesis in Hurler disease: dermatan sulfate accumulation linked to deficiency in elastin-binding protein and elastic fiber assembly. Am J Pathol 156(3):925–938
20. Hite SH, Peters C, Krivit W (2000) Correction of odontoid dysplasia following bone-marrow transplantation and engraftment (in Hurler syndrome MPS 1H). Pediatr Radiol 30(7):464–470
21. Hopwood JJ, Bunge S, Morris CP, Wilson PJ, Steglich C, Beck M, Schwinger E, Gal A (1993) Molecular basis of mucopolysaccharidosis type II: mutations in the iduronate-2-sulphatase gene. Hum Mutat 2(6):435–442
22. Horovitz DD, Magalhães Tde S, Pena e Costa A, Carelli LE, Souza e Silva D, de Linhares e Riello AP, Llerena JC Jr (2011) Spinal cord compression in young children with type VI mucopolysaccharidosis. Mol Genet Metab 104(3):295–300
23. Hughes DG, Chadderton RD, Cowie RA, Wraith JE, Jenkins JP (1997) MRI of the brain and craniocervical junction in Morquio's disease. Neuroradiology 39(5):381–385
24. Ingelmo P, Sahillioglu E (2010) Anaesthesia for children with mucopolysaccharidosis. In: Parini R, Andria G (eds) Lysosomal storage diseases, early diagnosis and new treatment, Mariani Foundation Paediatric Neurology Series. John Libbey Eurotext, Montrouge, p 23
25. Kachur E, Del Maestro R (2000) Mucopolysaccharidoses and spinal cord compression: case report and review of the literature with implications of bone marrow transplantation. Neurosurgery 47(1):223–228, discussion 228–9
26. Kaendler S, Bockenheimer S, Gräfin Vitzthum H, Galow W (1990) Cervical myelopathy in mucopolysaccharidosis type II (Hunter's syndrome). Neuroradiologic, clinical and histopathologic findings. Dtsch Med Wochenschr 115(36):1348–1352
27. Kakkis ED, Muenzer J, Tiller GE, Waber L, Belmont J, Passage M, Izykowski B, Phillips J, Doroshow R, Walot I, Hoft R, Neufeld EF (2001) Enzyme-replacement therapy in mucopolysaccharidosis I. N Engl J Med 344(3):182–188
28. Lachman R, Martin KW, Castro S, Basto MA, Adams A, Teles EL (2010) Radiologic and neuroradiologic findings in the mucopolysaccharidoses. J Pediatr Rehabil Med 3(2):109–118
29. Lipson SJ (1977) Dysplasia of the odontoid process in Morquio's syndrome causing quadriparesis. J Bone Joint Surg Am 59(3):340–344
30. Manara R, Priante E, Grimaldi M, Santoro L, Astarita L, Barone R, Concolino D, Di Rocco M, Donati MA, Fecarotta S, Ficcadenti A, Fiumara A, Furlan F, Giovannini I, Lilliu F, Mardari R, Polonara G, Procopio E, Rampazzo A, Rossi A, Sanna G, Parini R, Scarpa M (2011) Brain and spine MRI features of Hunter disease: frequency, natural evolution and response to therapy. J Inherit Metab Dis 34(3):763–780
31. Menezes AH (2008) Craniovertebral junction database analysis: incidence, classification, presentation, and treatment algorithms. Childs Nerv Syst 24(10):1101–1108
32. Miebach E, Church H, Cooper A, Mercer J, Tylee K, Wynn RF, Wraith JE (2011) The craniocervical junction following successful haematopoietic stem cell transplantation for mucopolysaccharidosis type I H (Hurler syndrome). J Inherit Metab Dis 34(3):755–761
33. Montano AM, Tomatsu S, Gottesman GS, Smith M, Orii T (2007) International Morquio A Registry: clinical manifestation and natural course of Morquio A disease. J Inherit Metab Dis 30(2):165–174
34. Muenzer J, Fisher A (2004) Advances in the treatment of mucopolysaccharidosis type I. N Engl J Med 350(19):1932–1934
35. Muenzer J, Gucsavas-Calikoglu M, McCandless SE, Schuetz TJ, Kimura A (2007) A phase I/II clinical trial of enzyme replacement therapy in mucopolysaccharidosis II (Hunter syndrome). Mol Genet Metab 90(3):329–337
36. Mut M, Cila A, Varli K, Akalan N (2005) Multilevel myelopathy in Maroteaux-Lamy syndrome and review of the literature. Clin Neurol Neurosurg 107(3):230–235
37. Nelson J, Crowhurst J, Carey B, Greed L (2003) Incidence of the mucopolysaccharidoses in Western Australia. Am J Med Genet A 123A(3):310–313
38. Northover H, Cowie RA, Wraith JE (1996) Mucopolysaccharidosis type IVA (Morquio syndrome): a clinical review. J Inherit Metab Dis 19(3):357–365
39. O'Brien DP, Cowie RA, Wraith JE (1997) Cervical decompression in mild mucopolysaccharidosis type II (Hunter syndrome). Childs Nerv Syst 13(2):87–90

40. Peter C, Steward CG (2003) Hematopoietic cell transplantation for inherited metabolic diseases: an overview of outcomes and practice guidelines. Bone Marrow Transplant 31:229–239
41. Pueschel SM, Scola FH (1987) Atlantoaxial instability in individuals with Down syndrome: epidemiologic, radiographic, and clinical studies. Pediatrics 80(4):555–560
42. Ransford AO, Crockard HA, Stevens JM, Modaghegh S (1996) Occipito-atlanto-axial fusion in Morquio-Brailsford syndrome. A ten-year experience. J Bone Joint Surg Br 78(2):307–313
43. Simmons MA, Bruce IA, Penney S, Wraith E, Rothera MP (2005) Otorhinolaryngological manifestations of the mucopolysaccharidoses. Int J Pediatr Otorhinolaryngol 69(5):589–595
44. Stevens JM, Kendall BE, Crockard HA, Ransford A (1991) The odontoid process in Morquio-Brailsford's disease. The effects of occipitocervical fusion. J Bone Joint Surg Br 73(5):851–858
45. Tandon V, Williamson JB, Cowie RA, Wraith JE (1996) Spinal problems in mucopolysaccharidosis I (Hurler syndrome). J Bone Joint Surg Br 78(6):938–944
46. Thorne JA, Javadpour M, Hughes DG, Wraith E, Cowie RA (2001) Craniovertebral abnormalities in Type VI mucopolysaccharidosis (Maroteaux-Lamy syndrome). Neurosurgery 48(4):849–852, discussion 852–3
47. Tierney RT, Maldjian C, Mattacola CG, Straub SJ, Sitler MR (2002) Cervical spine stenosis measures in normal subjects. J Athl Train 37(2):190–193
48. Vedolin L, Schwartz IV, Komlos M, Schuch A, Puga AC, Pinto LL, Pires AP, Giugliani R (2007) Correlation of MR imaging and MR spectroscopy findings with cognitive impairment in mucopolysaccharidosis II. AJNR Am J Neuroradiol 28(6):1029–1033
49. Vellodi A (2004) Lysosomal storage disorders. Br J Haematol 128:413–431
50. Vinchon M, Cotten A, Clarisse J, Chiki R, Christiaens JL (1995) Cervical myelopathy secondary to Hunter syndrome in an adult. AJNR Am J Neuroradiol 16(7):1402–1403
51. Visocchi M, Di Rocco F, Meglio M (2003) Craniocervical junction instability: instrumentation and fusion with titanium rods and sublaminar wires. Effectiveness and failures in personal experience. Acta Neurochir (Wien) 145(4):265–272, discussion 272
52. Weisstein JS, Delgado E, Steinbach LS, Hart K, Packman S (2004) Musculoskeletal manifestations of Hurler syndrome: long-term follow-up after bone marrow transplantation. J Pediatr Orthop 24(1):97–101
53. White KK, Steinman S, Mubarak SJ (2009) Cervical stenosis and spastic quadriparesis in Morquio disease (MPS IV). A case report with twenty-six-year follow-up. J Bone Joint Surg Am 91(2):438–442
54. Wraith JE, Alani SM (1990) Carpal tunnel syndrome in the mucopolysaccharidoses and related disorders. Arch Dis Child 65(9):962–963
55. Wright NM (2004) Posterior C2 fixation using bilateral, crossing C2 laminar screws: case series and technical note. J Spinal Disord Tech 17(2):158–162
56. Yamazaki M, Akazawa T, Koda M, Okawa A (2006) Surgical simulation of instrumented posterior occipitocervical fusion in a child with congenital skeletal anomaly: case report. Spine (Phila Pa 1976) 31(17):E590–E594

Pediatric Craniovertebral Junction Trauma

Mark E. Oppenlander, Justin C. Clark, Volker K.H. Sonntag, and Nicholas Theodore

Contents

M.E. Oppenlander, MD • J.C. Clark, MD • V.K.H. Sonntag, MD
N. Theodore, MD (✉)
Division of Neurological Surgery, Barrow Neurological Institute, St. Joseph's Hospital and Medical Center, 350 W Thomas Rd, Phoenix, AZ 85013, USA
e-mail: neuropub@dignityhealth.org

C. Di Rocco, N. Akalan (eds.), *Pediatric Craniovertebral Junction Diseases*, Advances and Technical Standards in Neurosurgery 40,
DOI 10.1007/978-3-319-01065-6_12, © Springer International Publishing Switzerland 2014

Abstract The craniovertebral junction consists of the occiput, atlas, and axis, along with their strong ligamentous attachments. Because of its unique anatomical considerations, trauma to the craniovertebral junction requires specialized care. Children with potential injuries to the craniovertebral junction and cervical spinal cord demand specific considerations compared to adult patients. Prehospital immobilization techniques, diagnostic studies, and spinal injury patterns among young children can be different from those in adults. This review highlights the unique aspects in diagnosis and management of children with real or potential craniovertebral junction injuries.

Keywords Craniovertebral junction trauma • Pediatrics

Introduction

The craniovertebral junction, also referred to as the upper cervical spine, consists of the occiput, atlas, and axis, along with their strong ligamentous attachments. This osseoligamentous complex surrounds the brainstem, upper cervical spine, and vertebral arteries. Because of its unique anatomical considerations, trauma to the craniovertebral junction requires specialized care.

Cervical spine trauma is rare in children and accounts for approximately 1.5 % of pediatric trauma admissions [65], but the medical and social expenses of severe pediatric cervical spine trauma may be widely disproportionate to this small percentage [91–93]. Injuries to the upper cervical spine in particular are associated with a high rate of neurologic injury and mortality in children. Early detection and treatment can significantly decrease mortality and improve overall outcomes.

Children with potential injuries to the craniovertebral junction and cervical spinal cord demand specific considerations compared to adult patients. Prehospital immobilization techniques [54], diagnostic studies [8, 71], and spinal injury patterns [48, 49] among young children can be different from those in adults. Understanding the unique anatomical and radiographic characteristics of the pediatric craniovertebral junction is therefore essential to treat these patients appropriately. This chapter highlights the unique aspects of diagnosis and management of children with real or potential craniovertebral junction injuries.

Demographics

Upper cervical spine injuries account for 56–73 % of all cervical spine injuries in children [3, 77]. They are most often the result of blunt trauma [65]. Males outnumber females by at least 1.5:1 [7, 23, 65]. Motor vehicle-related accidents are the most common mechanism of injury in children, accounting for 48–61 % of all pediatric cervical spine injuries [23, 65]. Of these, injuries to occupants of the motor vehicle predominate over those to pedestrians or bicycle riders [7, 23, 65].

Other mechanisms of injury to the craniovertebral junction in children include falls, sports injuries, nonaccidental trauma, and penetrating injuries [7, 23, 65]. Falls account for 18–30 % of cervical spine injuries in children less than 8 years old and 11 % in children older than 8 years [23, 65]. In contrast, sports-related injuries are more prevalent in the older-age group (20–38 %) and uncommon in the younger-age group (3 %) [23, 65]. Nonaccidental trauma is a less common cause of craniovertebral injury in very young children, and penetrating injuries occur but are uncommon in adolescents [7, 13].

A series of 1,098 pediatric cervical spine injury patients highlighted the prevalence and morbidity of upper cervical spine injuries [65]. Upper cervical spine injuries (C1–C4) were almost twice as common as lower cervical spine injuries (C5–C7). Younger (age ≤8 years) and older (age >8 years) children sustained almost equal rates of upper cervical spine injuries (42 % versus 58 %, respectively). Spinal cord injury occurred in 35 % of pediatric cervical spine injuries, but nearly half of these injuries demonstrated no radiographic evidence of bony injury. Seventy-five percent of spinal cord injuries were incomplete and 25 % were complete. The associated mortality rate of upper cervical spine injury was almost 6-fold greater than that of lower cervical injury. The highest mortality rate was associated with occipitoatlantal dislocation (48 %) [65].

Developmental Anatomy

Grasping the embryology and developmental anatomy of the pediatric upper cervical spine aids conceptualization of its biomechanical properties and interpretation of its imaging. The vertebral bodies undergo chondrification around the fifth or sixth week of gestation [9]. Ossification centers appear in the vertebral bodies by the fourth month, and ossification continues through adolescence. The body of each vertebra develops from fusion of the dorsal and ventral ossification centers, occurring by the 24th week of gestation [32].

In the atlas, ossification of the anterior arch begins by age 3 months in 33 % of children and by 1 year in 81 % of children [94]. Ossification of the posterior arch is complete by 3 years of age. The synchondroses between the body and the posterior elements fuse by age 7 years (Fig. 1) [27].

The axis is unique because two additional ossification centers are present and fuse in the midline to form the odontoid process. The body of C2 fuses to the odontoid between ages 3 and 6 years. The fusion line is often visible until the age of 11 years and remains visible throughout life in one-third of the population [27]. The C2 posterior arches fuse in the midline by age 2–3 years and fuse with the vertebral body by age 3–6 years. Secondary ossification centers appear at the apex of the odontoid, fusing with the dens around age 12 years, and at the inferior end plate of C2, fusing with the vertebral body by age 25 years (Fig. 2) [56].

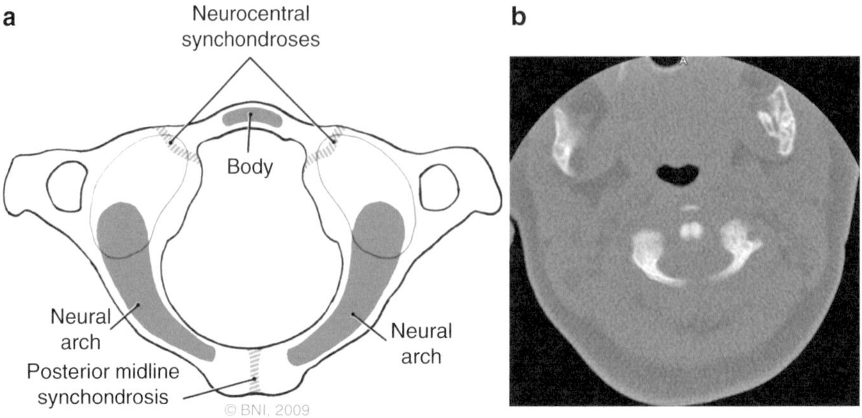

Fig. 1 (**a**) Illustration showing the ossification centers and synchondroses of the atlas. The neural arch ossification centers form during the seventh gestational week, whereas the ossification center within the body of C1 becomes visible during the first year of life. The posterior midline synchondrosis fuses at about the third year of life, while the neurocentral synchondroses about the atlas body fuse around the age of 7 years. (**b**) Correlative axial CT from a 24-week-old child (Used with permission from Barrow Neurological Institute)

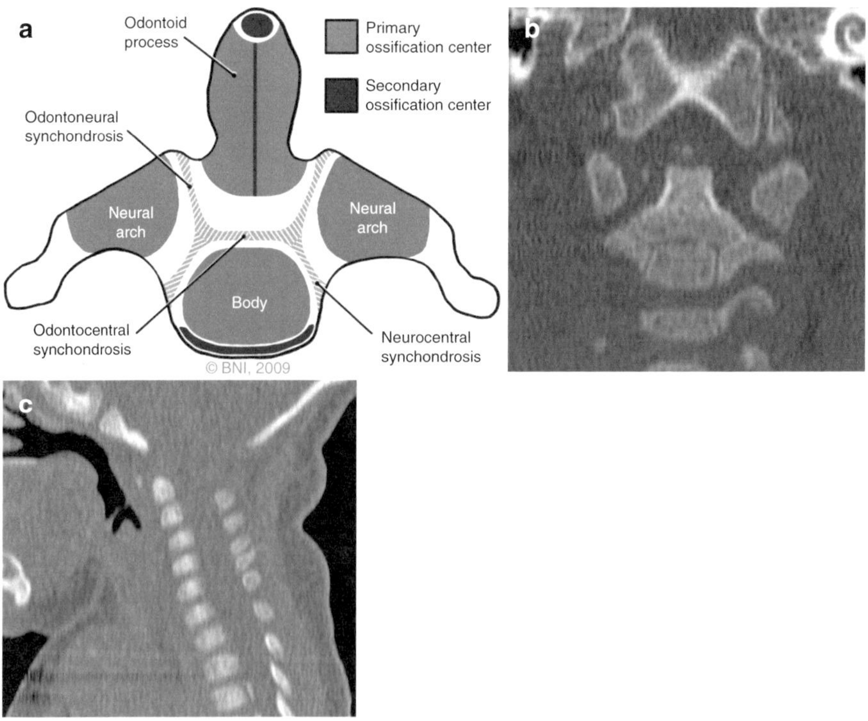

Imaging Characteristics of the Immature Craniovertebral Junction

Imaging findings of the immature craniovertebral junction can be confused for pathologic conditions, secondary to incomplete ossification and physiologic hypermobility in this region. The atlantodens interval (ADI), for example, should be <5 mm in the pediatric cervical spine [96], compared with the <3 mm guideline for the adult population. This exaggeration in the ADI may reflect incomplete ossification of the dens and laxity of the transverse ligament. Overriding of the arch of C1 on the dens during extension can also be mistaken for atlantoaxial instability, but this finding is normal in 20 % of children under 8 years old [11].

Physiologic C1 lateral mass displacement in the pediatric population may also be exaggerated. Up to 6 mm of C1 lateral mass displacement is common in children <4 years of age, and it may be present until the age of 7 years [47, 83]. A C1 lateral mass displacement >6.9 mm on open-mouth views may indicate transverse ligament disruption in adults, although magnetic resonance imaging (MRI) has demonstrated that the sensitivity of this technique is low [16, 79].

Synchondroses in the pediatric population can be mistaken for fracture lines, whereas fractures through synchondroses can be misinterpreted as within normal limits. The dens-C2 body synchondrosis can be mistaken for a type II dens fracture in children, but this synchondrosis is well corticated and lies below the level of the superior facets of C2. Conversely, a fracture through the dens-C2 body synchondrosis can be missed in pediatric patients [75], despite it being the most common injury to involve the odontoid process in children <7 years old [4, 73]. C1 synchondroses also can be misinterpreted as fractures or sites of abnormal separation [41].

Biomechanical Considerations in the Developing Craniovertebral Junction

The pediatric craniovertebral junction demonstrates an age-dependent hypermobility resulting from underdeveloped bony anatomy, ligaments, and musculature. Furthermore, a child's proportionally larger head enables a larger moment arm to

Fig. 2 (**a**) Illustration showing the ossification centers and synchondroses of the axis. Two ossification centers fuse in the midline to form the odontoid process by the seventh gestational month. The body of C2 fuses to the odontoid between ages 3 and 6 years. The neurocentral synchondroses also fuse between ages 3 and 6 years. The secondary ossification center at the apex of the odontoid appears between ages 6 and 8 years and fuses with the dens around the age of 12 years. (**b**) Correlative coronal CT from a 6-month-old child shows the synchondrosis between the odontoid and body of C2, the neurocentral synchondroses, and an early apical ossification center for the odontoid. (**c**) Correlative sagittal CT from a 24-week-old child shows the synchondrosis between the odontoid and body of C2. Note the absence of an apical ossification center (Used with permission from Barrow Neurological Institute) act on the underdeveloped spine. Biomechanical studies of the pediatric craniovertebral junction and upper cervical spine, however, are rare in comparison with the extensive published studies on biomechanics in the adult population.

Large series demonstrate that the occipitoatlantoaxial complex appears especially vulnerable in the young-age group (0–8 years), with a tendency toward pure ligamentous injuries rather than fractures [23, 65]. The craniovertebral junction is vulnerable in young children for several reasons:

1. The occipital condyles are smaller.
2. The occipital articulation with the lateral masses of C1 is more planar than cuplike, and it is biased toward the axial plane [24, 95].
3. The fulcrum of flexion is placed in the craniovertebral junction due to the relatively large head size and hypermobility of the upper cervical spine [27, 95].
4. The odontoid synchondrosis is susceptible to translational forces.

Because of these unique characteristics of the child's craniovertebral junction, care for the pediatric trauma patient must be provided with a high index of suspicion for injury to this region.

Patient Presentation and Evaluation

Presentation and Prehospital Immobilization

In pediatric patients with potential craniovertebral junction injury, immediate goals in the field are to establish an airway, obtain adequate ventilation, and provide cardiovascular support. Because considerable force is required to cause significant craniovertebral junction injury, patients may present with head, spinal cord, or multisystem traumatic injuries. Vertebral artery injury or cranial nerve deficits may be present. However, some patients with craniovertebral injury may have no neurologic deficits [38].

The primary goal of immediate spinal immobilization is to prevent further injury. Immobilization should be accomplished with the child's cervical spine in the neutral position. In children less than 8 years of age, consideration must be given to the relatively large head compared to the torso, which forces the neck into flexion when the child is placed supine on a flat surface. Of 40 children less than 8 years of age assessed by Nypaver and Treloar, all required elevation of the torso to achieve neutral alignment [54]. A cervical collar did not prevent the induced flexion when a flat spinal board was used [86]. Authors have therefore recommended either elevating the torso or placing the head in an occipital recess to achieve neutral position during immobilization of a pediatric patient [37, 54]. If occipitoatlantal dislocation is suspected, sandbags and tape should be used for initial immobilization of the head. Rigid cervical collars can lead to further distraction of the occipitoatlantal joint [18].

Clinical Clearance of the Cervical Spine

After the pediatric trauma victim has been immobilized and transported to an acute care facility, and following the initial clinical assessment and provision of cardiorespiratory support, evaluation of the cervical spine may begin. After a cervical collar has been placed on a child, formal clearance must be obtained before it can be removed. Certain low-risk children may not need imaging to exclude cervical spine injury [44, 90]. In 268 children with isolated head injuries, Laham et al. investigated the role of cervical 3-view (anteroposterior, lateral, and open mouth) spine x-rays [44]. Patients with isolated head injuries who were able to communicate and who had no neck pain or neurologic deficits were retrospectively classified as low risk ($n = 135$). High-risk patients were those incapable of verbal communication, because of either age (<2 years) or head injury, and those with neck pain ($n = 133$). After radiographic evaluation, no injuries were found in the low-risk group, but 10 injuries were discovered in the high-risk group. The authors concluded that cervical spine radiographs are not necessary in children with isolated head injuries who can communicate and have no neck pain or neurologic deficit [44].

Consistent with these results, Vicellio et al. prospectively evaluated the cervical spines of 3,065 children less than 18 years of age [90]. They identified 603 low-risk children, defined as those with the absence of each of the following criteria: midline cervical tenderness, evidence of intoxication, altered level of alertness or intubation, focal neurologic deficits, and painful distracting injury. After undergoing a three-view radiographic evaluation, none of these low-risk children had a documented cervical spine injury. The authors concluded that the collar may be clinically cleared without further imaging in patients meeting these low-risk criteria.

Imaging

Plain radiography has been used as the first imaging modality for the upper cervical spine, and pediatric patients who do not meet the above low-risk criteria should undergo at least anteroposterior and lateral x-rays. The utility of open-mouth odontoid views in pediatric trauma victims has been questioned [8, 84]. In young children, Swischuk et al. identified missed fractures on lateral views that were detected on open-mouth views at a rate of 0.007 per year per radiologist. They concluded that open-mouth view radiographs may not be needed routinely in young children (age <5 years) [84]. Buhs et al. found that open-mouth radiographs did not provide the diagnosis in any of 15 children less than 9 years of age who sustained cervical spinal injuries [8]. They concluded that open-mouth view radiographs are not necessary in children <9 years old.

Computed tomography (CT) provides superior detail of bony anatomy in comparison with plain radiography, but the role of CT in evaluating the cervical spines of pediatric trauma patients has not been well studied. Hutchings et al. retrospectively reviewed cervical spine clearance methods in 115 consecutive obtunded trauma patients <16 years old [40]. Both the sensitivity and specificity of CT for injury detection were 100 %, although a low incidence of injury in this population makes interpretation of these results difficult. When obtaining a CT, it is important to consider that most children younger than 10 years old with cervical spine injuries will have ligamentous injuries without a fracture [19, 34]. In older children with cervical spine injuries, the incidence of a ligamentous injury without fracture (20 %) is still significant, although less than the incidence of fracture (80 %) in this population [25, 90]. Therefore, normal osseous anatomy on CT imaging alone should not be used to exclude injury to the pediatric cervical spine.

As proposed by Pang, the condyle-C1 interval (CCI) as determined on CT is a sensitive diagnostic measurement of occipitoatlantal dislocation [60, 61]. Pang et al. analyzed the CCI from sagittal and coronal CT images of the craniovertebral junction from 89 children without occipitoatlantal dislocation and 16 children with occipitoatlantal dislocation. The abnormal CCI varied from 5 to 34 mm, and eight patients showed left-right joint asymmetry. Compared to "standard" tests on plain films with a sensitivity that ranged between 25 and 50 % and a specificity that ranged between 10 and 60 %, the CCI of 4 mm or greater had a sensitivity and specificity of 100 %. They concluded that the CCI criterion has the highest diagnostic sensitivity and specificity for occipitoatlantal dislocation among all radiographic methods [60].

MRI is superior to CT in delineating nonosseous anatomy. It can provide important information about ligamentous injury and influence surgical management. Keiper et al. reviewed their experience with MRI in the evaluation of children with clinical evidence of cervical spine trauma and no evidence of fracture on plain radiographs or CT, but who had persistent or delayed symptoms or instability [42]. In 52 children, 16 MRI examinations were abnormal. Of these 52 children, 4 underwent surgical treatment, and in each of these surgical cases, the MRI findings influenced the surgeon to stabilize more levels than would have otherwise been addressed. MRI can also provide prognostic information regarding existing neurological deficits. Davis et al. used MRI to evaluate pediatric spinal cord injury in 15 patients [15]. They found that MRI findings correlated with neurological outcome; hematomyelia was associated with permanent neurologic deficit [15].

We use MRI whenever a neurologic deficit is present and to assess the extent of ligamentous involvement of craniovertebral junction injuries. We have a low threshold for obtaining MRIs of the cervical spine in obtunded children with mechanisms of injury that are high risk for injury to the craniovertebral junction. However, MRI is a static test and does not necessarily predict cervical spine instability [39]. The extent of injury demonstrated on MRI can be used to guide management (Fig. 3).

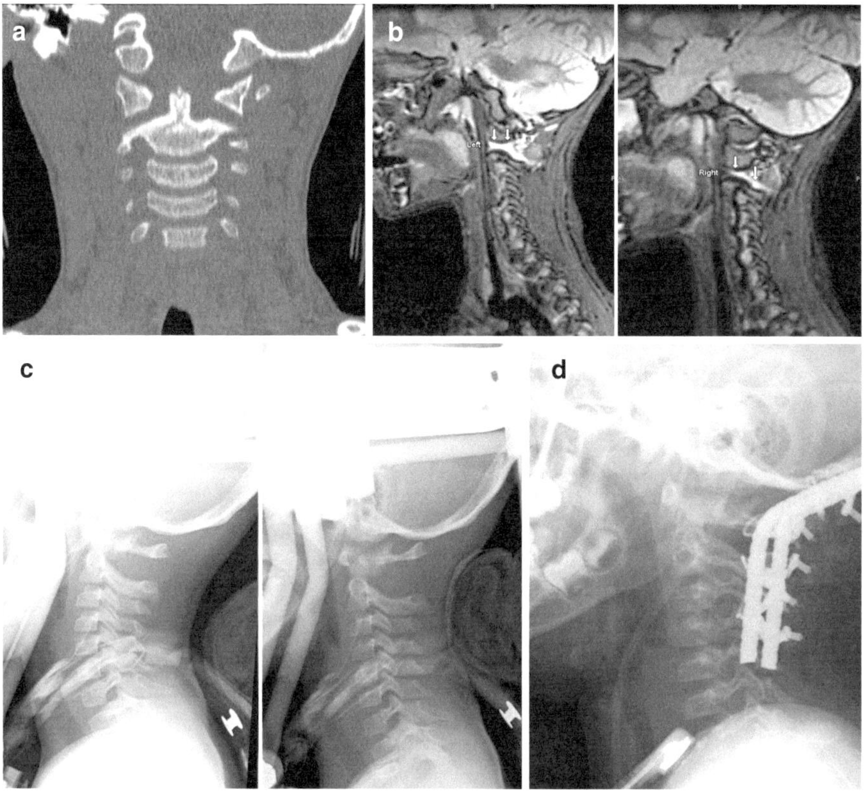

Fig. 3 (**a**) Coronal CT from a 4-year-old girl who was an unrestrained passenger in a motor vehicle accident, demonstrating widening of the bilateral atlantoaxial joints. (**b**) Sagittal MRI short T1-weighted inversion recovery (STIR) images show signal changes within the bilateral atlanto-axial joints and within the right occipitoatlantal joint. (**c**) Halo immobilization was unsuccessful as evidenced by persistent vertical translocation at C1–C2 between upright (*left*) and supine (*right*) films. (**d**) Surgical stabilization was achieved with occiput-to-C4 titanium rod fixation and autograft fusion (Used with permission from Barrow Neurological Institute)

Pediatric Spinal Cord Injury

The upper cervical spinal cord is particularly vulnerable to injury in children <8 years old, secondary to ligamentous injury often with no overt bony fractures [23, 65]. A thorough neurologic examination should be performed to identify the level of injury and to determine whether the injury is complete or incomplete. Sacral sparing should be tested, because it indicates continuity of long tracts and is associated with an improved likelihood for a return of neurologic function [50]. Upper cervical cord injuries may be fatal, and patients who do survive these injuries may be dependent on a respirator.

An acute nonoperative management consideration for pediatric spinal cord injury is maintenance of adequate mean arterial pressure. Hypotension should be avoided, and the mean arterial blood pressure should be elevated to protect spinal cord blood perfusion and to prevent ischemia [87]. Unlike blood pressure management, however, the use of high-dose steroids to treat spinal cord injury is controversial. There are few data on the use of methylprednisolone specific to pediatric patients. The National Acute Spinal Cord Injury study excluded all children younger than 13 years old, and based on the experience in adults, the use of methylprednisolone cannot be recommended [6, 33].

Spinal Cord Injury Without Radiographic Abnormality

The biomechanical properties of the craniovertebral junction in children <8 years old place them at risk for spinal cord injury without radiographic abnormality (SCIWORA) [23]. This syndrome was described by Pang and Wilberger in 1982 [63]. A meta-analysis conducted by Pang found the incidence of SCIWORA in pediatric patients with spinal cord injury to be about 35 % [58]. With more widespread use of MRI and with improvements in imaging quality, the incidence has been reported to be as low as 3 % [2]. The physiologic basis of SCIWORA is the hypermobility of the pediatric cervical spine. Traumatic hyperflexion, hyperextension, or distraction will cause the spine to recoil to its physiologic state, while the spinal cord sustains injury from temporary compression and deformation [58]. Children <8 years old are considerably more likely to sustain more rostral and severe SCIWORA than older children [20].

MRI is the modality of choice for patients with suspected SCIWORA. In the clinical setting of SCIWORA, injuries to extraneural structures as well as to the spinal cord have been documented on MRI. The patient's MRI examination may also be completely normal. Pang divided MRI findings within the spinal cord of 50 patients with clinical SCIWORA into the following categories: major hemorrhage, minor hemorrhage, edema, and no abnormality [58]. The severity of MRI findings correlated positively with severity of neurologic deficits. Pang also proposed the concept of "occult" instability of the spine in SCIWORA patients [58], which has been postulated to be a cause of delayed neurologic deterioration in these patients [57, 58]. Occult instability is also a possible cause of recurrent SCIWORA, in which minor trauma after an initial SCIWORA episode causes recurrent symptoms [67]. Presumably, weakened extraneural structures may facilitate recurrence, and the injured spinal cord is more vulnerable to repeat trauma.

Therapeutic immobilization of patients with SCIWORA is controversial. Pang and Pollack advocated 12 weeks of immobilization to allow ligamentous injuries to heal and to prevent recurrent SCIWORA [62]. Bosch et al., however, found that immobilization did not prevent SCIWORA recurrence [5]. A meta-analysis by Launay et al. showed that patients immobilized for 8 weeks had a 17 % chance of developing recurrent SCIWORA, but no patients immobilized for 12 weeks demonstrated SCIWORA recurrence [45]. These data suggest that 12 weeks of immobilization is appropriate for most cases of SCIWORA, followed by dynamic films to detect instability.

Neonatal Spinal Cord Injury

Birth injuries of the spinal cord occur in approximately 1 per 60,000 births [90]. The upper cervical spine is the most common level of injury, and neonates present with apnea and flaccid quadriplegia [48, 52]. Menticoglou et al. reported 15 neonates with birth-related upper cervical spinal cord injuries [52]. All were associated with cephalic presentation requiring rotational maneuvers with forceps, and all but one child was apneic at birth with quadriplegia. In another report, Mackinnon et al. described 22 neonates with birth-related spinal cord injuries; 14 of whom had upper cervical injuries [48]. Of the seven infants alive at last follow-up, six were dependent on mechanical ventilation. A thermoplastic molded device spanning the occiput to the thorax has been used for spinal immobilization in these difficult patients [35].

Osseoligamentous Injuries of the Pediatric Craniovertebral Junction

Occipitoatlantal and Atlantoaxial Dislocation

Traumatic occipitoatlantoaxial dislocations (OAAD) were once thought to be rare and predominantly fatal entities [53, 82]. Improvements in on-site resuscitation and transportation have increased the number of patients surviving these injuries [53, 64]. Often seen in young children involved in high-speed motor vehicle accidents, complete neurologic injury at this level usually results in rapid death. Therefore, neurologic deficits associated with OAAD are partial or absent.

In terms of distraction injuries, the occipitoatlantoaxial complex can be regarded as one unit [51]. Because the occipitoatlantoaxial ligaments span the occipital-C1 and the C1–C2 segments, instability should affect both segments. Neither the C0–C1 and C1–C2 joint capsules nor the atlantooccipital and atlantoaxial membranes contribute significantly to the vertical stability of the craniovertebral junction [96]. Rather, the tectorial ligament, alar ligaments, and surrounding musculature appear to have the largest roles in stabilizing this segment [21, 96]. As discussed earlier, younger children are uniquely predisposed to OAAD because their occipital articulation with the lateral masses of C1 is more planar than cuplike and because a young child has a relatively larger head and greater hypermobility of the upper cervical spine compared to older patients [27, 95].

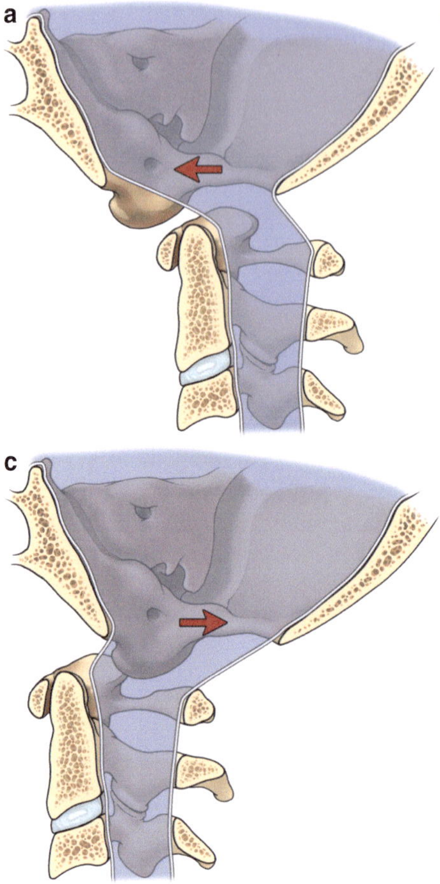

Fig. 4 Drawings representing the classification for occipitoatlantal dislocation. (**a**) Type I: anterior displacement (*arrow*) of the occiput with respect to the atlas. (**b**) Type II: distraction and vertical displacement (*arrow*). (**c**) Type III: posterior displacement (*arrow*) (Used with permission from Barrow Neurological Institute)

Traynelis et al. classically divided occipitoatlantal dislocation into three types (Fig. 4) [85]. The direction of dislocation of the occiput with respect to the atlas determines the type of injury. Type I injury describes an anterior displacement of the occiput with respect to the atlas. Type II injury is a distraction injury with vertical displacement. Type III injury involves posterior displacement of the occiput.

The diagnosis of OAAD requires a high index of suspicion, especially in a child involved in a high-speed motor vehicle accident or auto-pedestrian accident. None of the criteria for diagnosis of OAAD are failproof. Classic measurements on plain radiography to assess OAAD include Power's ratio [68], the basion-dens interval [97], basion-axial interval [36], and atlantodens interval [46]. The accuracy of these traditional radiographic criteria has been questioned. Reconstructed coronal and sagittal CT images can be used to assess the joint-space separation and symmetry at

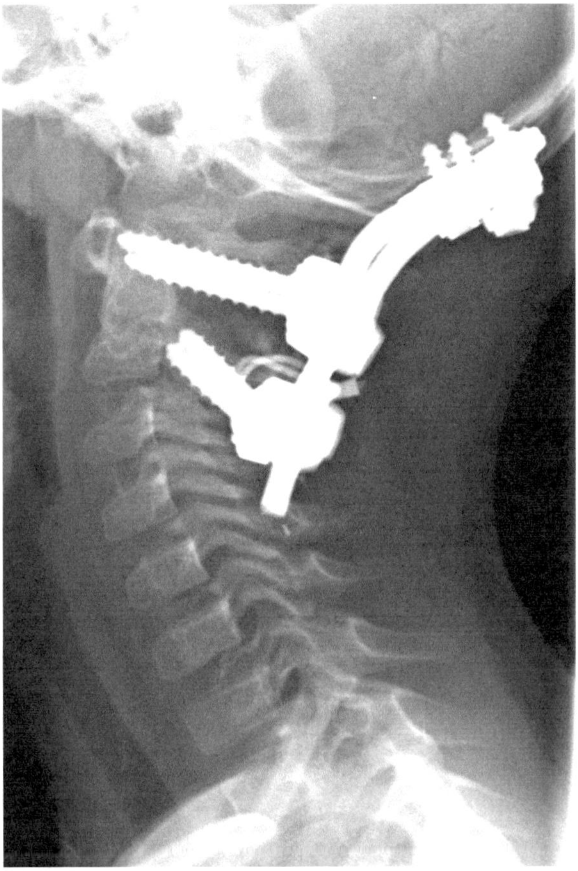

Fig. 5 Postoperative lateral radiograph of a 3-year-old girl with occipitoatlantoaxial dislocation, fixated with occipital keel screws, C1 lateral mass screws, and C2 pars interarticularis screws (Used with permission from Barrow Neurological Institute)

C0–C1 and C1–C2. A condyle-C1 interval (CCI) >4 mm as measured on CT may indicate occipitoatlantal dislocation [30, 60]. MRI can further define abnormalities of joints, ligaments, and soft tissues at C0–C1 and C1–C2. The integrity of the tectorial membrane on MRI may be a critical factor in determining severity of both occipitoatlantal and atlantoaxial joint injuries [82]. MRI also accurately depicts the anatomical integrity of the transverse ligament, which has been proposed as a criterion for early fusion for atlantoaxial instability [17].

Initial management of OAAD involves placement of the child into a halo vest. Traction and a cervical collar should be avoided, because these can lead to overdistraction and worsening of neurologic injury [18]. Definitive treatment of OAAD requires surgical fusion. Threaded contoured rods and wiring can be used from the occiput to C1 or C2, depending on the injury [74]. We have successfully used the rod-and-wire technique in children as young as 11 months [69]. Transarticular screws of C1–C2 or C2 pedicle screws, coupled with plate or rod constructs, have also been used in pediatric patients with excellent success [31, 74]. We have used occipital keel screws coupled with C1 lateral mass screws and C2 pars interarticularis screws to achieve occipitoatlantoaxial stabilization in young pediatric patients (Fig. 5).

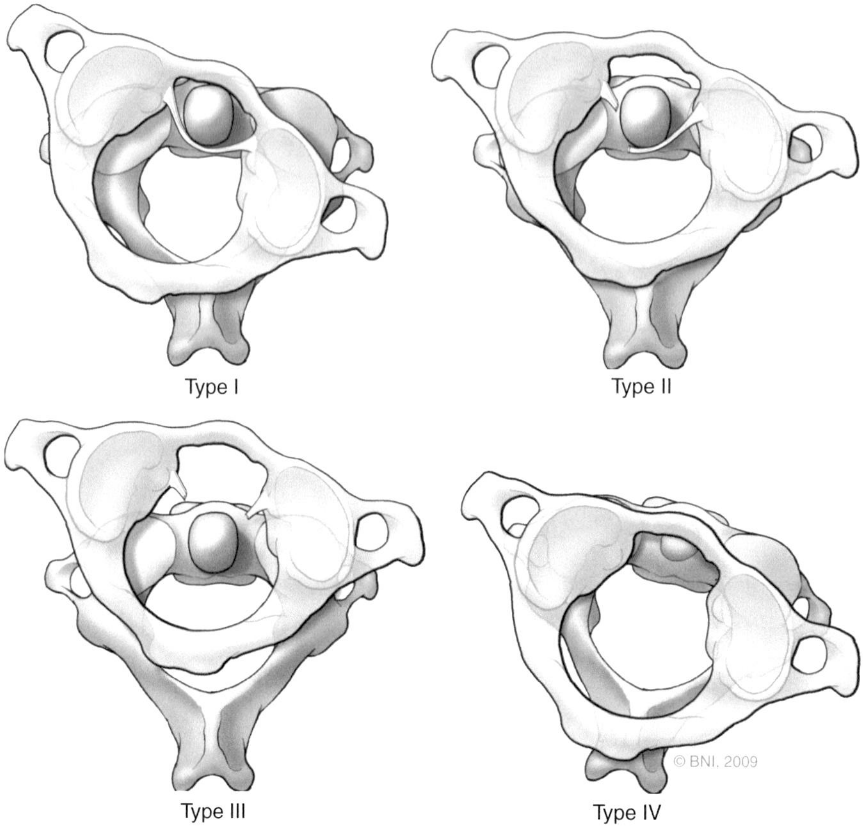

Fig. 6 Fielding and Hawkins classification scheme for atlantoaxial rotatory injuries. *Type I* is defined by an intact transverse ligament. *Types II* and *III* are defined by disruption of the transverse ligament alone and the transverse and alar ligaments, respectively. These injuries are associated with a progressively widened atlantodens interval. *Type IV* injury is a posterior rotatory displacement of the atlas on C2 in the setting of odontoid hypoplasia (Used with permission from Barrow Neurological Institute)

Atlantoaxial Rotatory Subluxation

Atlantoaxial rotatory subluxation is a frequent cause of torticollis in children. If it has persisted for more than 3 months, it is also known as atlantoaxial rotatory fixation. Trauma and upper respiratory infections are the main causes of this disorder, but iatrogenic and congenital causes also exist. The mechanism of injury is often trivial trauma resulting in subluxation of C1 on C2. Children present with a "cock-robin" appearance with the head tilted toward and rotated away from the side of the dislocation. With acute subluxation, a child presents with accompanying neck pain. If fixed persistent deformities are present, the pain often subsides.

Fielding and Hawkins presented the most commonly used classification scheme for these injuries (Fig. 6) [28]. Type I atlantoaxial rotatory injury is defined by an intact transverse ligament. Types II and III are defined by disruption of the transverse ligament alone and by the transverse and alar ligaments, respectively. These injuries are associated with a progressively widened atlantodens interval (ADI). Type IV injury is a posterior rotatory displacement of the atlas on C2 in the setting of odontoid hypoplasia.

Radiographs can be challenging to obtain and interpret because of the positioning in a patient with torticollis, but asymmetry of the lateral masses will be present on the open-mouth view. Dynamic CT and three-dimensional CT are the best means of demonstrating the condition [70, 72]. The atlas will be superimposed on the axis in a rotated position.

Several studies highlight the ease and success of nonsurgical management of these injuries when the subluxation is treated early rather than late [22, 34, 81]. Delays in treatment of atlantoaxial rotatory subluxation lead to worsening C1–C2 adherence [66]. Severity and chronicity of these injuries are associated with longer treatment, a greater chance of recurrence, higher rates of irreducibility, greater need for surgical stabilization, and higher rates of complete C1–C2 motion segment loss [59]. In cases of atlantoaxial rotatory subluxation that have endured more than 1 month, halo traction can be used to attempt reduction [10, 66]. After documentation of reduction by CT, the patient should remain in a halo vest for up to 3 months. First recurrences in the orthosis are treated with repeat traction and immobilization. During or after halo vest immobilization, irreducible deformity or recurrence is treated with posterior surgical fixation and fusion of C1–C2.

Odontoid Epiphysiolysis

The synchondrosis between the body of C2 and the dens may not fuse completely in children <7 years old and represents a vulnerable site of injury in young children [4, 76]. Falls and high-speed motor vehicle accidents, especially with children secured in forward-facing car seats, have been implicated in this injury pattern [55]. The lateral cervical spine radiograph will reveal an odontoid process angulated anteriorly or, rarely, posteriorly [76]. Reconstructed CT scans may show widening of the synchondrosis, and MRI can assist diagnosis of minimally displaced fractures by depicting bone and soft tissue edema at the fracture site (Fig. 7).

Treatment for C2 epiphyseal injuries is primarily via external immobilization [49, 55, 76]. Fassett et al. reported a meta-analysis of 55 odontoid synchondrosis fractures, in which closed reduction and immobilization were initially performed in 45 cases [26]. Stable fusion resulted in 42 (93 %) of these cases. Most of the patients were immobilized with a halo or Minerva jacket. Surgical fusion was performed in eight cases: four as initial treatment, three after failure of external orthosis, and one after a delayed diagnosis. The fusion procedures included 6 posterior C1–C2 fusions, one odontoid screw, and one temporary posterior wiring; all achieved stable fusion without complications. Therefore, closed reduction and immobilization offer the advantages of excellent results and preservation of the motion segment, but surgical fixation may be necessary when nonoperative treatment fails.

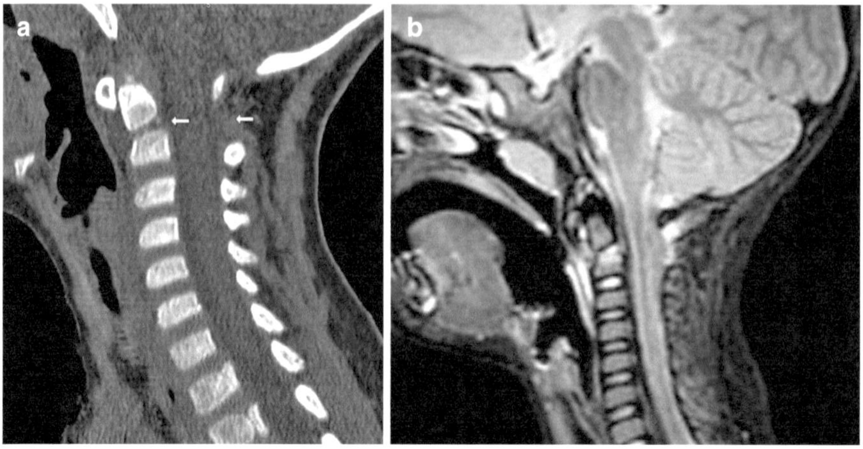

Fig. 7 (**a**) Sagittal CT of a 3-year-old boy who was a restrained passenger in a motor vehicle accident shows disruption of the synchondrosis between the odontoid process and body of C2. Note the widening of the posterior elements of C1 and C2. (**b**) Sagittal short T1-weighted inversion recovery (STIR) MRI confirms fracture across the odontoid synchondrosis and posterior ligamentous injury at C1–C2 (Used with permission from Barrow Neurological Institute)

Os Odontoideum

Os odontoideum is an ossicle of bone with smooth circumferential cortical margins separated from the foreshortened odontoid peg. Two anatomic types exist: orthotopic and dystopic [1, 88]. An orthotopic os moves in unison with the anterior arch of C1. It can therefore be reduced to be aligned normally with the dens. A dystopic os has migrated toward the clivus and is functionally fused to the basion. The etiology of os odontoideum has been documented as traumatic or congenital [14, 89]. Although controversy exists over the natural history of os odontoideum, this complex is believed to result in an incompetent cruciate ligament and subsequent atlantoaxial instability [1].

Patients can present within a wide spectrum of symptomatology. They may complain of occipitocervical pain, presumably from underlying atlantoaxial instability. Varying degrees of myelopathy can be found, ranging from transient symptoms to frank tetraplegia. The myelopathy is likely related to spinal cord compression secondary to the morphology of the foramen magnum and size of the upper cervical canal. A sagittal diameter of the spinal canal ≤13 mm on plain x-rays has been strongly associated with myelopathy [78, 80]. Patients with os odontoideum also may be asymptomatic and present incidentally.

The initial diagnosis can be made via plain cervical spine radiographs with open-mouth, anteroposterior, and lateral views. Flexion-extension films are useful for evaluation of atlantoaxial instability. CT best visualizes bony anatomy and can aid operative planning if needed. MRI will assess spinal cord compression and ligamentous anatomy [12, 14, 88].

The management of os odontoideum has been debated in the literature. Spierings and Braakman reported nonoperative management of 16 patients with os odontoideum without myelopathy [80]. At a median follow-up of 7 years, no patient had suffered neurologic deterioration. However, authors have documented a potential for neurologic injury, decompensation, and even death in asymptomatic children who have been followed conservatively [12, 29, 43]. Surgical decision making therefore requires careful consideration in these patients. Many authors agree that patients with an unstable os odontoideum or those with a fixed deformity compressing the spinal cord should be offered surgery for C1–C2 arthrodesis [1, 43].

Conclusions

Special consideration must be given to pediatric trauma victims suspected of sustaining injury to the craniovertebral junction. Understanding the unique anatomy, biomechanics, and imaging characteristics of the pediatric craniovertebral junction is essential to managing injuries involving this region. There are many areas for further investigation, including epidemiological data that could help improve methods of prevention, prospective analyses defining the indications and methods for cervical spine clearance in young children, and studies indicating the incidence and clinical significance of complications of craniovertebral junction injuries. Because of the relatively small number of pediatric craniovertebral junction injuries, future studies should be multi-institutional.

References

1. Arvin B, Fournier-Gosselin MP, Fehlings MG (2010) Os odontoideum: etiology and surgical management. Neurosurgery 66(3 Suppl):22–31
2. Bilston LE, Brown J (2007) Pediatric spinal injury type and severity are age and mechanism dependent. Spine (Phila Pa 1976) 32(21):2339–2347
3. Birney TJ, Hanley EN Jr (1989) Traumatic cervical spine injuries in childhood and adolescence. Spine (Phila Pa 1976) 14(12):1277–1282
4. Blauth M, Schmidt U, Otte D, Krettek C (1996) Fractures of the odontoid process in small children: biomechanical analysis and report of three cases. Eur Spine J 5(1):63–70
5. Bosch PP, Vogt MT, Ward WT (2002) Pediatric spinal cord injury without radiographic abnormality (SCIWORA): the absence of occult instability and lack of indication for bracing. Spine (Phila Pa 1976) 27(24):2788–2800
6. Bracken MB, Shepard MJ, Holford TR, Leo-Summers L, Aldrich EF, Fazl M et al (1997) Administration of methylprednisolone for 24 or 48 hours or tirilazad mesylate for 48 hours in the treatment of acute spinal cord injury. Results of the Third National Acute Spinal Cord Injury Randomized Controlled Trial. National Acute Spinal Cord Injury Study. JAMA 277(20): 1597–1604
7. Brown RL, Brunn MA, Garcia VF (2001) Cervical spine injuries in children: a review of 103 patients treated consecutively at a level 1 pediatric trauma center. J Pediatr Surg 36(8): 1107–1114

8. Buhs C, Cullen M, Klein M, Farmer D (2000) The pediatric trauma C-spine: is the 'odontoid' view necessary? J Pediatr Surg 35(6):994–997
9. Bullough PE, Boachie-Adjei O (1998) Atlas of spinal diseases. Lippincott Williams & Wilkins, New York
10. Burkus JK, Deponte RJ (1986) Chronic atlantoaxial rotatory fixation correction by cervical traction, manipulation, and bracing. J Pediatr Orthop 6(5):631–635
11. Cattell HS, Filtzer DL (1965) Pseudosubluxation and other normal variations in the cervical spine in children. A study of one hundred and sixty children. J Bone Joint Surg Am 47(7): 1295–1309
12. Choit RL, Jamieson DH, Reilly CW (2005) Os odontoideum: a significant radiographic finding. Pediatr Radiol 35(8):803–807
13. Cirak B, Ziegfeld S, Knight VM, Chang D, Avellino AM, Paidas CN (2004) Spinal injuries in children. J Pediatr Surg 39(4):607–612
14. Currarino G (2002) Segmentation defect in the midodontoid process and its possible relationship to the congenital type of os odontoideum. Pediatr Radiol 32(1):34–40
15. Davis PC, Reisner A, Hudgins PA, Davis WE, O'Brien MS (1993) Spinal injuries in children: role of MR. AJNR Am J Neuroradiol 14(3):607–617
16. Dickman CA, Greene KA, Sonntag VK (1996) Injuries involving the transverse atlantal ligament: classification and treatment guidelines based upon experience with 39 injuries. Neurosurgery 38(1):44–50
17. Dickman CA, Mamourian A, Sonntag VK, Drayer BP (1991) Magnetic resonance imaging of the transverse atlantal ligament for the evaluation of atlantoaxial instability. J Neurosurg 75(2):221–227
18. Dickman CA, Papadopoulos SM, Sonntag VK, Spetzler RF, Rekate HL, Drabier J (1993) Traumatic occipitoatlantal dislocations. J Spinal Disord 6(4):300–313
19. Dickman CA, Rekate HL, Sonntag VK, Zabramski JM (1989) Pediatric spinal trauma: vertebral column and spinal cord injuries in children. Pediatr Neurosci 15(5):237–255
20. Dickman CA, Zabramski JM, Hadley MN, Rekate HL, Sonntag VK (1991) Pediatric spinal cord injury without radiographic abnormalities: report of 26 cases and review of the literature. J Spinal Disord 4(3):296–305
21. Dvorak J, Schneider E, Saldinger P, Rahn B (1988) Biomechanics of the craniocervical region: the alar and transverse ligaments. J Orthop Res 6(3):452–461
22. El-Khoury GY, Clark CR, Gravett AW (1984) Acute traumatic rotatory atlanto-axial dislocation in children. A report of three cases. J Bone Joint Surg Am 66(5):774–777
23. Eleraky MA, Theodore N, Adams M, Rekate HL, Sonntag VK (2000) Pediatric cervical spine injuries: report of 102 cases and review of the literature. J Neurosurg 92(1 Suppl):12–17
24. Englander O (1942) Nontraumatic occipito-atlanto-axial dislocation. A contribution to the radiology of the atlas. Br J Radiol 15:341–345
25. Evans DL, Bethem D (1989) Cervical spine injuries in children. J Pediatr Orthop 9(5):563–568
26. Fassett DR, Clark R, Brockmeyer DL, Schmidt MH (2006) Cervical spine deformity associated with resection of spinal cord tumors. Neurosurg Focus 20(2):E2
27. Fesmire FM, Luten RC (1989) The pediatric cervical spine: developmental anatomy and clinical aspects. J Emerg Med 7(2):133–142
28. Fielding JW, Cochran GB, Lawsing JF III, Hohl M (1974) Tears of the transverse ligament of the atlas. A clinical and biomechanical study. J Bone Joint Surg Am 56(8):1683–1691
29. Fielding JW, Hensinger RN, Hawkins RJ (1980) Os odontoideum. J Bone Joint Surg Am 62(3):376–383
30. Gerlock AJ Jr, Mirfakhraee M, Benzel EC (1983) Computed tomography of traumatic atlanto-occipital dislocation. Neurosurgery 13(3):316–319
31. Gluf WM, Brockmeyer DL (2005) Atlantoaxial transarticular screw fixation: a review of surgical indications, fusion rate, complications, and lessons learned in 67 pediatric patients. J Neurosurg Spine 2(2):164–169
32. Grabb PA (1999) Spinal column trauma in children. In: Albright AL, Pollack IF, Adelson PD (eds) Principles and practice of pediatric neurosurgery. Thieme, New York, pp 935–953

33. Hadley MN, Walters BC, Grabb PA, Oyesiku NM, Przybylski GJ, Resnick DK et al (2002) Guidelines for the management of acute cervical spine and spinal cord injuries. Clin Neurosurg 49:407–498
34. Hamilton MG, Myles ST (1992) Pediatric spinal injury: review of 174 hospital admissions. J Neurosurg 77(5):700–704
35. Hanley PA (1990) Special problems of spinal stabilization in children. American Association of Neurological Surgeons, Park Ridge, IL
36. Harris JH Jr, Carson GC, Wagner LK (1994) Radiologic diagnosis of traumatic occipitovertebral dissociation: 1. Normal occipitovertebral relationships on lateral radiographs of supine subjects. AJR Am J Roentgenol 162(4):881–886
37. Herzenberg JE, Hensinger RN, Dedrick DK, Phillips WA (1989) Emergency transport and positioning of young children who have an injury of the cervical spine. The standard backboard may be hazardous. J Bone Joint Surg Am 71(1):15–22
38. Horn EM, Feiz-Erfan I, Lekovic GP, Dickman CA, Sonntag VK, Theodore N (2007) Survivors of occipitoatlantal dislocation injuries: imaging and clinical correlates. J Neurosurg Spine 6(2):113–120
39. Horn EM, Lekovic GP, Feiz-Erfan I, Sonntag VK, Theodore N (2004) Cervical magnetic resonance imaging abnormalities not predictive of cervical spine instability in traumatically injured patients. Invited submission from the Joint Section Meeting on Disorders of the Spine and Peripheral Nerves, March 2004. J Neurosurg Spine 1(1):39–42
40. Hutchings L, Atijosan O, Burgess C, Willett K (2009) Developing a spinal clearance protocol for unconscious pediatric trauma patients. J Trauma 67(4):681–686
41. Judd DB, Liem LK, Petermann G (2000) Pediatric atlas fracture: a case of fracture through a synchondrosis and review of the literature. Neurosurgery 46(4):991–994
42. Keiper MD, Zimmerman RA, Bilaniuk LT (1998) MRI in the assessment of the supportive soft tissues of the cervical spine in acute trauma in children. Neuroradiology 40(6):359–363
43. Klimo P Jr, Kan P, Rao G, Apfelbaum R, Brockmeyer D (2008) Os odontoideum: presentation, diagnosis, and treatment in a series of 78 patients. J Neurosurg Spine 9(4):332–342
44. Laham JL, Cotcamp DH, Gibbons PA, Kahana MD, Crone KR (1994) Isolated head injuries versus multiple trauma in pediatric patients: do the same indications for cervical spine evaluation apply? Pediatr Neurosurg 21(4):221–226
45. Launay F, Leet AI, Sponseller PD (2005) Pediatric spinal cord injury without radiographic abnormality: a meta-analysis. Clin Orthop Relat Res 433:166–170
46. Lui TN, Lee ST, Wong CW, Yeh YS, Tzaan WC, Chen TY et al (1996) C1-C2 fracture-dislocations in children and adolescents. J Trauma 40(3):408–411
47. Lustrin ES, Karakas SP, Ortiz AO, Cinnamon J, Castillo M, Vaheesan K et al (2003) Pediatric cervical spine: normal anatomy, variants, and trauma. Radiographics 23(3):539–560
48. MacKinnon JA, Perlman M, Kirpalani H, Rehan V, Sauve R, Kovacs L (1993) Spinal cord injury at birth: diagnostic and prognostic data in twenty-two patients. J Pediatr 122(3):431–437
49. Mandabach M, Ruge JR, Hahn YS, McLone DG (1993) Pediatric axis fractures: early halo immobilization, management and outcome. Pediatr Neurosurg 19(5):225–232
50. Marino RJ, Ditunno JF Jr, Donovan WH, Maynard F Jr (1999) Neurologic recovery after traumatic spinal cord injury: data from the Model Spinal Cord Injury Systems. Arch Phys Med Rehabil 80(11):1391–1396
51. Marshall KW, Koch BL, Egelhoff JC (1998) Air bag-related deaths and serious injuries in children: injury patterns and imaging findings. AJNR Am J Neuroradiol 19(9):1599–1607
52. Menticoglou SM, Perlman M, Manning FA (1995) High cervical spinal cord injury in neonates delivered with forceps: report of 15 cases. Obstet Gynecol 86(4 Pt 1):589–594
53. Montane I, Eismont FJ, Green BA (1991) Traumatic occipitoatlantal dislocation. Spine (Phila Pa 1976) 16(2):112–116
54. Nypaver M, Treloar D (1994) Neutral cervical spine positioning in children. Ann Emerg Med 23(2):208–211
55. Odent T, Langlais J, Glorion C, Kassis B, Bataille J, Pouliquen JC (1999) Fractures of the odontoid process: a report of 15 cases in children younger than 6 years. J Pediatr Orthop 19(1):51–54

56. Ogden JA (1984) Radiology of postnatal skeletal development. XII. The second cervical vertebra. Skeletal Radiol 12(3):169–177
57. Osenbach RK, Menezes AH (1989) Spinal cord injury without radiographic abnormality in children. Pediatr Neurosci 15(4):168–174
58. Pang D (2004) Spinal cord injury without radiographic abnormality in children, 2 decades later. Neurosurgery 55(6):1325–1342
59. Pang D, Li V (2005) Atlantoaxial rotatory fixation: part 3-a prospective study of the clinical manifestation, diagnosis, management, and outcome of children with alantoaxial rotatory fixation. Neurosurgery 57(5):954–972
60. Pang D, Nemzek WR, Zovickian J (2007) Atlanto-occipital dislocation – part 2: the clinical use of (occipital) condyle-C1 interval, comparison with other diagnostic methods, and the manifestation, management, and outcome of atlanto-occipital dislocation in children. Neurosurgery 61(5):995–1015
61. Pang D, Nemzek WR, Zovickian J (2007) Atlanto-occipital dislocation: part 1 – normal occipital condyle-C1 interval in 89 children. Neurosurgery 61(3):514–521
62. Pang D, Pollack IF (1989) Spinal cord injury without radiographic abnormality in children – the SCIWORA syndrome. J Trauma 29(5):654–664
63. Pang D, Wilberger JE Jr (1982) Spinal cord injury without radiographic abnormalities in children. J Neurosurg 57(1):114–129
64. Papadopoulos SM, Dickman CA, Sonntag VK, Rekate HL, Spetzler RF (1991) Traumatic atlantooccipital dislocation with survival. Neurosurgery 28(4):574–579
65. Patel JC, Tepas JJ III, Mollitt DL, Pieper P (2001) Pediatric cervical spine injuries: defining the disease. J Pediatr Surg 36(2):373–376
66. Phillips WA, Hensinger RN (1989) The management of rotatory atlanto-axial subluxation in children. J Bone Joint Surg Am 71(5):664–668
67. Pollack IF, Pang D, Sclabassi R (1988) Recurrent spinal cord injury without radiographic abnormalities in children. J Neurosurg 69(2):177–182
68. Powers B, Miller MD, Kramer RS, Martinez S, Gehweiler JA Jr (1979) Traumatic anterior atlanto-occipital dislocation. Neurosurgery 4(1):12–17
69. Rekate HL, Theodore N, Sonntag VK, Dickman CA (1999) Pediatric spine and spinal cord trauma. State of the art for the third millennium. Childs Nerv Syst 15(11–12):743–750
70. Rinaldi I, Mullins WJ Jr, Delaney WF, Fitzer PM, Tornberg DN (1979) Computerized tomographic demonstration of rotational atlanto-axial fixation. Case report. J Neurosurg 50(1): 115–119
71. Ruge JR, Sinson GP, McLone DG, Cerullo LJ (1988) Pediatric spinal injury: the very young. J Neurosurg 68(1):25–30
72. Scapinelli R (1994) Three-dimensional computed tomography in infantile atlantoaxial rotatory fixation. J Bone Joint Surg Br 76(3):367–370
73. Schippers N, Konings P, Hassler W, Sommer B (1996) Typical and atypical fractures of the odontoid process in young children. Report of two cases and a review of the literature. Acta Neurochir (Wien) 138(5):524–530
74. Schultz KD Jr, Petronio J, Haid RW, Rodts GE, Erwood SC, Alexander J et al (2000) Pediatric occipitocervical arthrodesis. A review of current options and early evaluation of rigid internal fixation techniques. Pediatr Neurosurg 33(4):169–181
75. Sherburn EW, Day RA, Kaufman BA, Park TS (1996) Subdental synchondrosis fracture in children: the value of 3-dimensional computerized tomography. Pediatr Neurosurg 25(5):256–259
76. Sherk HH (1978) Fractures of the atlas and odontoid process. Orthop Clin North Am 9(4):973–984
77. Sherk HH, Nicholson JT, Chung SM (1978) Fractures of the odontoid process in young children. J Bone Joint Surg Am 60(7):921–924
78. Shirasaki N, Okada K, Oka S, Hosono N, Yonenobu K, Ono K (1991) Os odontoideum with posterior atlantoaxial instability. Spine (Phila Pa 1976) 16(7):706–715
79. Spence KF Jr, Decker S, Sell KW (1970) Bursting atlantal fracture associated with rupture of the transverse ligament. J Bone Joint Surg Am 52(3):543–549

80. Spierings EL, Braakman R (1982) The management of os odontoideum. Analysis of 37 cases. J Bone Joint Surg Br 64(4):422–428
81. Subach BR, McLaughlin MR, Albright AL, Pollack IF (1998) Current management of pediatric atlantoaxial rotatory subluxation. Spine (Phila Pa 1976) 23(20):2174–2179
82. Sun PP, Poffenbarger GJ, Durham S, Zimmerman RA (2000) Spectrum of occipitoatlantoaxial injury in young children. J Neurosurg 93(1 Suppl):28–39
83. Suss RA, Zimmerman RD, Leeds NE (1983) Pseudospread of the atlas: false sign of Jefferson fracture in young children. AJR Am J Roentgenol 140(6):1079–1082
84. Swischuk LE, John SD, Hendrick EP (2000) Is the open-mouth odontoid view necessary in children under 5 years? Pediatr Radiol 30(3):186–189
85. Traynelis VC, Marano GD, Dunker RO, Kaufman HH (1986) Traumatic atlanto-occipital dislocation. Case report. J Neurosurg 65(6):863–870
86. Treloar DJ, Nypaver M (1997) Angulation of the pediatric cervical spine with and without cervical collar. Pediatr Emerg Care 13(1):5–8
87. Vale FL, Burns J, Jackson AB, Hadley MN (1997) Combined medical and surgical treatment after acute spinal cord injury: results of a prospective pilot study to assess the merits of aggressive medical resuscitation and blood pressure management. J Neurosurg 87(2):239–246
88. Vargas TM, Rybicki FJ, Ledbetter SM, MacKenzie JD (2005) Atlantoaxial instability associated with an orthotopic os odontoideum: a multimodality imaging assessment. Emerg Radiol 11(4):223–225
89. Verska JM, Anderson PA (1997) Os odontoideum. A case report of one identical twin. Spine (Phila Pa 1976) 22(6):706–709
90. Viccellio P, Simon H, Pressman BD, Shah MN, Mower WR, Hoffman JR (2001) A prospective multicenter study of cervical spine injury in children. Pediatrics 108(2):E20
91. Vogel LC, Krajci KA, Anderson CJ (2002) Adults with pediatric-onset spinal cord injuries: part 3: impact of medical complications. J Spinal Cord Med 25(4):297–305
92. Vogel LC, Krajci KA, Anderson CJ (2002) Adults with pediatric-onset spinal cord injury: part 1: prevalence of medical complications. J Spinal Cord Med 25(2):106–116
93. Vogel LC, Krajci KA, Anderson CJ (2002) Adults with pediatric-onset spinal cord injury: part 2: musculoskeletal and neurological complications. J Spinal Cord Med 25(2):117–123
94. Wang JC, Nuccion SL, Feighan JE, Cohen B, Dorey FJ, Scoles PV (2001) Growth and development of the pediatric cervical spine documented radiographically. J Bone Joint Surg Am 83-A(8):1212–1218
95. Ware ML (2006) Clinical biomechanics of the pediatric craniovervical junction and the subaxial spine. In: Brockmeyer DL (ed) Advanced pediatric craniocervical surgery. Thieme, New York, pp 27–42
96. White AA, Panjabi MM (1990) Clinical biomechanics of the spine, 2nd edn. Lippincott Williams and Wilkins, Philadelphia
97. Wholey MH, Bruwer AJ, Baker HL Jr (1958) The lateral roentgenogram of the neck; with comments on the atlanto-odontoid-basion relationship. Radiology 71(3):350–356

Author Index Volume 1–40

C. Di Rocco, N. Akalan (eds.), *Pediatric Craniovertebral Junction Diseases*, Advances and Technical Standards in Neurosurgery 40,
DOI 10.1007/978-3-319-01065-6, © Springer International Publishing Switzerland 2014

C

D

E

F

G

M

R

S

T

Y

Z

Subject Index Volume 1–40

C

Q

R

S

T

MIX
Papier aus verantwortungsvollen Quellen
Paper from responsible sources
FSC® C105338

If you have any concerns about our products,
you can contact us on
ProductSafety@springernature.com

In case Publisher is established outside the EU,
the EU authorized representative is:
Springer Nature Customer Service Center GmbH
Europaplatz 3, 69115 Heidelberg, Germany

Printed by Libri Plureos GmbH
in Hamburg, Germany